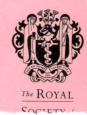

SENTINEL LYMPH NODE BIOPSY

This book is lovingly dedicated

to my wife, Myung-Hi,

to my daughters, Margaret, Elizabeth, and Vicky,

to my parents,

and to the memory of my great-grandfather,

Professor Henry S Jacoby

SENTINEL LYMPH NODE BIOPSY

Edited by

HIRAM S CODY III, MD

Breast Service, Department of Surgery
Memorial Sloan-Kettering Cancer Center
New York, NY
USA

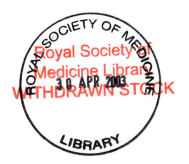
MARTIN DUNITZ

© 2002, Martin Dunitz Ltd, a member of the Taylor & Francis group

First published in the United Kingdom in 2002 by:
Martin Dunitz Ltd
The Livery House
7–9 Pratt Street
London NW1 0AE

Tel: +44-(0)20-7482-2202
Fax: +44-(0)20-7267-0159
E-mail: info.dunitz@tandf.co.uk
Website: http://www.dunitz.co.uk

Although every effort has been made to ensure that drug doses and other information are presented accurately in this publication, the ultimate responsibility rests with the prescribing physician. Neither the publishers nor the authors can be held responsible for errors or for any consequences arising from the use of information contained herein. For detailed prescribing information or instructions on the use of any product or procedure discussed herein, please consult the prescribing information or instructional material issued by the manufacturer.

A CIP catalogue record for this book is available from the British Library

ISBN 1-84184-034-3

Distributed in the USA by
Fulfilment Center
Taylor & Francis
7625 Empire Drive
Florence, KY 41042, USA
Toll Free Tel: 1-800-634-7064
Email cserve@routledge nv.com

Distributed in Canada by
Taylor & Francis
74 Rolark Drive
Scarborough
Ontario M1R 4G2, Canada
Toll Free Tel: 1-877-226-2237
Email: tal fran@istar.ca

Distributed in the rest of the world by
ITPS Limited
Cheriton House
North Way, Andover
Hampshire SP10 5BE, UK
Tel: +44 (0)1264 332424
Email: reception@itps.co.uk

Composition by Wearset Ltd, Boldon, Tyne and Wear
Printed and bound in Singapore by Kyodo Printing Pte. Ltd.

Contents

Preface

The best ideas in clinical medicine are often simple ones, and the sentinel node hypothesis—that the first lymph node draining a cancer could predict the status of the remaining nodal basin—is one of these. Over the final decade of the twentieth century, sentinel lymph-node biopsy has entered clinical practice with astonishing rapidity. This intuitive, ingenious, and powerful technique represents a new standard of care for melanoma and breast cancer patients, and shows great promise for the treatment of urologic, colorectal, gynecologic, and head and neck cancers as well.

Like many scientific breakthroughs, sentinel node biopsy is not an entirely new idea, but represents the coalescence of existing knowledge accumulated over the last 120 years from a diversity of fields, encompassing the anatomy and physiology of the lymphatic system, radiographic lymphography, radionuclide lymphoscintigraphy, operative instrumentation, surgical technique, and pathologic methodology.

This book aims to present a comprehensive overview of sentinel lymph-node biopsy, organized into broad categories. The first comprises an overview of the subject, including lymphatic anatomy, the history of lymphatic mapping, the role of nuclear medicine, and instrumentation. The second and third parts review the use of sentinel lymph-node biopsy in the treatment of the diseases for which it may be considered the new standard of care: melanoma and breast cancer. The final chapters explore its emerging role in cancers of other sites.

Sentinel lymph-node biopsy is a robust technique, and it has produced strikingly similar results despite wide variations in methodology during its rapid evolution. Many of these technical nuances remain the subject of lively controversy, and a major goal of this book is to present as concisely as possible the techniques used by those institutions with the largest experience. For those who wish to start a sentinel node biopsy program (nuclear medicine physicians, surgeons, and pathologists), we hope to provide the tools to do so. For all those who care for the cancer patient, we hope to provide direction in interpreting the results. To the extent that "God is in the details," we aim to define the details, and to the extent that consensus is possible, we aim to find it.

Sentinel lymph-node biopsy demonstrates simultaneously the truth of the classic "Halstedian" model of tumor biology (that the local spread of cancer is mechanistic, anatomically defined, and limited by the regional nodes) and the more recent "Fisher hypothesis" (that micrometastases are frequently present and that systemic dissemination can occur early in the course of disease). What sentinel lymph-node biopsy cannot do is to explain the biologic heterogeneity of cancer or the profound mystery of tumor invasion and metastasis. What it can do, quite simply, is to demonstrate with increased clarity the *presence of metastasis*, thereby defining with unprecedented accuracy the risk posed by each cancer and allowing an ever more precise adjustment of therapy, local and systemic, to each patient's disease.

Hiram S Cody III

Acknowledgements

This book, like the subject of sentinel node biopsy itself, represents a coalescence of effort, present and past, for which the editor can take little personal credit, but for which he is very grateful.

Alexandra MacDonald of our own Editorial Division has overseen all of the elements of this project, corresponding with the authors, reading and editing every chapter, and assembling the final manuscript. To the extent that this work has continuity and flow, she is largely responsible. This volume could not have been completed without her invaluable assistance. I wish to thank her colleagues, Denise Haller-Buckley and Daniel Kellum, for their help as well.

Our publisher, Martin Dunitz, expressed early enthusiasm for this work. Despite my having missed many meetings with him, he has never lost interest. Loss of momentum must be a common phenomenon, particularly in the later stages of preparing multiauthored texts. Our collaboration with Managing Editor, Alison VM Campbell, and Senior Production Controller, Ian Stoneham, at Martin Dunitz Ltd has been a pleasure, and thanks to their able professionalism, all elements of production have proceeded smoothly and ahead of schedule.

One's education never ends, and my indebtedness to those who have taught me can never be fully repaid. For my residency years at The Roosevelt Hospital, I am particularly grateful to Drs Walter Wichern, J Beall Rodgers, Chin Bor Yeoh, Thomas Royster, Stuart Quan, and Richard Marks. My fellowship at Memorial Hospital was particularly memorable for my rotations with Dr Alan Turnbull, to this day a 'compleat' surgical oncologist. I am especially grateful to Dr Jerome A Urban, who gave me my start in breast cancer surgery. An early proponent of the extended radical mastectomy, but one who never hesitated to offer his patients less radical surgical options as they became available, he would have been especially pleased to see the development of sentinel node biopsy.

Final and very special thanks must go to my present colleagues, Drs Patrick Borgen, Chief of the Breast Service, and Murray Brennan, Chairman of the Department of Surgery, at Memorial Sloan-Kettering Cancer Center. I deeply appreciate their unfailing mentorship, support, collegiality, and friendship over the last 6 years.

HSC III

Contributors

Charles M Balch, MD
Department of Surgery and Oncology
Johns Hopkins University Medical Institute
550 North Broadway
Suite 1003
Baltimore, MD 21205
USA

Anton Bilchik, MD
2200 Santa Monica Blvd
Santa Monica, CA 90404
USA

Patrick I Borgen, MD
Breast Service
Department of Surgery
Memorial Sloan-Kettering Cancer Center
1275 York Avenue
New York, NY 10021
USA

Mary Sue Brady, MD
Gastric and Mixed Tumor Service
Department of Surgery
Memorial Sloan-Kettering Cancer Center
1275 York Avenue
New York, NY 10021
USA

Ramon M Cabanas, MD
Department of Surgery
Victory Memorial Hospital
699 92nd Street
Brooklyn, NY 11228
USA

Mathew H Chung, MD, MAJ
Division of Surgical Oncology
John Wayne Cancer Institute
St John's Health Center
2200 Santa Monica Blvd
Santa Monica, CA 90404
USA

Dayalan Clarke, MD
Department of Surgery
University of Wales College of Medicine
Heath Park
Cardiff CF14 4XN
UK

Alistair J Cochran, MD, FRCPath
Department of Pathology & Laboratory
Medicine (13-145 CHS)
Division of Surgical Pathology
UCLA School of Medicine
10833 Le Conte Avenue
Los Angeles, CA 90095-1732
USA

Hiram S Cody III, MD
Breast Service
Department of Surgery
Memorial Sloan-Kettering Cancer Center
1275 York Avenue
New York, NY 10021
USA

Daniel G Coit, MD
Gastric and Mixed Tumor Service
Department of Surgery
Memorial Sloan-Kettering Cancer Center
1275 York Avenue
New York, NY 10021
USA

Charles E Cox, MD
Department of Surgery
H Lee Moffitt Cancer Center
and Research Institute
University of South Florida
12901 Magnolia Drive
Tampa, FL 33612-9497
USA

C Wayne Cruse, MD
Cutaneous Oncology Program
Department of Surgery
H Lee Moffitt Cancer Center
and Research Institute
University of South Florida
12901 Magnolia Drive
Tampa, FL 33612-9497
USA

Kambiz Dowlatshahi, MD
Department of General Surgery
Rush-Presbyterian-St Luke's Medical Center
Rush University
653 West Congress Parkway
Chicago, IL 60612-3833
USA

Richard Essner, MD
Roy E Coats Research Laboratories
John Wayne Cancer Institute
St John's Health Center
2200 Santa Monica Blvd
Santa Monica, CA 90404
USA

Viviana Galimberti, MD
Division of Breast Cancer
European Institute of Oncology
Via Ripamonti 435
Milan 20141
Italy

Wolfgang Gatzemeier, MD
Division of Breast Cancer
European Institute of Oncology
Via Ripamonti 435
Milan 20141
Italy

Jeffrey E Gershenwald, MD
Departments of Surgical Oncology and Cancer
Biology
University of Texas MD Anderson Cancer
Center
1515 Holcombe Blvd, Box 444
Houston, TX 77030
USA

Armando E Giuliano, MD
Joyce Eisenberg Keefer Breast Center
Division of Surgical Oncology
John Wayne Cancer Institute
St John's Health Center
2200 Santa Monica Blvd
Santa Monica, CA 90404
USA

Arnold DK Hill, MCh, FRCSI
Department of Surgery
St Vincent's University Hospital
Elm Park
Dublin 4
Ireland

Robert Howman-Giles MD, FRACP
Department of Medicine
University of Sydney
Nuclear Medicine & Diagnostic Ultrasound
Royal Prince Alfred Hospital Medical Center
100 Carillon Avenue
Newton NSW 2042
Australia

Dennis Kraus, MD
Head & Neck Surgery Service
Department of Surgery
Memorial Sloan-Kettering Cancer Center
1275 York Avenue
New York, NY 10021
USA

Bin BR Kroon, MD, PhD
Department of Surgery
Antoni van Leeuwenhoek Hospital
The Netherlands Cancer Institute
Plesmanlaan 121
1066 CX Amsterdam
The Netherlands

Julie Lange, MD
Department of Surgery and Oncology
Johns Hopkins University Medical Institute
550 North Broadway
Suite 1003
Baltimore, MD 21205
USA

Charles Levenback, MD
Department of Gynecologic Oncology
University of Texas MD Anderson Cancer
Center
1515 Holcombe Blvd, Box 440
Houston, TX 77030
USA

Laura Liberman, MD
Department of Radiology
Memorial Sloan-Kettering Cancer Center
1275 York Avenue
New York, NY 10021
USA

Kelly M McMasters, MD, PhD
Division of Surgical Oncology
Department of Surgery
University of Louisville
James Graham Brown Cancer Center
529 South Jackson Street
Louisville, KY 40202
USA

Robert E Mansel, FRCS
Department of Surgery
Division of Hospital Based Specialties
University of Wales College of Medicine
Heath Park
Cardiff CF14 4XN
UK

Donald L Morton, MD
Roy E Coats Research Laboratories
John Wayne Cancer Institute
St John's Health Center
2200 Santa Monica Blvd
Santa Monica, CA 90404
USA

Omgo E Nieweg, MD, PhD
Department of Surgery
Antoni van Leeuwenhoek Hospital
The Netherlands Cancer Institute
Plesmanlaan 121
1066 CX Amsterdam
The Netherlands

Michael P Osborne, MD, FRCS, FACS
Strang Weill Cornell Breast Center
425 East 61st Street
New York, NY 10021
USA

Giovanni Paganelli, MD
Division of Breast Cancer
European Institute of Oncology
Via Ripamonti 435
Milan 20141
Italy

Snehal Patel, MD, FRCS
Fellow, Head and Neck Surgery Service
Department of Surgery
Memorial Sloan-Kettering Cancer Center
1275 York Avenue
New York, NY 10021
USA

Douglas Reintgen, MD
Department of Surgery
H Lee Moffitt Cancer Center
and Research Institute
University of South Florida
12901 Magnolia Drive
Tampa, FL 33612-9497
USA

Sharon M Rosenbaum Smith, MD
Division of Breast Cancer
St Luke's-Roosevelt Hospital Center
425 West 59th Street, Suite 7A
New York, NY 10019
USA

Merrick I Ross, MD
Department of Surgical Oncology
University of Texas MD Anderson Cancer
Center
1515 Holcombe Blvd, Box 444
Houston, TX 77030
USA

Emiel J Rutgers, MD, PhD, FRCS
Department of Surgery
Antoni van Leeuwenhoek Hospital
The Netherlands Cancer Institute
Plesmanlaan 121
1066 CX Amsterdam
The Netherlands

Virgilio Sacchini, MD
Breast Service
Department of Surgery
Memorial Sloan-Kettering Cancer Center
1275 York Avenue
New York, NY 10021
USA

Matthew A Sadlier, MB, BCh, BSc
Department of Surgery
St Vincent's University Hospital
Elm Park
Dublin 4
Ireland

Sukamal Saha, MD
3500 Calkins Road, Suite A
Flint, MI 48532
USA

Christopher Salud, BA
Department of Surgery
H Lee Moffitt Cancer Center
and Research Institute
University of South Florida
12901 Magnolia Drive
Tampa, FL 33612-9497
USA

Lisa Schneider, MD
Fellow, Department of Radiology
Memorial Sloan-Kettering Cancer Center
1275 York Avenue
New York, NY 10021
USA

Hans Starz, MD
Department of Dermatology & Allergology
Klinikum Augsburg
D-86156 Augsburg
Germany

Deena Thayer, DO
Gastric and Mixed Tumor Service
Department of Surgery
Philadelphia College of Osteopathic Medicine
4170 City Avenue
Philadelphia, PA 19131
USA

John F Thompson, MD, FRACS, FACS
Department of Surgery
University of Sydney
Sydney Melanoma Unit
Royal Prince Alfred Hospital Medical Center
Missenden Road
Camperdown NSW 2050
Australia

Alessandro Testori, MD
Melanoma Unit
Division of General Surgery
European Institute of Oncology
Via Ripamonti 435
Milan 20141
Italy

Roderick R Turner, MD
Department of Pathology
St John's Health Center
1328 Twenty-Second Street
Santa Monica, CA 90404
USA

Roger F Uren, MD, FRACP
Department of Medicine
University of Sydney
Nuclear Medicine & Diagnostic Ultrasound
Royal Prince Alfred Hospital Medical Center
100 Carillon Avenue
Newton NSW 2042
Australia

Umberto Veronesi, MD
Division of Breast Cancer
European Institute of Oncology
Via Ripamonti 435
Milan 20141
Italy

David Wiese, MD
McLaren Regional Medical Center
401 South Ballenger Highway
Flint, MI 48532
USA

Sandra L Wong, MD
Division of Surgical Oncology
Department of Surgery
University of Louisville
James Graham Brown Cancer Center
529 South Jackson Street
Louisville, KY 40202
USA

William R Wrightson, MD
Division of Surgical Oncology
Department of Surgery
University of Louisville
James Graham Brown Cancer Center
529 South Jackson Street
Louisville, KY 40202
USA

Pat Zanzonico MD, PhD
Nuclear Medicine Service
Memorial Sloan-Kettering Cancer Center
1275 York Avenue
New York, NY 10021
USA

Part I
Overview of Sentinel Lymph-Node Biopsy

1

The historic background of lymphatic mapping

Michael P Osborne and Sharon M Rosenbaum Smith

The treatment of breast cancer has evolved from the radical, disfiguring mastectomy described by Halsted in the late nineteenth century to the less invasive, less debilitating lumpectomy and axillary lymph-node dissection (ALND) as new discoveries have been made into the mechanism of the spread of breast cancer. Independent of the method of treatment of the primary cancer, accurate assessment of the status of the axillary lymph nodes has remained an integral part of the management of breast cancer. The status of the axillary lymph nodes is the single most important predictor for survival, and the presence of lymph-node metastasis dictates the need for adjuvant chemotherapy.

Complete ALND has significant associated potential morbidity that may negatively affect quality of life. Morbidity from ALND includes lymphedema, pain, numbness, and restricted arm movement.[1] A less invasive means of assessing axillary nodal status that would eliminate unnecessary ALNDs and decrease associated morbidity was desired. A technique was developed in the 1970s using radioisotope-labeled agents in an attempt to identify the primary regional lymph node draining a breast

cancer. This technique consisted of injecting a radioisotope into the breast. Images were obtained, and the level of isotope uptake was correlated with the primary regional node uptake and the nodal pathology.[2] In the 1980s, a new technique for examining the axillary nodal basin for metastases emerged, called the sentinel lymph-node biopsy technique. This technique is based on the concept that the pathological status of the sentinel lymph node (SLN), the first lymph node to receive drainage from the breast, reflects the status of the entire axilla. Therefore, if the SLN is negative for metastases, it can be presumed that the entire axilla will be negative for disease, and no further surgery in the axilla is warranted. The ability to identify the SLN has enabled surgeons to eliminate ALNDs in patients with node-negative disease and will therefore have a major impact on the management of breast cancer.

THE ORIGINS OF LYMPHATIC MAPPING

The origins of lymphatic mapping date to 1622 with Aselius's discovery of the lacteals in a recently fed dog.[3] Pecquet demonstrated the cisterna chyli in animals in 1654,[4] and Bartholin confirmed this in the human.[5] It was not until 1786, however, that Cruikshank described the lymphatic anatomy of the human breast in detail. He described two pathways of lymphatic drainage, one accompanying the external thoracic artery and vein, the other accompanying the internal thoracic vein: the "external absorbents arise from the nipple and from the external part of the mamma, from the integuments and the tubuli lactiferi. They run outwards towards the axilla and sometimes pass through small glands halfway between the nipple and the axilla ... The internal mammary absorbents arise from the posterior part of the mamma and perforate in many places the intercostal muscles."[6]

Mascagni described a similar arrangement of the lymphatics in his book in 1787.[7] Sappey, in 1883, further described the lymphatics of the breast. Using mercurial injections into the lactating breast, he detailed a superficial group of lymphatics that originated at the nipple (Sappey's plexus) and drained the skin over the breast, and a deep group of lymphatics that drained the breast tissue itself.[8] He wrongly believed, however, that there was no lymphatic drainage either outside the posterior surface of the breast or to the internal mammary chain.

Compiling the work from previous studies, Poirer, Cuneo, and Delamere described four distinct pathways of lymphatic drainage of the breast.[9] These consisted of the main pathway of Sappey, which extends from the subareolar plexus to the axilla; the interpectoral pathway, originally described by Grossman in 1896 and Rotter in 1899;[10,11] the internal mammary pathway illustrated by Cruikshank in 1786 and Mascagni in 1787;[6,7] and, lastly, a group of inconsistent vessels that extend from the parenchyma of the breast and pass directly to the axilla.

Stibbe, in 1918, described the anatomical arrangement of the internal mammary chain in great detail.[12] He saw the internal mammary chain as originating from the anterior prepericardial lymph nodes lying on the upper surface of the diaphragm. In addition to receiving lymphatic drainage from portions of the liver, diaphragm and rectus abdominis muscle, and rectus sheath, this group of lymph nodes receives lymphatic drainage from the lower quadrants of the breast. The major efferent lymphatics of the inner quadrants of the breast pierce the pectoral fascia to enter the pectoralis major muscle, and then pass medially through the intercostal muscles at the medial end of each intercostal space to join the internal mammary lymphatics. The internal mammary lymphatics empty into the great vein either directly, or indirectly via the thoracic duct on the left and via the lymphatic duct on the right. Rouvière, in 1932, summarized the existing anatomical knowledge of the human breast lymphatics.[13]

The importance of the lymphatic system in the dissemination of malignant cells has been well documented. Actius of Amida in the sixth century stated that "the disease of the female breast consists of a large tumor ... and gives rise to malignant phlegmons in the armpits." Valsalva, in 1704, and Le Dran, in 1757, clinically described the local spread of breast cancer to the regional lymph nodes.[14,15] Virchow, in 1860, documented the histopathological spread of breast cancer to the regional lymph nodes. Heidenhain in 1888, Stiles in 1892, and Handley in 1907 described the involvement of the retromammary lymphatics in the spread of cancer cells, and the theory of tumor dissemination by the "lymphatic of the deep fascial plexus" was formulated.[16–18] Grossman, in 1896, identified a group of lymph nodes lying between the pectoral muscles.[10] Rotter, in 1899, showed that the retromammary lymphatics penetrated the pectoralis major muscle to reach the interpectoral nodes and that these nodes were a potential site for breast cancer metastases.[11]

Pickren, in 1956, examined in detail the spread of breast cancer cells into the axilla.[19] He found that a central group of axillary lymph nodes was involved in 90% of the cases, and that this group was exclusively involved 38% of the time. The mammary, scapular, and interpectoral groups of lymph nodes were rarely exclusively involved. Haagensen, in 1971, further investigated the spread of breast-cancer cells into the axillary lymph nodes.[20] In over

1000 radical mastectomy specimens, he found a 56% incidence of axillary nodal metastases. The incidence increased to 65% when serial sectioning of apparently node-negative specimens was performed.

THE TECHNIQUE OF LYMPHOSCINTIGRAPHY

The technique of lymphangiography and the use of radioisotope injections further advanced our knowledge of the lymphatic anatomy. Morl, in 1952, used India ink injected ante-mortem to demonstrate that all quadrants of the breast drained into the sternal lymph nodes.[21] Haagensen, in 1972, illustrated axillary node uptake of vital blue dye during mastectomy.[22]

A number of radiolabeled compounds were developed as potential lymphoscintigraphic agents. Sherman and Ter-Pogossian, in 1953,[23] introduced the selective localization of regional lymph nodes with interstitially injected radioactive colloid gold, marking the beginning of lymphoscintigraphy (LSG). Then Hultborn, Larsson, and Ragnhult, in 1955, used radioisotope injections into the breast to detect the direction of the flow of lymph.[24] They injected radioactive colloid gold intraparenchymally, and performed a radical mastectomy several days later. By studying the uptake by the lymph nodes postoperatively, they concluded that 97–99% of the isotope was taken up by the axillary lymph nodes and only 1–3% drained into the internal mammary nodes. Turner-Warwick, in 1959, used a combination of radioactive colloidal gold and Patent Blue-V dye to outline the anatomy of the breast.[25]

In addition, radioactive colloid gold was used by zum Winkel (1963)[26] to visualize the retroperitoneal and ilioinguinal nodes, by Schwab (1965)[27] for the cervical nodes, by Bethune (1978)[28] for the mediastinal nodes, and by Rossi and Ferri (1966),[29] Schenck (1966),[30] and Matsuo (1974)[31] for the internal mammary nodes. Matsuo was the first to confirm that the internal mammary LSG results correlated with internal mammary lymph-node pathology. In 106 cases, preoperative scans were examined

and correlated with the pathological analysis of an internal mammary lymph node that was obtained during radical mastectomy. In 90% of the cases a positive diagnosis for metastases by LSG correlated with the pathological findings, and in 100% a negative scan correlated with pathological findings. Less than 50% of the LSG scans deemed "suspicious" correctly predicted internal mammary node metastases. Although these results seemed promising, interest in radioactive colloid gold waned in the late 1970s owing to the high level of radiation emitted by this isotope.[32]

Further advancements in LSG came with the development of technetium-99m by Harper et al.[33] Derived from molybdenum, Tc-99m has the advantage of a short half-life and low-energy gamma emission. Hauser et al, in 1969, used Tc-99m-sulfur colloid (Tc-99m-SC) for lymph-node imaging,[34] but Aspegren et al found a poor correlation between LSG and pathological findings for this agent.[35] Garzon and associates developed a modification in the method of preparing the sulfur colloid that yielded a smaller particle size.[36] Ege, in 1977, used this modified Tc-99m-antimony sulfur colloid (TC-99m-ASC) to study the internal mammary lymph nodes.[37]

Other substances to be used experimentally for LSG included Tc-99m-labeled stannous phytate,[38] mercury-197-sulfide labeled colloid,[39] indium-111-labeled colloid,[40] and Tc-99m-labeled liposomes.[41] Experimental studies did not prove these substances to be superior to Tc-99m-ASC.[42]

THE EMERGENCE OF THE SENTINEL LYMPH NODE CONCEPT

Direct LSG of the breast was the indirect predecessor of the SLN concept. Kett, in 1970, demonstrated that one node, the "Sorgius node," typically received the drainage from the breast first, before it progressed through to the remaining axillary lymph nodes.[43] Other studies using LSG described a "primary draining node,"[2,44,45] but the significance of this node was not appreciated at the time.

The term "sentinel node" was first coined by Gould in 1960, based on the anatomical position of a lymph node found during a radical neck dissection during parotidectomy.[46] Cabanas, however, is credited with the first physiologic description of the "sentinel lymph node" in 1977, when he described the existence of a specific lymph-node center that drained the penis.[47] In his landmark paper, Cabanas performed lymphangiograms on 100 patients via lymphatics on the dorsum of the penis, the dorsum of the foot, or both. When the lymphangiogram was performed using the dorsal lymphatics of the penis, Cabanas found that the drainage was consistently to a lymph node located at the anterior or medial aspect of the superficial epigastric vein. This corresponded to the superficial epigastric lymph-node group. Cabanas confirmed that this group of lymph nodes was not only the first site of metastases from penile carcinomas, but that it might be the only lymph node to be involved. He further suggested that for the treatment of penile carcinoma, if this first draining lymph node—termed the "sentinel lymph node"—was negative for metastases, no further therapy was indicated. Only if the SLN was positive for metastasis should further dissection be performed.

PIONEERS IN SLN BIOPSY

Morton (Figure 1.1) and his colleagues expanded the SLN concept by applying it to use in clinical Stage I cutaneous melanomas.[48] Morton observed that 90% of patients with melanoma have no clinical evidence of metastasis in the regional lymph nodes. Prophylactic elective lymph-node dissection in these patients is controversial, because it affords no survival benefit to patients with negative lymph nodes. Studies have shown, however, that melanoma patients with lymph-node metastasis who undergo a therapeutic lymph-node dissection have a 27% higher survival rate.[48] In 1977, Robinson et al successfully used cutaneous LSG with colloidal gold to identify the regional lymph-node basin of primary drainage for

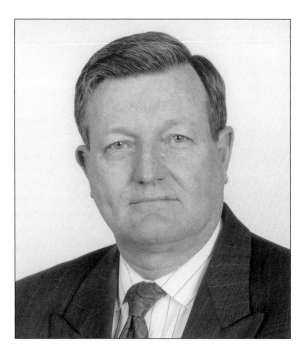

Figure 1.1 Donald L Morton, MD, Medical Director and Surgeon-in-Chief, Roy E Coats Research Laboratories of the John Wayne Cancer Institute at St John's Health Center, Santa Monica, California.

melanomas located in ambiguous sites on the body.[49] Morton then postulated that if the SLN could be identified intraoperatively, patients with negative lymph nodes could be spared a lymph-node dissection and its associated potential morbidity. Morton first demonstrated the feasibility of this technique using a feline model. He injected a vital dye intradermally in the lower extremity and identified the SLN. This technique was then applied to humans. In 223 patients with clinical Stage I melanoma, a vital blue dye was injected intradermally around the melanoma. An incision was made directly overlying the expected lymphatic basin and all blue lymphatic channels were traced to the SLN. Overall, an SLN was identified in 82% of patients. Metastases were detected in 21%; in 12% by routine hematoxylin-and-eosin (H&E) staining, and in 9% by immunohistochemical (IHC) technique alone. A 1% false-negative rate was found in this study, and no false-positive finding occurred. Based on his findings, Morton concluded that for patients with clinical Stage I melanomas, the identification and examination of the SLN is an accurate means of assessing the lymph-node basin and that patients with a negative SLN could therefore be spared a total lymphadenectomy. Additionally, it was noted that the use of IHC-staining techniques improved the pathological detection of metastases compared with routine H&E staining alone. It was therefore suggested that both techniques be routinely employed in the examination of the SLN.

Osborne et al showed that a "primary regional lymph node" draining the breast could be identified and correlated with the axillary lymph-node status.[50] This technique could not reliably predict the presence or absence of axillary node metastases,[51,52] however, and it was not until 1993 that interest in this procedure for breast cancer patients developed. In 1993, Krag (Figure 1.2) and colleagues applied the technique of gamma-probe localization of radiolabeled lymph nodes to identify the SLN in order to determine the axillary lymph-node status.[53] This technique was shown to be successful in preclinical trials using a feline model.[54] Technetium-99m-sulfur colloid was injected intradermally into the lower extremity of the cat. Gamma-probe localization of the SLN was found to be highly accurate and sensitive. This study suggested that gamma-probe localization of the SLN is advantageous because it permits the surgeon to determine, on the surface of the skin, the precise location of the underlying lymph node, allowing a smaller skin incision to be used. Also, the gamma probe can guide the surgeon to the SLN intraoperatively and confirm that the correct lymph node is removed. The use of the gamma probe also permits verification that no residual SLNs remain.

Krag et al then applied radiolocalization to the staging of breast cancer.[55] They attempted to determine if the SLN could be identified in breast-cancer patients, and if this node was predictive of the status of the entire axillary lymph-node basin. His trial consisted of injecting Tc-99m-SC into the breast tissue either surrounding a tumor or around the biopsy cavity if the tumor had been removed previously.

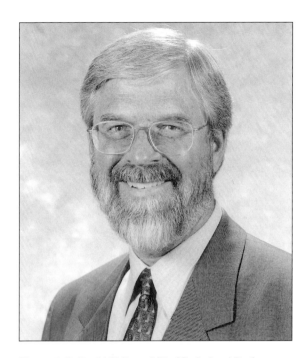

Figure 1.2 David N Krag, MD, SD, Ireland Professor of Surgery, Department of Surgery, College of Medicine, University of Vermont, Burlington, Vermont.

A hand-held gamma probe was used during the surgery to identify the lymph node (or nodes) that received the drainage from the breast. In Krag's study, an SLN was identified in 18 of 22 consecutive patients (82%). Of these 18 patients, the SLN was positive for metastatic cancer in 7 patients, and in 3 of these patients, the SLN was the only lymph node containing metastatic cancer. No patient in Krag's study had a falsely negative SLN. This and subsequent larger studies concluded that the radiolocalization and selective resection of the SLN are possible, and that the SLN correctly predicts the status of the remaining axilla.[55–57]

Giuliano (Figure 1.3) and colleagues in 1994 modified Morton's technique of intraoperative lymphatic mapping using vital blue dye and applied it to breast cancer.[58] Giuliano injected isosulfan blue dye into the breast cancer and the surrounding breast parenchyma in 174 patients. An incision was made in the axilla, and all blue lymphatic channels were identified and traced to a blue node. In his study,

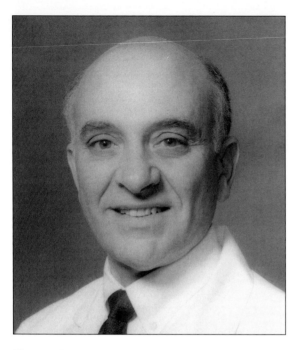

Figure 1.3 Armando E Giuliano, MD, Director, Joyce Eisenberg Keefer Breast Center Associate Director and Chief of Surgical Oncology, John Wayne Cancer Institute.

Giuliano successfully identified the SLN in 114 of 174 patients (66%). A sensitivity of 88% and a false-negative rate of 6.5% were found. Subsequently, large studies have shown that using both a vital dye and radioisotope together improved both the SLN detection rate to greater than 90%, and the false-negative rate to less than 5%.[59]

THE CURRENT IMPACT OF SLN BIOPSY

A prospective study by Giuliano and colleagues confirmed the feasibility of SLN biopsy alone in patients whose SLNs were found to be tumor-free.[60] This study enrolled 133 patients with invasive breast cancer clinically less than or equal to 4 cm in size and no axillary lymphadenopathy. Patients underwent SLN biopsy using vital blue dye. Sentinel lymph nodes were histologically evaluated using standard techniques and IHC. Patients whose SLNs were found to be tumor-free underwent no further axillary surgery. Completion ALND was performed only in patients whose SLNs contained metastatic disease or in patients in whom no SLN could be identified. The SLN identification rate was 99%. Of the 133 patients, 8 were excluded from further evaluation because they were treated with mastectomy for multifocal carcinoma or they refused completion ALND. Of the 125 patients remaining, 57 (46%) had SLNs containing metastatic disease, 67 (54%) had tumor-free SLNs, and 1 patient had an unsuccessful mapping procedure. The median follow-up period for the patients was 39 months. At that time, there were no reported axillary recurrences in the 57 patients who underwent SLN biopsy alone. Additionally, the complications reported in the ALND group were significantly higher than in the SLN biopsy-only group (35% and 3%, respectively). This study demonstrates not only the decrease in morbidity associated with this procedure compared with ALND, but also the efficacy of SLN biopsy alone in patients with tumor-free SLNs. The lack of axillary recurrences suggests that patients with tumor-free SLNs do not need an ALND.

The defining of the lymphatics of the breast and the development of the SLN mapping technique are having a major impact on the management of patients with breast cancer. This technique enables an accurate assessment of the axillary lymph-node basin while minimizing the potential risks associated with complete ALND. The results of current clinical trials will determine the precise role of the SLN biopsy technique in the management of breast cancer.

REFERENCES

1. Schrenk P, Rieger R, Shamiyeh A, Wayand W, Morbidity following sentinel lymph node biopsy versus axillary lymph node dissection for patients with breast carcinoma. *Cancer* 2000; **88**:608–14.
2. Osborne MP, Payne JH, Richardson VJ et al, The preoperative detection of axillary lymph node metastases in breast cancer by isotope imaging. *Br J Surg* 1983; **70**:141–4.

3. Aselius G, *De Lactibus.* Apud Jo. Baptistam Bidellium: Mediolani, 1627.

4. Pecquet J, *De Veinis Taur Lacteis Thoracis.* Geneva, 1654.

5. Bartholin T, *Vasa Lymphatica, Nupa Hafnae in Animantibus Inventa et Hepatis Exqhiae.* Copenhagen: Petri Hakii, 1653.

6. Cruikshank W, The anatomy of the absorbing vessels of the human body. London, 1786.

7. Mascagni P, *Vasorum Lymphaticorum Corporis Humani Historia et Ichnographia.* Italy, 1787.

8. Sappey PC, *Anatomie, physiologie et pathology, des vaisseaux lymphatiques consideres chez l'homme et les vertebres.* Paris, 1883.

9. Poirier P, Cuneo B, Delamere G, *The Lymphatics.* London, 1903.

10. Grossman F, *Ueber die axillaren Lymphdrusen.* Berlin, 1896.

11. Rotter J, Concerning the topography of mammary carcinoma. *Arch F Klin Chir* 1899; **58**:346.

12. Stibbe EP, The internal mammary lymphatic glands. *J Anat* 1918; **52**:257.

13. Rouvière H, *Anatomie des lymphatiques de l'homme.* Paris, 1932.

14. Valsalva AM, *Deaure humana troatatus.* Bononrae, 1704.

15. Le Dran HF, Memoires avec un precis de plusieurs observations sur le cancer. *Mem Acad R Chir* 1757; **3**:1.

16. Heidenhain L, Concerning the cause of the local recurrence of cancer after amputatio mammae. *Arch F Klin Chir* 1888; **39**:97.

17. Stiles HJ, Contributions to the surgical anatomy of the breast. *Edinb Med J* 1892; **37**:1099.

18. Handley S, *Cancer of the Breast and its Operative Treatment.* London, 1907.

19. Pickren JW, Lymph node metastasis in carcinoma of the female mammary gland. *Roswell Park Bull* 1956; **1**:79.

20. Haagensen CD, The natural history of breast carcinoma. In: Haagensen CD, ed, *Diseases of the Breast*, 2nd edn, 635–718. WB Saunders: Philadelphia, 1971.

21. Morl F, *Chirug* 1952; **23**:238.

22. Haagensen CD, Lymphatics of the breast. In: Haagensen CD, Feind CR, Herter FP, Slanetz CA, Weinberg JA, eds, *The Lymphatics in Cancer*, 300–98. WB Saunders: Philadelphia, 1972.

23. Sherman AI, Ter-Pogossian M, Lymph node concentration of radioactive colloidal gold following interstitial injection. *Cancer* 1953; **6**:1238–40.

24. Hultborn KA, Larsson LG, Ragnhult I, The lymph drainage from the breast to the axillary and parasternal lymph nodes, studied with the aid of colloidal Au 198. *Acta Radiol* 1955; **43**:52–64.

25. Turner-Warwick RT, The lymphatics of the breast. *Br J Surg* 1959; **46**:574–82.

26. zum Winkel K, Zur Technik der indirekten abdominellen Lymphknotenszintigraphie mit 198-Au-colloidale. *Nucl Med* 1963; **3**:148.

27. Schwab W, Scheer KE, zum Winkel K, Szintigraphy des zervikalen Lymphsystems. *Strahlentherapie* 1965; **130**:504.

28. Bethune DC, Mulder DS, Chiu RC, Endobronchial lymphoscintigraphy (EBLS). New diagnostic modality. *J Thorac Cardiovasc Surg* 1978; **76**:446–52.

29. Rossi R, Ferri O, La visualizzazione della catena mammaria interna con [198]Au. Presentazione di una nuova metodica; la linfoscintigrafia. *Minerva Med* 1966; **57**:1151–5.

30. Schenck P, Scintigraphische dasstellung des parasternalen Lymphsystems. *Strahlentherapie* 1966; **130**:504.

31. Matsuo S, Studies on the metastasis of breast cancer to lymph nodes-II, diagnosis of metastasis to internal mammary nodes using radiogold. *Acta Med Okayama* 1975; **28**:361–71.

32. Zum Winkel K, Hermann HJ, Scintigraphy of lymph nodes. *Lymphology* 1977; **10**:107–14.

33. Harper PV, Lathrop KA, Jiminez F et al, Technetium 99m as a scanning agent. *Radiology* 1965; **85**:101–8.

34. Hauser W, Atkins HL, Richards P, Lymph node scanning with ^{99m}Tc-sulfur colloid. *Radiology* 1969; **92**:1369–71.

35. Aspegren K, Strand SE, Persson BRR, Quantitative lymphoscintigraphy for detection of metastases to the internal mammary lymph nodes; biokinetics of 99mTc-sulfur colloid uptake and correlation with microscopy. *Acta Radiol Oncol Radiat Phys Biol* 1978; **17**:17–26.

36. Garzon OL, Palcof NC, Radicella R, A preparation of ^{99m}Tc-labelled colloid. *Int J Appl Radiat Isot* 1965; **16**:613.

37. Ege GN, Internal mammary lymphoscintigraphy in breast carcinoma: a study of 1072 patients. *Int J Radiat Oncol Biol Phys* 1977; **2**:755–61.

38. Osborne MP, Jeyasingh K, Jewkes RF, Burn I, The preoperative detection of internal mammary lymph node metastases in breast cancer. *Br J Surg* 1979; **66**:813–18.

39. Cox PH, The kinetics of macromolecule transport in lymph and colloid accumulation in lymph nodes. In: Cox PH, ed, *Progress in*

Radiopharmacology, volume II, pp. 267–92. Elsevier/North Holland: Amsterdam, 1981.

40. Goodwin DA, Finston RA et al, ^{111}In for imaging: lymph node visualization. *Radiology* 1970; **94:** 175–8.

41. Osborne MP, Richardson VJ, Jeyasingh K, Ryman BE, Radionuclide-labelled liposomes—a new lymph node imaging agent. *Int J Nucl Med Biol* 1979; **6:**75–83.

42. Osborne MP, Meijer WS, DeCosse JJ, Lymphoscintigraphy in the staging of solid tumors. *Surg Gyn Obstet* 1983; **156:**384–91.

43. Kett K, Varga G, Lukacs L, Direct lymphography of the breast. *Lymphology* 1970; **1:**3–12.

44. Agwunobi TC, Boak JL, Diagnosis of malignant breast disease by axillary lymphoscintigraphy: a preliminary report. *Br J Surg* 1978; **65:**379–83.

45. Christensen B, Blichert-Toft M, Sieminssen OJ, Nielsen SL, Reliability of axillary lymph node scintiphotography in suspected carcinoma of the breast. *Br J Surg* 1980; **67:**667–8.

46. Gould EA, Winship T, Philbin PH, Hyland Kerr H, Observations on a "sentinel node" in cancer of the parotid. *Cancer* 1960; **13:**77–8.

47. Cabanas RM, An approach for the treatment of penile carcinoma. *Cancer* 1977; **39:**456–66.

48. Morton DL, Wen DR, Wong JH et al, Technical details of intraoperative lymphatic mapping for early stage melanoma. *Arch Surg* 1992; **127:**392–9.

49. Robinson DS, Sample WF, Fee HJ et al, Regional lymphatic drainage in primary malignant melanoma of the trunk determined by colloidal gold scanning. *Surg Forum* 1977; **28:**147–8.

50. Osborne, MP, Payne, JH, Richardson VJ et al, The preoperative detection of axillary lymph node metastases in breast cancer by isotope imaging. *Br J Surg* 1983;**70:**141–4.

51. Peyton JWR, Crosbie J, Bell TK et al, High colloidal uptake in axillary nodes with metastatic disease. *Br J Surg* 1981; **68:**507–9.

52. Christensen B, Blichert-Toft M, Siemssen OJ, Nielsen SL, Reliability of axillary lymph node scintigraphy in suspected carcinoma of the breast. *Br J Surg* 1980; **67:**667–8.

53. Krag DN, Weaver DL, Alex JC, Fairbank JT, Surgical resection and radiolocalization of the sentinel node in breast cancer using a gamma probe. *Surg Onc* 1993; **2:**335–40.

54. Alex JC, Krag DN, Gamma-probe guided localization of lymph nodes. *Surg Onc* 1993; **2:**137–43.

55. Krag D, Weaver D, Ashikaga T et al, The sentinel node in breast cancer—a multicenter validation study. *N Engl J Med* 1998; **339:**941–6.

56. Cox CE, Pendas S, Cox JM et al, Guidelines for sentinel node biopsy and lymphatic mapping of patients with breast cancer. *Ann Surg* 1998; **227:**645–53.

57. Hill ADK, Tran KN, Akhurst T et al, Lessons learned from 500 cases of lymphatic mapping for breast cancer. *Ann Surg* 1999; **229:**528–35.

58. Giuliano AE, Kirgan DM, Guenther JM, Morton DL, Lymphatic mapping and sentinel lymphadenectomy for breast cancer. *Ann Surg* 1994; **220:**391–401.

59. Albertini JJ, Lyman GH, Cox C et al, Lymphatic mapping and sentinel node biopsy in the patient with breast cancer. *JAMA* 1996; **276:**1818–22.

60. Giuliano AE, Haigh PI, Brennan MB et al, Prospective observational study of sentinel lymphadenectomy without further axillary dissection in patients with sentinel-node-negative breast cancer. *J Clin Oncol* 2000; **18:**2553–9.

2

The anatomy and physiology of the lymphatics of the breast

Arnold DK Hill and Matthew A Sadlier

CONTENTS   **Anatomy**   •   **Physiology**

ANATOMY

The breasts are best described as paired modified sweat glands that extend from the second to the sixth rib and from the lateral border of the sternum to the midaxillary line.[1] The breast lies mainly in the superficial fascia, with the axillary tail piercing the deep fascia at the lower border of the pectoralis major muscle, and comes into close contact with the axillary vessels.

The lymphatics of the breast have been shown to be the same as lymphatics elsewhere in the body, in that they follow the vascular supply.[2] The inner quadrants of the breast are supplied by a number of perforating branches of the internal thoracic artery or internal mammary artery. These arteries perforate the intercostal space and the origin of the pectoralis major muscle along the lateral sternal border.[3]

The axillary artery supplies the breast via the lateral thoracic and thoracoacromial branches. Both are branches of the second part of the axillary artery.[1] The thoracoacromial artery runs inferiorly, pierces the clavipectoral fascia, and divides into terminal branches. The lateral thoracic artery runs along the lower border of the pectoralis minor and runs around the lateral border of the pectoralis major. The outer quadrants of the breast receive their supply from the lateral cutaneous branches of the posterior intercostal arteries.[2] Within the breast, these arteries interconnect in an anastomotic network.[3]

The venous drainage does not parallel the arterial supply exactly. In the periareolar region, the veins form an anastomotic circle around the areola in the subcutaneous tissue. This plexus drains via large-diameter subcutaneous veins in a centrifugal manner towards the periphery and connects with the veins that accompany the arteries.[3] Eventually, the venous drainage reaches the axillary or the internal thoracic veins.[1]

Lymphatic drainage to the axilla

The majority of the lymph drainage of the breast runs to the axilla (Figure 2.1). The main axillary lymphatics arise in the lobules of the breast. These lymphatics run a course within the substance of the breast, in the interlobular connective tissue, rather than on its deep or superficial surface. On their journey to the axilla, they are joined by many tributaries. Within the axillary tail, they pass through the deep fascia and come to lie on the medial wall of the axilla.[2] These lymph vessels run alongside the lateral thoracic vessels and course inferomedially and then anteriorly to the axillary vein. Although most of the lymph drainage of the breast runs into the lateral thoracic group of lymph nodes, some passes into the subscapular group of nodes.[2]

The axillary lymph nodes are the most important nodes draining the breast. These nodes have been divided by anatomists into five groups, not wholly distinct from one another. Four of these groups can be seen as intermediary pathways, with the apical group seen as the terminal group of nodes.[1] For simplicity's sake, the axilla can be seen as a three-sided pyramid with lymph nodes located along each edge, at the apex of the pyramid, and in the center. The five groupings are as follows:

1. *Lateral (brachial) node group*: these nodes are few in number and are concerned with lymph drainage of the arm. They are found

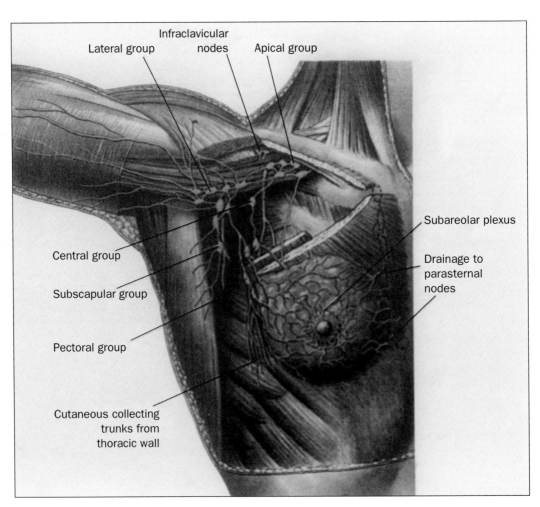

Figure 2.1 The lymphatics of the breast. (Reprinted with permission from Williams PL, Gray H, eds, *Gray's Anatomy*, 37th edn. Churchill Livingstone: London, 1989.)

posteromedially to the axillary vein and drain into the apical nodes.[1]

2. *Anterior (pectoral) node group*: these are found along the inferior border of the pectoralis major and drain the anterior body wall as well as the centrolateral portion of the breast.[1]

3. *Posterior (subscapular) node group*: these nodes are found on the posterior wall of the axilla in association with the subscapular vessels. They drain mainly the posterior aspect of the inferior neck, as well as the dorsal aspect of the trunk to the level of the iliac crest.[1]

4. *Central node group*: this group consists of three or four large nodes found buried within the axillary fat. They receive lymph from the previous node groupings. The efferent lymph drains into the apical nodes.[1]

5. *Apical (terminal) node group*: these nodes are found in the apex of the axilla partly posterior to the pectoralis major and partly superior to its upper border. These glands receive some lymph directly from the arm as well as some from the upper peripheral regions of the breast. These glands mainly serve to drain the four previously mentioned nodal groupings.[1] The efferents from these nodes form the subclavian trunk, which drains into the great veins of the neck either via the thoracic duct and right lymphatic trunk or independently of these vessels.[4]

Most surgeons group the axillary nodes into three levels. Level I comprises those nodes found below the lateral border of the pectoralis minor. Level II comprises the nodes lying behind the pectoralis minor, and Level III consists of the nodes lying above the pectoralis minor.[4]

Most lymph from the breast passes to the external mammary group of nodes (of Rouvière), which extend from the axillary tail all the way to the apex of the axilla. The lymph vessels that accompany the thoracoacromial vessels first pass through the interpectoral nodes, which lie between the pectoralis major

and minor, before entering the higher axillary nodes.[2]

Intrathoracic lymphatic drainage

Hultborn, in 1955, showed that only 1–3% of the lymph drainage entered the internal mammary nodes;[5] however, lymph entered this system from injections to all areas of the breast. In the same study, Hultborn claimed that the ipsilateral axillary chain received 98% of the lymphatic drainage of the breast.[5]

A small amount of the lymphatic drainage of the medial breast runs to the internal mammary lymph nodes that are found accompanying the internal thoracic artery and vein. They receive lymph from vessels that accompany the anterior perforating arteries of the internal thoracic artery. They may also receive lymph from vessels that accompany the lateral perforating branches of the upper intercostal arteries.[2] The nodes are found in the intercostal spaces and posterior to the costal cartilages close to the sternum. In 1972, Donegan found an average of 3.8 of these nodes in extended radical mastectomy specimens.[6] The nodes were found mostly in the upper parasternal areas near bifurcations of the intercostal and internal mammary veins. Efferent lymphatics connect these nodes and terminate above in the various lymphatics that enter the jugular veins.[3]

Most lymphatics that leave the posterior surface of the breast pass through the pectoralis major to reach the internal mammary chain and axilla. The pectoralis minor muscle has lymphatics in front of it, above it, and below it. No significant pathway crosses it, however.[2]

This intrathoracic route of lymph spread has important clinical and therapeutic importance for breast carcinoma. Thomas et al, in 1979, showed that the main route of spread of breast carcinoma to the thorax was lymphatic and not hematogenous, as was believed at the time.[7] This, they claimed, would explain why pleural effusions that develop in association with breast carcinomas tend to occur ipsilateral to the primary lesion. They suggested that carcinoma spreads via the lymphatic route from the internal mammary nodes to lymph nodes on both sides of the mediastinum, and from there to the thoracic solid organs.

The lymphatic spread of breast carcinoma to other solid organs has been questioned. In 1922, Handley described lymphatic connections between the breast and the liver via the prepericardial nodes on the anterior surface of the diaphragm.[8] Lymphatic drainage of the upper portions of the liver to the lowermost internal mammary nodes is well documented. The localization of bone metastases, however, is credited to the connections between intercostal and paravertebral veins described by Batson in 1940.[9]

The subareolar lymphatic plexus

Sappey, in 1885, described the subareolar lymphatic plexus (see Chapter 1). Many authors since have believed that the majority of lymph from the breast drains centripetally through this area before draining to the axilla.[2] In the subareolar region, there is a subcutaneous pathway that communicates with ducts draining the lactiferous ducts.[3] These ducts are important in absorbing secretions, especially during pregnancy. The subareolar plexus is in continuation with the subepithelial and subdermal plexuses.[3] The lymphatics that accompany the lactiferous ducts lie in the loose connective tissue just outside the myoepithelial layer of the duct wall.[10]

Turner-Warwick in 1959 and Halsell in 1965, however, refuted the idea that lymph flows centripetally into the subareolar plexus, suggesting that lymph flows via valvular lymphatics from superficial to deep tissue and then on towards regional nodes.[2,11]

The clinical significance of the subareolar plexus of lymphatics is exemplified by the work of Borgstein and Meijer, who inject blue dye into the subareolar plexus of lymphatics for sentinel lymph node (SLN) mapping in all cases of breast cancer, regardless of the location of the primary tumor within the breast.[12]

The subcutaneous lymphatics

The subcutaneous network of lymphatics lies in the same plane as the superficial venous plexus, which can become visible during pregnancy. This network, which is no different from the subcutaneous lymphatic plexus in other areas of the body, extends across the midline, over the clavicles, and down into the anterior abdominal wall. This network anastomoses with the deeper lymphatics of the breast, especially with the subareolar plexus.[2] It does not contain valves, thus allowing lymph drainage in all directions.[13]

The subcutaneous network of lymphatics drains very little of the lymph of the body but is very important in the spread of carcinoma. Considerable spread of radioactivity in the subcutaneous tissues beyond the area of simple diffusion has been shown following intramammary injection of colloid gold.[2]

Intramammary lymph nodes

In 1956, during correlation of histopathologic changes in the breast with radiologic findings, a number of apparently benign lesions were shown to be lymph nodes within the breast itself.[14] In a study published in 1982, Egan and McSweeney demonstrated the presence of lymph nodes within the breast in 28% of pathologic breast specimens.[14] The nodes were found in all quadrants of the breast and were not associated with the usual drainage pathway of the breast lymphatics. The true prevalence of intramammary lymph nodes is difficult to estimate, however, as there is no clear anatomical division between the end of the tail of the breast and the beginning of the axilla.

PHYSIOLOGY

The lymphatic system has a number of important functions in normal physiology. It is involved in the production and destruction of blood cells, and performs the immunologic function of defending against invading pathogens.[15] It also has a circulatory function as a drainage system for the interstitium of the breast.[16]

The lymphatic system is a necessary byproduct of our highly evolved, closed-circuit, high-pressure circulatory system. Less complex species lack lymphatics, having instead open circulations that allow direct drainage of the interstitium to the venous system.[16] The lymphatic system's purpose is to carry away large molecules, such as proteins, as well as cells and particulate molecules that occur in the interstitium in both health and disease.[15] Most of our understanding of the functions of the lymphatics as a drainage system comes from Starling's work at the turn of the last century.[16]

Organization

Lymphatics are thin-walled vessels that converge upon the neck, where they drain into the venous system. The vessels encountered from the tissues to the neck are classified and named according to their size and position. The smallest lymphatic vessels are the capillaries, which exist in every region of the body that has a vasculature. Unlike their cardiovascular equivalents, the lymphatic capillaries are blind-ending, resembling the fingers of a glove. The postcapillary lymphatic vessels have valves projecting into the lumen and smooth muscle in the intimal layer of the wall. The prenodal collecting vessels terminate at the subcapsular sinus in the lymph node.[16]

The next level in the organization of the drainage system is the lymph node. Under normal circumstances, all lymph traverses at least one set of nodes prior to entering the venous system.[16]

The efferent vessels from the lymph nodes branch and divide before either entering more nodes, or congregating to enter larger lymph vessels, the lymphatic trunks, and the ducts. The lymphatic trunks are a few large, named vessels that drain the major groups of lymph nodes. They may enter the bloodstream themselves or empty into one of the two lymphatic ducts. The right lymphatic duct lies in front of the scalenus anterior muscle and receives the lymphatic drainage from the upper-right part of the body. It rarely extends beyond 1 cm, and drains into the right subclavian or internal jugular veins. The thoracic duct runs from the cisterna chyli in the abdomen through the thorax to drain into the left subclavian vein. It receives lymph from all but the upper-right part of the body.[16]

Function

The flow in lymphatics is dependent on the following three components:

- valves
- compression of the vessels by movement of neighboring tissues
- smooth muscle in the walls of the vessels themselves.[15]

Valves are found in all lymphatics above the level of capillaries with the exception of those in the parenchyma of certain organs such as thyroid and lungs.[13] The subdermal network of lymphatics is also deficient in valves; thus flow can occur in all directions.[15] Retrograde flow in these vessels is only possible in the presence of the dilatation that normally accompanies obstruction to flow. Frequently, however, the valvular lymphatics will rupture before they allow any reverse flow.

The valves are bicuspid in structure, and the absolute distance separating the valves is dependent on the diameter of the vessel in question, the distance being shorter in the smaller vessels. The almost universal presence of valves in the lymphatic system results in a fixed direction of flow, which, along with the aggregation of lymphatic trunks from areas of tissue, allows us to predict the specific route of flow of lymph—from a particular area of the body to a specific group of nodes.[13] The route of lymph flow does not adhere to an absolute law, however, as each area of the body has subsidiary lymphatics that form anastomoses and can drain to a different set of nodes. Normally, these subsidiary lymphatics play a small role in the lymphatic drainage, but the subsidiary channels may enlarge and multiply if the main pathways become blocked for any reason.[13]

The force that drives the flow in lymphatics is similar to that in veins. It depends on contractility of surrounding structures, including muscle and other tissues such as arterial pulsations.[15] Spontaneous contractility of the lymphatics of other species is a well-documented phenomenon, having been seen by Heller in 1869 in the mesenteric vessels of guinea pigs.[15]

Evidence of inherent contractility of human lymphatics was first seen in 1956, when Kinmouth and Taylor reported seeing it in the thoracic duct of adults.[17] The muscular coat found in the tunica media of the larger lymphatics provides the kinetic force for the forward propulsion.[16] Rhythmic contractions have

also been demonstrated in the lymphatic capillaries, although they lack a muscular coat.[18] The presence of many cytoplasmic filaments and heavy meromyosin is believed to be responsible for producing this contraction. Contractility of lymphatics has been documented in the periphery as well as in the larger lymphatic ducts.[19] More recent observations indicate that it is this intrinsic contractility of the lymphatic vessels that is largely responsible for the perfusion of lymph toward the thoracic duct.[20]

For the lymphatic capillaries to function as a drainage system of the interstitium, there must be a preferential pathway for proteins and cells to the lymphatic capillaries. The major pathway is the intercellular junction, although endocytosis does occur. There are specialized intercellular junctions resembling flap valves on the

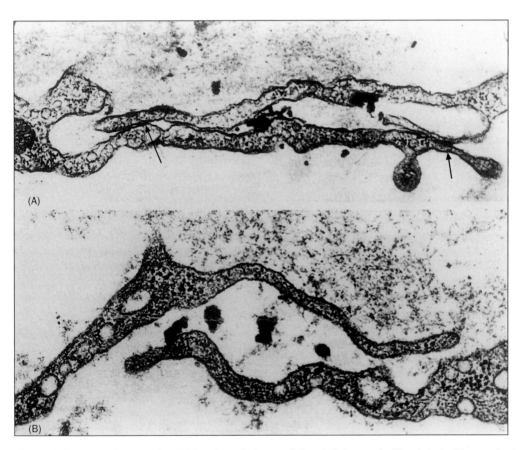

Figure 2.2 (A, B) Passage of colloid carbon via intercellular cleft (arrows). (Reprinted with permission from Abramson DL, Dobrin PB, eds, *Blood Vessels and Lymphatics in Organ Systems*. Academic Press: Orlando, 1984.)

lymphatic capillary endothelial structure that allow for rapid transport of fluid, macromolecules, and cells. These valves open and close in response to the pressure differential between the lumen of the capillary and the interstitial space, allowing them to open when the connective-tissue pressure outside the vessel exceeds that inside (Figure 2.2).

Lymph collects in the capillaries because of the ability of the capillaries to create a "suction" effect. This ability is due, in turn, to the intrinsic contractility of the lymphatic vasculature. Also, the lymphatic capillaries are well fixed to the surrounding interstitium via anchoring filaments; expansion of the interstitium with the collection of fluid leads to the expansion of the lymphatics. This creates a negative suction pressure within them that causes the flap valves to open and a net influx of cells, protein, and fluid to occur.[15]

Finally, it has been noted that adrenergic fibres have been found in the walls of the large lymphatics in close association with the smooth-muscle cells. This implies regulation by the sympathetic nervous system of the rhythmic contractions of the lymphatics.[21]

Sentinel lymph-node mapping is based on an understanding of the physiology of the lymphatic system. Particles of the blue dye or isotope need to be 50–100 nm in size to be taken up by the lymphatics and trapped in the lymph node. Hence, methylene blue is not useful for the procedure owing to its small particle size, which allows it to pass on into second-tier lymph nodes.

REFERENCES

1. Williams PL, Gray H, eds, *Gray's Anatomy*, 37th edn. Churchill Livingstone: London, 1989.
2. Turner-Warwick RT, The lymphatics of the breast. *Br J Surg* 1959; **46:**574–82.
3. Donegan WL, Spratt JS, eds, *Cancer of the Breast*, 4th edn. Saunders: Philadelphia, 1995.
4. Jamieson GG, Carter ML, Block dissection of axillary lymph nodes: the anatomy of the axilla. In: Jamieson GG, ed, *The Anatomy of General Surgical Operations*. Churchill Livingstone: New York, 1992.
5. Hultborn KA, Larsson LG, Ragnhult I, The lymph drainage from the breast to the axillary and parasternal nodes, studied with the aid of colloid Au[198]. *Acta Radiol* 1955; **43:**52–64.
6. Donegan WL, Mastectomy in the primary management of invasive mammary carcinoma. In: Hardy JD, ed, *Advances in Surgery*, vol. 6, 1–101. Mosby Year Book: St Louis, 1972.
7. Thomas JM, Redding WH, Sloane JP, The spread of breast cancer: the importance of the intrathoracic lymphatic route and its relevance to treatment. *Br J Cancer* 1979; **40:**540–7.
8. Handley WS, *Cancer of the Breast and its Treatment*, 2nd edn. John Murray: London, 1922.
9. Batson OV, The function of the vertebral veins and their role in the spread of metastases. *Ann Surg* 1940; **122:**138.
10. Bonser GM, Dossett JA, Jull JW, *Human and Experimental Breast Cancer*. Pitman: London, 1961.
11. Halsell JT, Smith JR, Bentlage CR et al, Lymphatic drainage of the breast demonstrated by vital dye staining and radiography. *Ann Surg* 1965; **162:**221.
12. Borgstein P, Meijer S, Historical perspective of lymphatic tumour spread and the emergence of the sentinel node concept. *Eur J Surg Oncol* 1998; **24:**85–9.
13. Gray JH, The relation of lymphatic vessels to the spread of cancer. *Br J Surg* 1938; **26:**462–95.
14. Egan RD, McSweeney MB, Intramammary lymph nodes. *Cancer* 1983; **51:**1838–42.
15. Kinmouth JB, *The Lymphatics—Diseases, Lymphography, and Surgery*, 2nd edn. Edward Arnold: London, 1982.
16. Abramson DL, Dobrin PB, eds, *Blood Vessels and Lymphatics in Organ Systems*. Academic Press: Orlando, 1984.
17. Kinmouth JB, Taylor GW, Spontaneous rhythmic contractility in human lymphatics. *J Physiol (Lond)* 1956; **133:**3P.
18. Leak LV, Studies on the permeability of lymphatic capillaries. *J Cell Biol* 1971; **50:**300–23.
19. Szegvari M, Lakos A, Szontagh F, Foldi M, Spontaneous contraction of the lymph vessels in man. *Lancet* 1963; **i:**1329.
20. Hall JG, Morris B, Woolley G, Intrinsic rhythmic propulsion of lymph in the unanaesthetized sheep. *J Physiol (Lond)* 1965; **180:**336–49.
21. Todd GL, Bernard GR, Functional anatomy of the cervical lymph duct of the dog. *Anat Rec* 1971; **169:**443A.

3

The role of nuclear medicine

Roger F Uren and Robert Howman-Giles

Nuclear medicine is one of three major specialties that must be integrated in the sentinel lymph-node biopsy method to ensure its successful application. These three major specialties are nuclear medicine, surgical oncology, and histopathology.

The importance of nuclear medicine in this biopsy method lies in the contribution of high-quality lymphoscintigraphy, with which accurate mapping of the pattern of lymphatic drainage from the primary tumor site to its draining lymph nodes, the sentinel nodes, can be obtained preoperatively. Any lymph node that receives lymph drainage directly from the primary tumor site is a sentinel lymph node (SLN), and in all patients, all such nodes must be identified for the SLN biopsy procedure to be successful. Lymphoscintigraphy allows all SLNs to be identified in each patient, regardless of the location of these nodes. Failure to identify some SLNs because they lie in an unusual location outside of recognized node fields will lead to an incomplete SLN biopsy in that patient.

THE DEVELOPMENT OF LYMPHOSCINTIGRAPHY

In 1953, Sherman and Ter-Pogossian described a new technique called lymphoscintigraphy (LSG), which allowed the physiology of lymph flow in individual patients to be accurately studied following interstitial injection of a radiocolloid.[1] When this technique was applied to patients with melanoma and other malignancies of the trunk, it soon became clear that long-held beliefs about the expected patterns of lymphatic drainage from different parts of the skin, based mainly on Sappey's original work, did not hold true in many patients. Many subsequent workers confirmed the extreme variability of the lymphatic drainage from the skin of the trunk.[2–5] Norman et al defined and expanded new zones of ambiguity based on this increasing store of knowledge,[6] and Eberbach and Wahl combined data from several authors to further illustrate the extensive overlap of areas that drain to the various node fields.[7] Likewise, when the lymphatic drainage of the mammary glands was studied using LSG, it was shown that, as in the skin, the patterns of drainage in individual patients can be quite variable and are not clinically predictable based simply on the site of the breast cancer within the gland.

Increasing experience with LSG has shown many variations in the lymphatic drainage of the skin and breast in humans, and very few sites in the body have been shown to produce clinically predictable drainage.

LYMPHOSCINTIGRAPHY TECHNIQUE

The performance of high-quality LSG for SLN biopsy relies on several important factors:

- radiocolloid entry into the lymphatic system
- movement of the tracer along the lymphatic vessel to the draining SLN
- retention of the radiocolloid in the SLN
- distinction of SLNs from second-tier nodes
- establishment of appropriate imaging protocols that ensure the identification of all SLNs
- accurate demarcation of the surface location of the SLN.

Radiocolloid entry into the lymphatic system

The success of LSG as part of the SLN biopsy procedure revolves around its ability to show the lymphatic vessels passing from the tumor site to the draining lymph nodes (Figure 3.1). These are the same vessels that the surgeon sees staining blue at operation when preoperative blue dye is used. It is the visualization of such channels entering a node that unequivocally identifies it as an SLN, and this should be achieved during dynamic LSG. The interface between the interstitial fluid and the lymphatic system is the initial lymphatic capillary. The radiocolloid being used must gain ready access to the lumen of this initial lymphatic in sufficient quantity for the lymph vessels to be seen on the dynamic scans. The particle size of the radiocolloid is a critical factor in the ease with which these tracers enter the lymphatic system.

Particles up to 1–2 nm in diameter tend to enter the venous blood system directly. Particles between 5 nm and 25 nm in size enter lymphatic capillaries via the gaps between cell junctions and the intercellular clefts formed by overlapping cells, which measure 10–25 nm across. Particles up to 75 nm in diameter may gain entry into the lymphatic lumen by pinocytosis.[8] Particles greater than 75 nm in diameter will find the connective-tissue lattice increasingly difficult to penetrate, causing most of the injected tracer to remain at the injection site.

The entry of radiocolloid into the initial lymphatic capillary can be increased with the use of massage[9] and larger volumes of injectate. Both of these interventions cause large gaps to open up between the lymphatic endothelial cells because of the effects of movement and tension in the soft tissues. These effects can be employed to overcome in part the disadvantages of using colloids with large particle sizes, such as technetium-99m-sulfur colloid (Tc-99m-SC). There is, however, a potential problem when large injection volumes are used, as new lymph channels may be forced open, draining tracer to nodes that would not receive lymph flow from the primary tumor site under physiological conditions. To avoid this, we recommend that injection volumes in the skin not exceed 0.1 ml (cc)—and in the breast, 1.0 ml—at each injection site.

The first technetium-labeled radiocolloid used for LSG was Tc-99m-SC, with a range of particle size of 50 nm to 2000 nm and an average size of 300 nm. Because of the large particles, this tracer had poor clearance from the injection site; this encouraged the development of Tc-99m colloids with a smaller particle size. Kaplan et al studied two radiocolloids, Tc-99m-stannous phytate and Tc-99m-antimony sulfur colloid, as agents for LSG in humans.[10] They concluded that Tc-99m-antimony sulfur colloid was the agent of choice for LSG. It gains ready access to the lymphatic vessels and migrates rapidly through the vessels to the draining node field, yet there is excellent retention in the lymph nodes for up to 24 hours. Antimony sulfur colloid has particles of relatively uniform size, most 10–15 nm in diameter, ranging up to 40 nm. These particles are an ideal size to pass

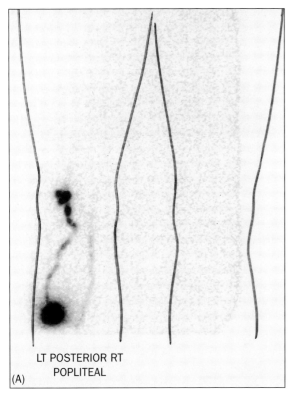
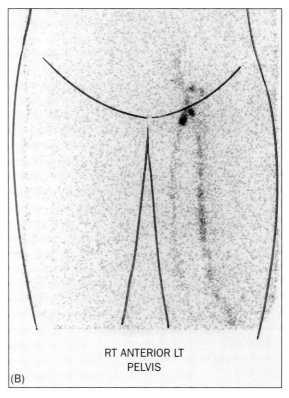

Figure 3.1 Summed dynamic-phase LSG performed posteriorly over the legs (A) and anteriorly over the thighs and groins (B) shows two lymphatic vessels passing up the leg from the injection site on the lateral left midcalf. One channel passes laterally up to an SLN in the popliteal fossa, while a second channel passes medially up the leg directly to the groin where it enters a separate SLN, which is the medial of the two nodes seen at this time in the groin. The other node seen just lateral to this receives drainage via the channel that has already passed through the popliteal SLN; thus, it is a second-tier node. High-resolution LSG is needed to clarify such complex situations.

freely into the lymphatic capillaries via the 10-nm to 25-nm clefts between overlapping cells and the intercellular gaps. Similarly, Tc-99m-nanocolloidal albumin migrates well following intradermal injection, and its use produces excellent scans in most patients. This tracer has a wide range of particle sizes (3–80 nm), but 77% are less than 30 nm.[11]

Thus, it appears that the ideal radiocolloid for LSG is any colloid with particles in the 5-nm to 75-nm range. Both Tc-99m-nanocolloidal albumin and Tc-99m-antimony sulfur colloid have particles that fall in this range, and both are excellent for LSG and SLN biopsy. They also both have specific regulatory approval for LSG in humans.

Variations in the drug approval regimens in different countries have led to some nations having no direct clinical access to these desirable radiocolloids. This situation is the case particularly in the USA, where there is no Food and Drug Administration approval for such agents, and clinicians use Tc-99m-SC by default.

The size distribution of Tc-99m-SC can be significantly altered by the method of preparation,[12] and by filtering the radiocolloid. Particles over 200 nm can be removed by the use of 0.2 μm filters; however, the colloid must be used soon after filtering as the particle size increases slowly over a 5-hour period. Such filtered sulfur colloid is favored by some, as owing to its larger size it tends to be retained well by the SLN.[13]

Despite filtering, the size of the Tc-99m-SC particles does limit movement of this tracer into the lymphatic capillaries, and in practice this means that, during dynamic LSG using Tc-99m-SC, the lymphatic vessels will often not be visualized. This removes one of the key pieces of information used to identify an SLN by LSG (i.e., the identification of a lymphatic vessel entering the node on dynamic imaging).

Extensive clinical experience, however, has been gained using filtered Tc-99m-SC, and it appears in clinical practice to be adequate to identify the SLNs on LSG in most patients.[12] A recent study by Wong and colleagues suggested that particle size is not important in identifying the SLN and stated a preference for Tc-99m-SC because there was less movement of this colloid onward to second-tier lymph nodes when compared with Tc-99m-human serum albumin (HSA), the other tracer they studied.[14] When Tc-99m-SC has been directly compared with the smaller colloids, however, such as antimony sulfur or nanocolloidal albumin, fewer channels have been seen on dynamic images with sulfur colloid, fewer draining nodes fields have been seen per patient, and fewer SLNs have been seen per node field.[15] We remain concerned, therefore, that although an apparently "successful" SLN biopsy procedure may be completed using microfiltered Tc-99m-SC, not all true SLNs will be detected in all patients.

Technetium-99m-human serum albumin (Tc-99m-HSA) is frequently used in the USA for LSG. Its nonparticulate nature means that it enters the lymphatic capillaries rapidly via the intercellular clefts and gaps and shows rapid movement through the lymphatic channels.[16] However, its nonparticulate nature also means that it may proceed rapidly from the SLN to second-tier nodes,[13] which is a significant disadvantage, given that the purpose of LSG is to locate the SLNs. Furthermore, it may pass completely through the SLN, so that on delayed LSG scans, no activity is seen in the SLNs at all.[12]

Whichever tracer is used for SLN biopsy, it is important that each institution develop optimal protocols for LSG, blue-dye injection, and gamma-probe use during surgery to maximize the rate of success of locating the SLN. It is also important that physiological interventions, such as massage, for example, be used whenever possible to improve the entry of the radiocolloid into the lymphatic system.

If either antimony sulfur colloid or nanocolloidal albumin is available at your institution, we recommend these be used in preference to sulfur colloid, as there remains some doubt whether all true SLNs will be identified when using the latter agent.

Movement of tracer along the lymphatic vessel to the draining SLN

Once particles gain entry to the lumen of a lymphatic capillary, they move freely and uniformly toward the draining lymph nodes. There is very little if any retrograde flow of lymph, as the valves in the lymphatic vessels ensure unidirectional flow. Sometimes transient focal accumulations of tracer are seen along the course of a lymphatic vessel. These are "lymphatic lakes" and usually clear in a matter of minutes, rendering them invisible on delayed scans (Figure 3.2). The movement of tracers along lymphatic capillaries in the skin is surprisingly fast. Nathenson and colleagues have measured the rate of flow of Tc-99m-HSA in lymphatics following intradermal injection. They found the average rate of flow of this nonparticulate tracer in a total of 17 patients was 10.4 ± 7.3 cm/min.[16] The movement of Tc-99m-antimony sulfur colloid through the lymphatic capillaries following intradermal injection has also been measured in 198 patients with primary melanoma sites on various parts of the body: an average flow rate of 4.4 cm/min was found.[17] The most important factor affecting flow is the site of intradermal injection of the tracer. The fastest average flow rates were 10 cm/min in the leg and foot, 5.5 cm/min in the forearm and hand, and 4.2 cm/min in the thigh. Flow averaged 3.9 cm/min on the posterior trunk and 2.8 cm/min on the anterior trunk. The slowest average flow rates were seen on the head and neck (1.5 cm/min). An absence of flow on the early dynamic images was most

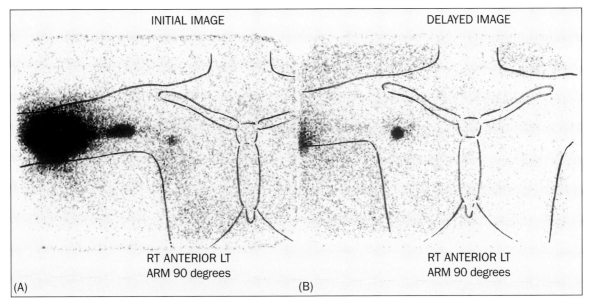

Figure 3.2 Dynamic and delayed LSG in a patient with a melanoma on the right arm. During the dynamic phase (A), a lymphatic lake appears as a focal accumulation of tracer along the path of the lymph vessel, fading completely on the delayed scan (B). A single SLN is seen in the right axilla.

common for the shoulder or arm, the head and neck, and the thigh.

Inflammation, commonly present in the skin when LSG is performed following excision-biopsy of the primary melanoma, will increase the production and rate of lymph flow. Experience suggests that this inflammation does not cause any change in the ability of LSG to detect the true SLN. In fact, there may be an advantage to performing LSG in this situation, as the enhanced lymph flow may actually facilitate identification of the SLN.

The breast is not as richly supplied with lymphatic capillaries as the skin, and movement through the lymphatic vessels is slower in the breast. It is not uncommon to see no drainage on the early dynamic phase of mammary LSG, while this phenomenon is rare in the skin. Massage following intramammary injection of the tracer is vital to the success of lymphatic mapping in the breast, as it enhances entry into the lymph vessel and movement along the channel to the SLNs.

Partial or complete blockage of the lymphatic channels by metastatic tumor deposits will decrease the flow of radiocolloid through the system and may decrease the number of nodes visualized on delayed scans and induce collateral lymph flow through other vessels that do not normally drain the primary tumor site. This problem is usually not encountered when performing LSG to locate SLNs, as this procedure is only performed in patients who have no clinically palpable metastatic lymph nodes.

Previous lymphatic or lymph node surgery has a profound effect on lymphatic drainage. There may simply be a decrease in the number of lymph channels and lymph nodes seen, through to overt lymphedema with no channels, dermal backflow and no uptake whatsoever in lymph nodes. In patients with melanoma on the lower limbs, previous surgery on the groin lymph nodes may induce lymphatic flow across the pubic area to nodes in the contralateral groin.[18,19] These nodes then become the SLNs in such patients.

It has been appreciated for some time that LSG following wide-local excision in patients with melanoma is unreliable, often resulting in no migration of the radiocolloid in the disrupted lymphatics. It is preferable to perform LSG prior to wide-local excision of the biopsy site, as the excision will have an unpredictable effect on the patterns of lymphatic drainage, and a wide-local excision performed the day after LSG removes the skin that has received the highest dose of radiation from the radiocolloid. This can be as high as 0.45 Gy if there is no migration of the tracer.

Mammary LSG is usually performed after needle biopsy of the cancer but before lumpectomy. This is important as the lymphatic vessels may become clogged with postoperative debris following lumpectomy, which will cause failure of the tracer to migrate from the injection site and, thus, nonvisualization of the SLNs. The incidence of false-negative SLN biopsies is also increased after lumpectomy or radiation therapy, presumably because these procedures disrupt the physiology of the lymphatic system.[20]

Retention of the radiocolloid in the SLN

Any foreign particles present in the interstitial space will eventually enter the lymphatic capillaries and be carried with the lymph flow to the draining lymph nodes where they are phagocytosed.[21] The uptake and retention of radiocolloids in the draining lymph nodes is a complex physiological process, and it is important to emphasize that lymph nodes are not simply mechanical filters. This misconception can lead to the erroneous conclusion that large particles, over 100–200 nm, will be trapped in SLNs and that small particles, 5–75 nm in diameter, will not be trapped and will pass on rapidly to other lymph nodes. This is not the case. The phagocytic cells that trap the radiocolloid are macrophages, and they are concentrated especially in the subcapsular and medullary sinuses.[22]

The highest levels of uptake in the draining lymph nodes have been achieved with colloidal gold and Tc-99m-antimony sulfur colloid. Two hours following interstitial injection, uptake in lymph nodes averaged 8% and 6% of the injected dose, respectively, for these two agents.[23] Using Tc-99m-nanocolloidal albumins,

Kapteijn et al found an average of 0.69% of the injected dose in SLNs and 0.23% in nonsentinel second-tier nodes 24 hours following intradermal injection.[11]

The colloids with larger particles such as Tc-99m-sulfur colloid show poor uptake in the lymph nodes because very little of the injected tracer leaves the injection site.[21]

The retention of Tc-99m-antimony sulfur colloid in the SLN is excellent, and at 24 hours following injection, the SLNs usually remain the most radioactive nodes by far.[24]

Distinction of SLNs from second-tier nodes

A second-tier lymph node is any node that receives lymph flow that has previously passed through the physiological filter function of an SLN (see Figure 3.1).

There is a variable incidence of tracer movement onward from the SLNs to second-tier nodes. This correlates directly with the speed of lymph flow.[25] Rapid lymph flow is associated with an increased incidence of activity in second-tier nodes.

Second-tier nodes tend to be located either in the same node field as the SLN but at a more central position within it, or in a separate node field located more centrally on the lymphatic pathway to the thoracic duct.

Any node seen on delayed scans that is more peripheral to an SLN seen on dynamic imaging must be considered to be another SLN and marked as such, since retrograde flow of lymph does not occur. Likewise, a node that is seen only on delayed imaging but that lies lateral to or medial to a known SLN (e.g., in the groin) must be considered another SLN. When in doubt, it is best to mark a second-tier node as a potential SLN; during surgery, with the lymphatics and nodes on view, and with the use of blue dye, the surgeon can determine whether this node receives the dye after it has passed through an SLN or directly from the primary tumor site.

Sometimes, the anatomic arrangement of the afferent lymphatic vessel and the lymph node means that the lymph is only partially subjected to the physiological filter function of the node and that some of the lymph fluid will pass on to the next node without passing through the SLN.[26] This will be seen on LSG as the rapid appearance of a second node more centrally in the node field after an apparent single channel has entered an SLN. When this is seen on LSG the second node must also be marked as a potential second SLN. The resolution limitations of LSG mean that these situations can be confirmed only at operation.

In the breast, activity in second-tier nodes in the axilla is sometimes seen but is always significantly less than that seen in the sentinel lymph node or nodes. Often the only radioactive node in the axilla is the SLN, a situation that facilitates the use of the gamma probe.

The combined use of the above techniques will ensure minimal likelihood of a second-tier node being mistaken for an SLN.

Establishment of appropriate imaging protocols that ensure the identification of all SLNs

Injection of tracer
The tracer should be injected around the primary tumor or the excision-biopsy site. For cutaneous LSG, the chosen radiopharmaceutical is administered by intradermal injection, and in mammary LSG, by peritumoral injection at the depth of the tumor in the 3, 6, 9, and 12 o'clock positions. Most patients will require four intradermal or intramammary peritumoral injections. We perform this under ultrasound guidance, and this has been shown to improve the success rate of the procedure. The study should be performed in an air-conditioned environment with the temperature maintained at no less than 21–22 °C. If the room is cold, lymph flow will be decreased and the likelihood of an unsuccessful study increased.

Gloves should always be worn during the injection procedure. The specific activity we use is 5 MBq (135 μCi) in 0.05 ml for the skin and 5–10 MBq (135–270 μCi) in 0.2 ml for the breast. Volumes of up to 1 ml per injection in the breast appear to produce reliable results, but volumes

above this may radiolabel non-SLNs. A fine 25- or 27-gauge needle is used after the skin is cleaned with an alcohol wipe. There is usually pain at the site of injection. When the injection is commenced, a small bleb appears or the skin blanches at the site of injection due to the very high interstitial pressure that is generated. A gauze swab is placed over the needle before it is withdrawn from the skin to prevent the skin around the injection site being sprayed with tracer and the patient's interstitial fluid. It is also advisable to place a large, impervious incontinence sheet containing a cut-out window over the lesion site prior to injection to help avoid contamination of the patient's surrounding skin, as this could confound later interpretation.

Imaging the patient
Injection of tracer should be completed as quickly as possible and a dynamic acquisition commenced. For cutaneous LSG, ten frames at 1 minute per frame are adequate to allow the rate of lymph flow to be measured in cm/min. The early dynamic study is an essential part of LSG prior to SLN surgery, because it allows confident identification of SLNs as lymphatic channels drain directly to them (see Figure 3.1). The lymph channels should be followed until they reach the draining node field or fields. Lateral views of the head and neck and the axilla are often helpful at this stage in order to identify multiple SLNs. Dynamic images are usually acquired for a total of 20 minutes. The lymphatic channels are best appreciated by summing the individual dynamic frames to produce a composite dynamic image, or by performing a separate 5-minute static acquisition at the end of the dynamic phase.

For mammary LSG, after the 5-minute postinjection massage, a 5 to 10-minute static anterior dynamic-phase image is acquired to display any lymphatic vessels that may be present. A lateral or anterior oblique view of the axilla is also often useful at this time to identify multiple axillary SLNs. In some patients, no movement of tracer will be seen in this early phase, and the SLNs will need to be identified on the delayed scans. When this occurs, it is worthwhile having the patient perform a further 5 minutes of rotary massage over the injection sites before leaving the imaging suite.

Delayed scans are then performed at 2.5 hours following injection of tracer. These delayed scans should include all node fields that can possibly receive drainage from the injection site. It is important in cutaneous LSG that, during this phase of the study, even unusual drainage pathways are detected. These are listed in Table 3.1.

In the breast, anterior and lateral views of the chest will usually be adequate to visualize all SLNs. Sometimes an anterior oblique view of the axilla is useful to separate tracer injected around a primary tumor in the upper outer quadrant from an axillary SLN lying close by. If the breast cancer is in a lower outer quadrant, a posterior view should be performed, as it is possible for lymph to flow to posterior intercostal nodes from this part of the breast. Sentinel lymph nodes in breast cancer may be seen in the axilla, internal mammary chain, supraclavicular or infraclavicular regions, or interpectoral region; they may also be intramammary interval nodes.[20] When the primary site is in the upper outer quadrant, the activity at the injection site may obscure SLNs in the axilla in the anterior view. In addition to a lateral view, an anterior view with the patient upright is often helpful in this situation, as the activity in the breast tissue will then fall downwards, away from the axillary SLN (Figure 3.3).

Each static acquisition should be 5–10 minutes in length to ensure that even very faint SLNs are detected. Most workers use a transmission source to outline the patient during delayed imaging (Figure 3.4). This provides some anatomic guidelines for the surgeon when viewing the scans in the operating room the following day.

Accurate demarcation of surface location of node

Once all the appropriate node fields have been scanned, the SLNs in each node field should be marked. This is done by finding the surface location of the node with the help of a surface marker and then permanently marking this location using a pinpoint tattoo of carbon black ink and a small cross of Castellani's paint or other indelible ink. It is important that the marking be performed with the patient in exactly the same position as that anticipated for use during surgery. Failure to ensure this will mean that the skin mark will not overlie the node. The depth of the node beneath the skin can also be measured using an orthogonal view and by briefly imaging with a small radioactive point source placed on the skin at the site of the surface mark. The depth can then be measured electronically on the acquisition computer system or manually on the film.

Table 3.1 Unusual lymphatic drainage pathways from the skin

- The triangular intermuscular space from the skin of the back
- Paravertebral nodes from the skin of the back
- Costal margin interval node from periumbilical skin
- Supraclavicular fossa nodes from the forearm and wrist
- Interpectoral nodes from the forearm
- Postauricular nodes from the face and anterior scalp
- Level IV and V cervical nodes from the scalp
- Nodes across the midline, especially on the back and the face
- Occipital, parotid, and Level II cervical nodes from the base of the neck
- Axillary nodes from the base of the neck
- Retroperitoneal nodes from the skin of the loin

Data adapted from Uren RF, Thompson JF, Howman-Giles RB. *Lymphatic Drainage of the Skin and Breast: Locating the Sentinel Nodes*. Harwood: Amsterdam, 1999.

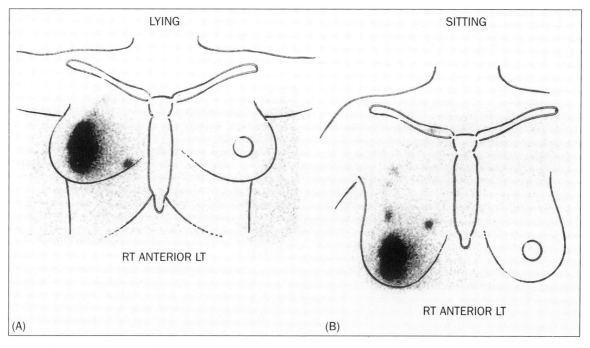

Figure 3.3 Delayed breast LSG in a woman with cancer in the right upper outer quadrant. With the patient supine, the injection site obscures the right axillary SLN (A), but this is easily identified on the anterior upright view (B). The patient also has a second SLN, an intramammary interval node inferiorly and medially.

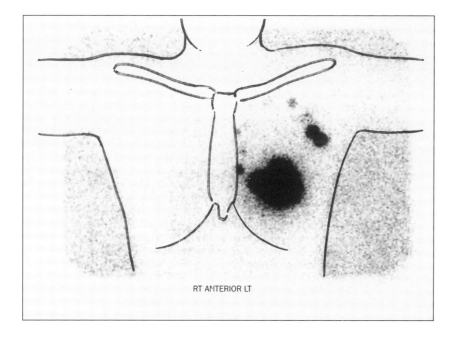

Figure 3.4 Breast LSG in a patient with cancer in the 12 o'clock position just above the nipple. Drainage is to two SLNs in the left axilla and a single SLN in the left internal mammary chain. The transmission source placed behind the patient for this anterior acquisition outlines the patient for anatomic reference. Note faint second-tier nodes in both the axilla and internal mammary chain.

Radiation dosimetry

When Tc-99m radiopharmaceuticals are injected into the interstitial space, the radiation dosimetry depends upon the rate of clearance of the tracer from the point of injection. Clearance of radiocolloids from the interstitial space is quite slow; thus, a significant radiation dose is delivered to the site of injection. A lesser dose is received by the lymph nodes that drain the point of injection, and a very small dose is received by the reticuloendothelial system, particularly the liver, which ultimately traps the colloid particles after they reach the bloodstream.

Bronskill found a biological half-clearance time from this injection site of 20.6 hours following intramuscular injection of Tc-99m-antimony sulfur colloid (Tc-99m-ASC) in the subcostal area.[27] He calculated that this half-time delivered a dose at the injection site of 0.456 Gy for the injected activity of 20 MBq (45.6 rad for 0.5 mCi). He also estimated the absorbed dose for a typical lymph node to be less than 0.2 Gy. Bronskill did not specifically measure the absorbed dose for the intradermal injection of this tracer.

Glass et al measured the washout half-times after intradermal injection for Tc-99m nanocolloidal albumin, Tc-99m-HSA, and Tc-99m-SC (both of the colloids had been filtered through a 0.2-μm filter).[28] They found half-times from the injection site averaged 7.5 ± 6.4 hours, 4.3 ± 1.4 hours, and 13.9 ± 12.7 hours, respectively, for the three agents. These clearance half-times imply lower doses at the injection site than those calculated by Bronskill.

If one assumes a "worst-case scenario" of no migration of tracer from the injection site after intradermal or intramammary injection, maximum absorbed dose using 5 MBq of Tc-99m-ASC at each injection site would be in the order of 0.45 Gy assuming a volume of distribution of 1 ml. This is below the threshold dose for deterministic radiation effects; thus, no erythema or other effect should be observed.

In our institution, the injections are given intradermally around the excision-biopsy site, for melanoma patients, or peritumorally around the breast cancer the day before

surgery. Surgery entails wide-local excision of the biopsy site for melanoma patients and lumpectomy with a good margin of normal breast tissue for breast cancer patients. The radiation dose at the injection site, which accounts for the majority of the absorbed dose, thus becomes irrelevant, as this tissue is excised within 24 hours of tracer injection in both of these scenarios.

There is no risk to the surgical team or histopathologists handling the surgical specimens, as these activities usually take place the day after LSG, by which time several physical half-lives for Tc-99m have expired. Sometimes breast surgery is performed in the afternoon following a morning LSG. Handling the breast cancer with surgical forceps rather than with the fingers reduces the finger dose the surgeon receives by a factor of 30. Using the hands alone, without forceps, and operating on the same day as LSG, a surgeon would need to perform in the order of 270 procedures a year to approach the limits of allowed radiation dose to the fingers.

THE "SENTINEL" LYMPH NODE

Definition of an SLN

A sentinel node was defined by Morton and colleagues as "the first lymph node to receive drainage from a lesion site."[29] This definition is open to misinterpretation, especially if there is more than one SLN. We prefer the definition, "any lymph node receiving direct lymphatic drainage from a lesion site,"[30] as this essentially describes the physiology of the sentinel node concept itself as seen on dynamic LSG and includes all possible scenarios including multiple SLNs and interval nodes. This also removes the concept of time from the definition, as this can become confusing if one SLN receives tracer rapidly and another SLN receives tracer slowly. They both remain SLNs if they receive the tracer directly from the lesion site (Figure 3.5).

There is usually only one SLN in node fields that drain the skin of the trunk, although there may be multiple node fields draining certain parts of the skin of the trunk. The axilla and groin both average 1.3 SLNs when drainage occurs from the skin of the trunk. In breast-cancer patients, we have found an average of 1.4 SLNs in the axilla.[20]

Multiple SLNs are more likely to occur in the groin with lower-limb lesion sites and in the cervical, occipital, preauricular, and postauricular node fields with lesion sites on the head and neck. With lesion sites on the lower limbs, there are on average 3.3 SLNs in the groin. For the head and neck, there are on average 2.7 SLNs per patient, and 85% of patients have multiple SLNs.

These multiple SLNs in individual node fields reflect the varying physiology of the lymphatic system in different parts of the body and are not an artifact caused by the use of a particular colloid.

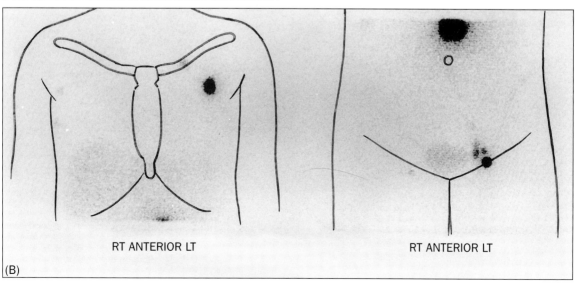

Figure 3.5 Dynamic (A) and delayed (B) LSG in a man with melanoma on the midback, just to the left of midline. The dynamic study shows three lymph channels, a dominant channel passing to the left axilla and left groin and a faint channel passing to the right groin, which it reaches slowly. On the delayed scans a single SLN is seen in the left axilla and left groin with faint second-tier activity, and there is a single, faint SLN in the right groin.

(A)

LT POSTERIOR RT

(B)

RT ANTERIOR LT

RT ANTERIOR LT

Interval nodes

Interval nodes are lymph nodes that drain a lesion site and lie between that lesion site and a recognized node field. If they receive lymphatic drainage from the lesion site directly, they are, by definition, sentinel nodes. When such interval nodes are sentinel nodes, they have the same likelihood of harboring micrometastases as SLNs located in standard node fields,[31] and an SLN biopsy procedure that ignores interval nodes will be incomplete, regardless of whether the procedure is concerned with the skin or the breast (Figure 3.6).

PATTERNS OF LYMPHATIC DRAINAGE OF THE SKIN

The SLNs that receive direct lymphatic drainage from the skin may lie in any of the node fields listed in Table 3.2.

The patterns of flow are not predictable in any individual, but some useful information

---

Table 3.2 Lymph node fields draining the skin

- Axillary
- Epitrochlear
- Interpectoral
- Paravertebral
- Retroperitoneal
- Triangular intermuscular space
- Right costal margin
- Internal mammary
- Groin (superficial inguinal, femoral, obturator, and external iliac)
- Popliteal
- Cervical (Levels I–V) and supraclavicular (part of Level V)
- Preauricular
- Postauricular
- Occipital

Data adapted from Uren RF, Thompson JF, Howman-Giles RB. *Lymphatic Drainage of the Skin and Breast: Locating the Sentinel Nodes*. Harwood: Amsterdam, 1999.

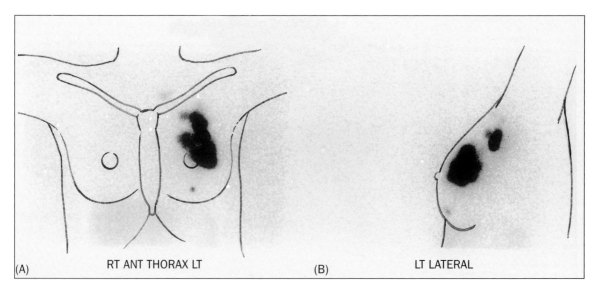

(A) RT ANT THORAX LT (B) LT LATERAL

Figure 3.6 Breast LSG in a woman with cancer in the left upper outer quadrant. The SLN in the axilla is obscured in the anterior view (A) but easily visible in the left lateral view (B). The patient also has a small intramammary interval node in the lower part of the breast which is also an SLN.

can be obtained by looking at the frequency with which lymph flows from particular parts of the skin to the various node fields.

Trunk

The patterns of lymphatic drainage in a series of 731 patients with primary sites on the trunk, 610 of these sites on the posterior trunk and 121 on the anterior trunk, are shown in Table 3.3.

Interval nodes in the subcutaneous tissue of the trunk are most commonly found low in the midaxillary line, along channels passing towards the axilla. They are also found along the back, as channels pass up and toward the midline before passing through the body wall to paravertebral nodes.[20] Interval nodes are also often seen along the path of channels passing up toward posterior triangle (cervical Level V) nodes from sites on the upper back, and on the posterior buttocks in the line of channels heading toward groin nodes from sites on the low back.

Posterior trunk
In this group of patients with posterior trunk primary sites, of those patients who showed drainage to the axilla, 186 (33.5%) showed bilateral axillary drainage. Of those who showed drainage to groin nodes, 16 (26.2%) had bilateral groin node drainage.

In some patients, lymphatics drain from the skin of the back to nodes in the triangular intermuscular-space node field.[32] This drainage can be unilateral or bilateral. Drainage to this node field is perhaps the most important unusual pathway to look for when performing LSG to locate the SLNs. The incidence of drainage from the posterior trunk to the triangular intermuscular space lymph nodes is about 9% overall; however, this underestimates the true incidence of drainage to this node field, as the earlier studies were performed using an imaging protocol that did not look for SLNs in this node field.

Occasional patients have lymphatic channels that pass from the skin of the posterior loin superiorly toward the midline, then through

Table 3.3 Patterns of lymphatic drainage for melanoma of the trunk

Draining node field	Anterior trunk (*N* = 121) (%)	Posterior trunk (*N* = 610) (%)
Axilla	81	91
Groin	18	10
Triangular intermuscular space	0	9
Paravertebral	0	2.5
Cervical Level II	<1	0
Cervical Level III	2.5	<1
Cervical Level IV	<1	1
Cervical Level V	6	21
Supraclavicular (part of Level V)	6	14
Occipital	0	<1
Costal margin	4	0
Interval nodes	5	9

Data adapted from Uren RF, Thompson JF, Howman-Giles RB. *Lymphatic Drainage of the Skin and Breast: Locating the Sentinel Nodes*. Harwood: Amsterdam, 1999.

the body wall to paravertebral lymph nodes, and then upwards toward the thoracic duct. A lymph channel may also be seen to pass directly through the body wall in the posterior loin to nodes in the retroperitoneal space, with onward drainage from there to paravertebral nodes.[33] Most of these patients also have some drainage to the usual node fields of the axilla and groin, but occasionally there is exclusive drainage to paravertebral nodes, with no drainage at all to the axilla or groin[34] (Figure 3.7). It is important to be aware of this drainage in individual patients as the presence of metastatic melanoma in such intra-abdominal nodes represents local–regional disease, not systemic spread.

Eight of the patients with drainage to the triangular intermuscular space showed drainage to these nodes bilaterally, and 10 patients showed drainage to the supraclavicular nodes bilaterally. Five of the 40 patients with drainage to posterior triangle nodes (cervical Level V) had bilateral drainage to these nodes.

Anterior trunk

In patients with anterior-trunk primary sites who showed drainage to the axilla, 21 (21.4%) had bilateral drainage, while only one patient had bilateral drainage to the supraclavicular fossa. A noticeable difference between the anterior and posterior trunk drainage is the significantly smaller percentage of patients with anterior trunk primary sites who show drainage to the supraclavicular fossa; 6% for the anterior trunk versus 14% for the posterior trunk. Drainage from the anterior trunk to the triangular intermuscular space was not expected and was not found. No drainage was seen to Level V cervical nodes (except for the supraclavicular fossa) or occipital nodes, and it appears that direct drainage to paravertebral nodes does not occur from the anterior trunk. Drainage from the skin of the anterior trunk directly to internal mammary nodes appears to be rare and was not observed in this particular series. In 20% of patients, lymphatics drain from the periumbilical area to a right or left costal margin interval node before passing toward the midline and then through the chest

wall to internal mammary nodes.[35] Interval nodes were seen less often on the anterior trunk compared with the posterior trunk.

Base of the neck

The skin around the base of the neck is an area that has particularly unpredictable drainage patterns. Drainage can occur to supraclavicular nodes, occipital nodes, cervical nodes (Levels II, III, IV, and V), triangular intermuscular-space nodes, and axillary nodes.[20] It is not uncommon for lymph channels to pass over the shoulder from the back to supraclavicular nodes (cervical Level V nodes). The drainage pattern from the area at the base of the neck usually involves multiple draining node fields.

The findings in a series of 154 patients with primary melanoma sites in this area are shown in Table 3.4. In 24 patients (15.6%), drainage was to both axillae, while 11 had bilateral drainage to the supraclavicular fossae, three had bilateral drainage to Level V cervical nodes, one had bilateral drainage to Level IV cervical nodes, and one had bilateral drainage to triangular intermuscular-space SLNs. Thus a total of 26% of patients with primary sites in this region showed bilateral drainage to particular node fields. Drainage from the posterior base of the neck to both supraclavicular fossae was possible from only a very small area of the skin of the upper back around the midline. In 124 patients, the primary site was on the posterior aspect of the base of the neck, and 53 of these patients (43%) showed drainage over the shoulders to SLNs in the supraclavicular fossa. Seven of these patients (6%) had drainage over the shoulders to anterior cervical nodes at Level III or IV. There was drainage across the midline in 40 patients (32%) to SLNs in a total of 53 node fields.

In the 30 patients who had primary sites on the base of the neck anteriorly, there were 6 (20%) who showed drainage across the midline. Five (17%) showed drainage up the neck to cervical Level II or III nodes, and 25 (83%) showed drainage down to the axilla. Axillary drainage was bilateral in 3 patients, while 1 patient had bilateral drainage to supraclavicular nodes, and 1 had bilateral drainage to cervical Level III nodes.

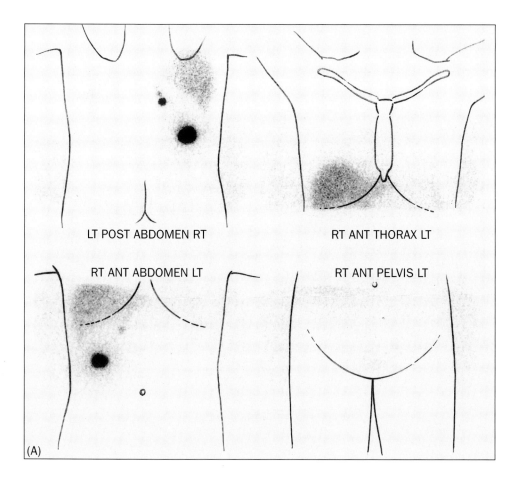

LT POST ABDOMEN RT

RT ANT THORAX LT

RT ANT ABDOMEN LT

RT ANT PELVIS LT

(A)

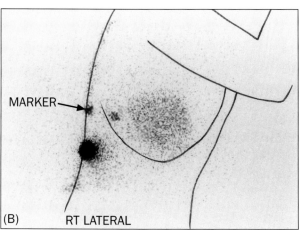

MARKER

(B)

RT LATERAL

Figure 3.7 Lymphoscintigraphy in a man with melanoma on the right posterior loin shows anterior and posterior views of the abdomen, axillae, and groins (A), and a right lateral view of the abdomen (B). There is exclusive drainage from the skin of the back to a paravertebral SLN in this patient, with no drainage to nodes in either groin or either axilla. The marker on the skin of the back shows the node to be about 6 cm deep to the skin in the paravertebral region on the right.

Table 3.4 Patterns of lymphatic drainage for melanoma of the head and neck		
Draining node field	**Head and neck (*N* = 205) (%)**	**Base of neck (*N* = 154) (%)**
Preauricular (parotid)	39	0
Postauricular	13	0
Occipital	11	<1
Cervical Level I	18	0
Submental (part of Level I)	2	0
Cervical Level II	62	1
Cervical Level III	14	3
Cervical Level IV	17	5
Cervical Level V	32	62
Supraclavicular (part of Level V)	14	44
Axilla	3	87
Triangular intermuscular space	0.5	7
Interval nodes	3.5	6

Data adapted from Uren RF, Thompson JF, Howman-Giles RB. *Lymphatic Drainage of the Skin and Breast: Locating the Sentinel Nodes.* Harwood: Amsterdam, 1999.

Head and neck

In the past, guidelines have been proposed for clinical prediction of lymphatic drainage patterns from the skin of the head and neck.[36,37] When LSG was used to examine lymphatic flow patterns in the head and neck, however, it was found that lymphatic drainage was discordant with clinical prediction in 33 (34%) of 97 patients studied.[38] A total of 21 patients (22%) had drainage to nodes other than the parotid and the five standard neck levels. In 13 patients, this was to postauricular nodes, and in 5 this was to occipital nodes. The postauricular nodes are not usually resected in an elective radical node dissection for malignant disease of the head and neck, and the occipital nodes are only resected when the primary site is on the posterior scalp or upper neck.

The draining node fields in 205 patients with primary melanoma sites on the head and neck are shown in Table 3.4.

Drainage occurred across the midline in 30 patients (15%), and the coronal line across the head, defined by the position of the ears, was crossed in 27 patients (13%). Direct drainage down the neck to SLNs beyond those normally expected occurred in 42 patients (21%). Unexpected drainage also occurred from primary sites low in the neck up to SLNs in the occipital, preauricular, postauricular, Level I cervical, or Level II cervical nodes in 28 patients (14%).

Clearly, therefore, any attempt to make clinical predictions about lymphatic drainage pathways in patients with head and neck melanomas is unrealistic (Figure 3.8). If these predictions are used to determine the site and extent of lymph-node surgery, the surgeon will fail to remove nodes potentially containing metastatic disease in 1 in 3 patients.[20]

Upper limb

On LSG, most skin sites on the upper limb drain to the axilla. As in other parts of the body, lymph drainage from the upper limb is extremely variable, with channels passing directly to SLNs in many parts of the axilla.

There is most commonly only one SLN in the axilla (average 1.3 SLNs with upper-limb injections).[20]

Some patients have direct drainage from the arm to supraclavicular nodes and, in rare cases, to cervical nodes. Drainage from the forearm is usually exclusively to the axilla, although in some patients there is also direct drainage to supraclavicular nodes.[39]

Drainage to epitrochlear nodes occurs perhaps less often than had previously been thought;[40] however, it is important to perform a full delayed acquisition over the epitrochlear region during LSG to ensure that any SLNs in this field are detected. One can expect drainage to the epitrochlear node group in up to 20% of patients with melanoma sites on the hand or forearm. SLNs in the epitrochlear region will be

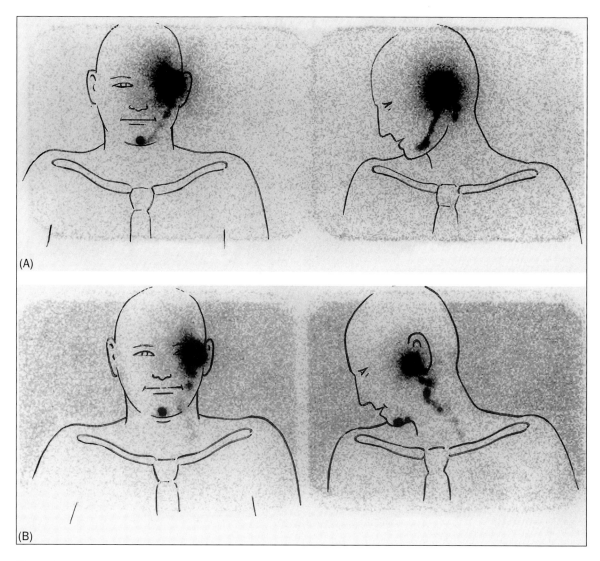

Figure 3.8 Dynamic (A) and delayed (B) LSG in a man with melanoma on the tragus of the left ear. Lymph flows to SLNs in the left upper cervical region but also via a separate channel to an SLN in the submental area in the midline. Note some second-tier nodes are also seen in the left cervical area.

missed unless this area is carefully scanned in all patients with hand and forearm primary melanoma sites.

Drainage from the skin of the forearm to an interpectoral or inferior clavicular node[20] is rare.

In a series of 298 patients with primary melanoma sites on the upper limbs and shoulders (using a vertical line in a sagittal plane through the axilla to define the limits of the upper limb and shoulder versus the trunk), there were 205 patients with lesion sites on the anterior upper limb or shoulder and 92 with posterior lesion sites. The draining node fields seen in these patients are summarized in Table 3.5.

Of the 21 patients who had drainage to an SLN in the supraclavicular fossa, there were four whose primary site was on the forearm.

Lower limb

As expected, lymphatic drainage from the lower limb is exclusively to the ipsilateral groin except when the patient has had prior surgery on the groin nodes; in this situation, lymphatic channels may be seen passing across the pubis to the contralateral groin nodes.[18,19]

Table 3.5 Patterns of lymphatic drainage for melanoma of the upper limb

Draining node field	Upper limb (N = 205) (%)
Axilla	97
Supraclavicular	7
Epitrochlear	4
Interpectoral	<1
Triangular intermuscular space	<1
Cervical Level V	<1
Interval nodes	5

Data adapted from Uren RF, Thompson JF, Howman-Giles RB. *Lymphatic Drainage of the Skin and Breast: Locating the Sentinel Nodes.* Harwood: Amsterdam, 1999.

In LSG, there is a general tendency for the lymph channels to pass medially, but there is a great variation in the path taken by these channels in different patients. Lymphatic channels from the leg commonly pass both medially and laterally up the lower limb (see Figure 3.1). Drainage to the popliteal nodes has been observed from the skin of the dorsum of the foot, the sole of the heel, the medial heel, and the lower calf on the medial side. This is a considerably more extensive distribution of sites than that suggested by Clouse, who found popliteal drainage only from the skin of the posterolateral heel.[41]

As is the case with drainage to the epitrochlear region, drainage to the popliteal fossa will be missed unless a full 10-minute acquisition is performed over this node field on delayed imaging. Relying on the presence of tracer in this area on the persistence scope is inadequate. Drainage to the popliteal fossa can be expected in approximately 15% of patients with melanoma sites on the leg and foot.

The frequency with which second-tier lymph nodes are seen,[25] often on the early dynamic-phase component of the study, is another consistent feature of lymphatic mapping in the lower limbs. This is in contrast to the situation in the axilla, where SLNs are often the only nodes seen to contain tracer and, even at 24 hours, can remain the only significantly radioactive nodes. The high incidence of second-tier lymph nodes in the groin is associated with high lymph-flow velocities, as mentioned earlier, and it has already been mentioned that lymph-flow rates from the lower limb are the highest seen in the skin.[17]

Drainage to multiple node fields

Multiple node fields draining a single skin site are common on the trunk and also in lesion sites around the base of the neck and around the midline of the body, both anteriorly and posteriorly (see Figure 3.5). The skin sites that drain to two or more node fields tend to be congregated around the midline of the trunk, in a band around the waist, across the shoulders posteriorly, and in the head and neck region. Drainage to three node fields is seen in a similar distribution over the posterior trunk and in the periumbilical area anteriorly as well as the head and neck, but drainage to four or more node fields is seen only occasionally in the head and neck and from very restricted areas of the trunk.[20] These truncal areas lie between the scapulae and at L2 level near the midline (where Sappey's lines cross) on the back, and in the periumbilical area on the anterior trunk.

LYMPHATIC DRAINAGE OF THE BREAST

Lymphatic drainage from the breast following intramammary injection may occur to the axilla, the internal mammary chain, clavicular nodes (usually supraclavicular), interpectoral nodes, and intramammary interval nodes (see Figure 3.6).[20,42] Drainage from the lower outer quadrant is said to be possible to posterior intercostal nodes,[43] although we have not yet observed this in our breast-cancer patients.

The pattern of lymphatic drainage following intramammary peritumoral injections that we have observed in breast-cancer patients is shown in Table 3.6. We studied 217 patients, but there was no movement of tracer from the

injection site in 14 (6%). This occurred early in our experience when we were using a smaller volume of 0.1 ml injectate per injection site and were not using postinjection massage. Since changing to a volume of 0.2 ml per injection and using postinjection massage, we have seen only three patients who showed no movement of the injected tracer. One of these patients had undergone lumpectomy, which is known to increase the incidence of unsuccessful SLN biopsy procedures, and two patients had nodes replaced by metastatic deposits, one in the axilla and the other in a large intramammary interval node, which presumably caused the failure of the test in these two patients.

The locations of the primary breast cancers in our patients are shown in Table 3.7.

In 203 patients who showed drainage from the injection site, drainage to one node field occurred in 104 (51%) patients, to two node fields in 85 (42%) patients, and to three node fields in 13 (6%) patients.

It is important to note that 101 (50%) patients had drainage to SLNs outside the axilla and that in 14 (7%) the SLNs were all outside the axilla. Thus, any SLN biopsy protocol that ignores nonaxillary SLNs has the potential to understage the node status of about half of the patients with breast cancer. Sentinel lymph nodes found outside standard node fields in melanoma patients have been shown to have the same chance of harboring micrometastases as any other SLN.[31,44] There is evidence that this is also the case for internal mammary nodes and is likely to be the situation for all SLNs in breast-cancer patients. Therefore, an SLN biopsy procedure that ignores SLNs outside the axilla will be incomplete in about half of patients with breast cancer. This is incompatible with the principles of the SLN biopsy method, which demand that a successful SLN biopsy involves the removal of all SLNs followed by specific, targeted histologic examination of all such nodes. In this way only can the true node status of the patient be determined.

Our experience confirms the fact that most patients with breast cancer have lymphatic drainage which includes the axilla, and we found this in 93% of our patients. Thus, nodal

Table 3.6 Patterns of lymphatic drainage for breast cancer	
Draining node field	Breast cancer patients ($N = 203$) (%)
Axilla	93
Internal mammary	47
Supraclavicular	12
Interpectoral	2
Intramammary interval nodes	12

Data adapted from Uren RF, Thompson JF, Howman-Giles RB. *Lymphatic Drainage of the Skin and Breast: Locating the Sentinel Nodes.* Harwood: Amsterdam, 1999.

Table 3.7 Locations of primary breast cancers in 217 patients

Location	Right breast (n = 104)	Left breast (n = 113)
UO quadrant	33	41
UI quadrant	17	10
LO quadrant	12	10
LI quadrant	6	6
Juncture UO-UI	15	16
Juncture UI-LI	3	4
Juncture LI-LO	6	9
Juncture LO-UO	9	13
Subareolar	3	4

I, inner; L, lower; O, outer; U, upper.

staging of axillary nodes is an important part of a successful SLN biopsy in most patients; however, as mentioned above, it does not follow that SLNs in other node fields should be ignored.

In the 189 patients who showed SLNs in the axilla, one SLN was seen in each of 128 patients (67.5%), two SLNs were seen in 55 patients (29%), three SLNs were seen in 4 patients (2%), and four SLNs were seen in 3 patients (1.5%). Thus, in the vast majority of patients (96.5%), a successful SLN biopsy in the axilla involves the surgical removal of only one or two axillary nodes. This ensures minimal postsurgical morbidity with a low likelihood of developing the more serious postoperative complications such as lymphedema and frozen shoulder.

Like others, we have found that the site of the cancer in the breast cannot be used to clinically predict the pattern of lymphatic drainage. In 46 patients with cancers confined to the inner quadrants of the breast, lymph drainage was seen to the axilla in 33 patients (72%) (Figure 3.9). In 120 patients with cancers confined to the outer quadrants of the breast, drainage to internal mammary nodes occurred in 45 patients (37%). In our patients, 47% of cancers

showed lymphatic drainage across the centerline of the breast. We have not observed direct lymphatic drainage across the midline of the patient to SLNs on the contralateral side, though we have seen internal mammary sentinel nodes on one side drain on to second-tier nodes in the contralateral internal mammary chain (Figure 3.10). When drainage to internal mammary lymph nodes was seen, it was common for a series of nodes to be radiolabeled, and it may be that the internal mammary nodes do not retain the radiocolloid as well as other lymph nodes (Figure 3.11).

When peritumoral injections are used, the SLNs will not be identified in some patients because of nonmigration of the tracer. This problem is more common in patients with either large primary tumors or large, fatty breasts. The patients with large primary tumors may have impaired lymphatic drainage due to clusters of metastatic cells blocking the lymphatic capillaries or replacing the SLNs, while in patients with large, fatty breasts, there seems to be a paucity of lymphatic vessels per unit of breast volume, and this may cause failure of the tracer to enter a lymphatic capillary.

Faced with this phenomenon, which is also

more common when large-particle colloids are used, some have tried alternatives to the peritumoral injection method. There have been recent reports that a successful SLN biopsy of the axilla can be achieved in close to 100% of patients with the use of an intradermal injection of radiocolloid in the skin over the site of the breast cancer.[45] Other reports have stated that the SLN found in the axilla is the identical SLN that would be found in that patient if peritumoral injections were used instead. Others, however, have reported that when tracer is injected in these two different locations in the same patient, different lymph nodes are radiolabeled in the axilla. We would caution against the intradermal injection method, as it is plausible that the lymphatic drainage of the tumor differs from that of the overlying skin in some patients and, therefore, that the radiolabeled axillary node will not be the true SLN.

It is true from our experience in melanoma patients that close to 100% of patients who receive intradermal injections over the anterior chest will show drainage to SLNs in the axilla; however, in 62 patients we have studied in this way, we have never seen direct lymphatic drainage to nodes in the internal mammary chain. This means that although an intradermal injection in the skin over a breast cancer will radiolabel a lymph node in the axilla, and even assuming that this is the identical SLN that would be seen if peritumoral injections had been given, intradermal injections will not display the complete pattern of lymphatic drainage of the tumor. Sentinel lymph nodes in the internal mammary chain, supraclavicular area, and interpectoral region will be missed, as will intramammary interval SLNs. As mentioned earlier, failure to identify and biopsy these other SLNs defeats the purpose of the SLN biopsy method.

Studies of the patterns of lymphatic drainage

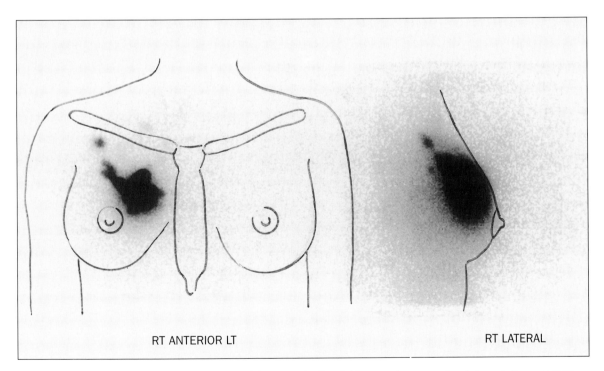

Figure 3.9 Lymphoscintigraphy in a woman with cancer in the right upper inner quadrant. Lymph flows across the centerline of the right breast to an SLN high in the apex of the right axilla in the subclavian area. The direction of lymphatic drainage cannot be predicted based on the location of the cancer in the breast.

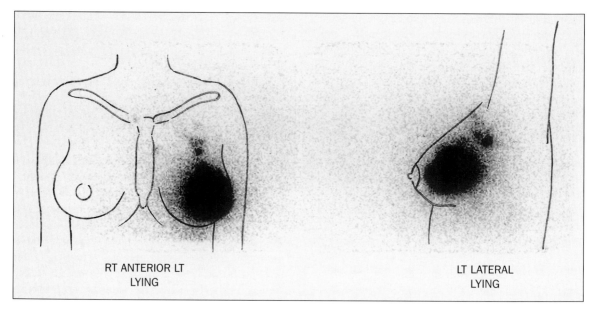

RT ANTERIOR LT
LYING

LT LATERAL
LYING

Figure 3.10 Breast LSG in a woman with cancer in the left upper outer quadrant near the nipple. Two SLNs are seen in the left axilla, and there is a single SLN in the left internal mammary chain. Tracer then passes on to a node high in the right internal mammary chain behind the manubrium. This latter node is a second-tier node, and we have not yet observed direct drainage to an SLN across the midline of the patient.

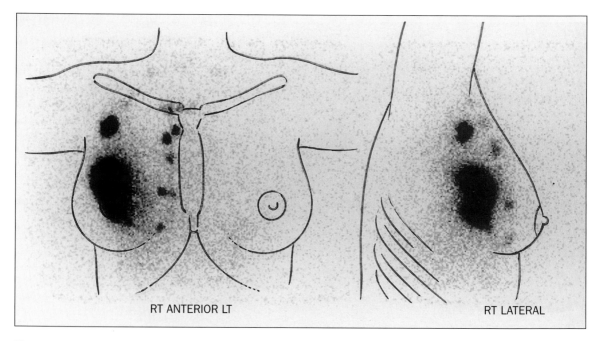

RT ANTERIOR LT

RT LATERAL

Figure 3.11 Breast LSG in a woman with cancer in the right breast at the 12 o'clock position just above the areola. Lymph drainage is to a bright right-axillary SLN and also to right-internal mammary SLNs. Internal mammary nodes are often seen as a chain of "hot" nodes, even when only one lymph vessel passes to this area. They appear not to retain the radiocolloid as well as lymph nodes elsewhere in the body. The channel passing in a curvilinear fashion to the first right-internal mammary node is seen regularly on mammary LSG.

of the breast tissue that have involved intra-mammary injections of tracer have consistently shown that about 90–95% of sites in the breast will include some axillary drainage.[20,42,46] Thus, if a technique such as the intradermal injection of tracer is used, which produces a 100% incidence of drainage to axillary nodes, such drainage will be irrelevant in about 5–10% of patients, as peritumoral lymphatic drainage in these patients would not have included the axilla. Injection around the site of the tumor remains the sensible approach.

THE FUTURE

New Tc-99m-labeled tracers for lymphatic mapping

The ideal radiocolloid for LSG would migrate completely from the intradermal injection site and be retained completely by the SLNs. Such an agent is not yet available.

In a recent effort to further improve visualization of lymphatic channels and SLNs, some novel approaches have been described. New radiotracers using receptor-binding agents[47] or surface-engineered nanospheres to increase phagocytosis in the regional lymph nodes[48] have been developed. Vera et al have developed a nonparticulate receptor-binding radiotracer that has excellent retention in the SLNs, thus potentially offering the advantages of both rapid flow through lymph channels of the nonparticulate agents such as human serum albumin and the good node retention of the particulate agents such as antimony sulfur colloid.[47] Moghimi et al have used copolymers to sterically stabilize nanospheres.[48] This dramatically increases the opsonization of these agents in the lymph nodes, so that up to 40% of the injected dose is trapped in SLN macrophages. The high percentage of injected dose that reaches draining lymph nodes also suggests that clearance from the injection site has been enhanced, perhaps by an increase in lymphatic capillary uptake of these agents through their opsonization and active transport into the capillary by pinocytosis. Developments such as these may lead to better tracers for LSG in the future.

Collimators

High-resolution collimators are best for LSG, and microcast collimators are preferable to folded metal collimators as they have less star artifact caused by septal penetration of high activity from the injection site. Ideally, septal penetration should be less than 1% at 140 keV energy. This will prevent the occurrence of star artifact.

Other cancers

Reports are already appearing attesting to the usefulness of the SLN biopsy approach in cancer of the penis, vulva, prostate, bowel, pancreas, and thyroid (see Chapters 30–32).

CONCLUSION

Lymphatic mapping using high-resolution LSG is an essential first step for accurate biopsy of the SLNs in patients with melanoma and breast cancer. It ensures that SLNs will not be overlooked, even if they are in unusual node fields or are interval nodes lying along the path of the lymphatic vessel. Micrometastases are present in such SLNs, with an incidence similar to that seen with SLNs in standard node fields. This is the key to the importance of LSG in SLN biopsy. It ensures that all true SLNs are identified in each patient and that SLNs are not overlooked because they might lie in an unusual location. There is no logic in a surgical SLN biopsy procedure that targets sentinel nodes seen in one node field but not those seen in another. The practice of performing only an axillary SLN biopsy in patients with breast cancer while ignoring SLNs outside the axilla, either those in the internal mammary chain or clavicular area, or intramammary interval nodes, is likely to be discontinued as surgeons realize that this practice potentially understages the node status of about half of their breast-cancer patients.

Knowledge of the accurate surface location of the SLNs prior to surgery simplifies the surgical procedure and shortens the time required under anesthesia. If preoperative LSG is not performed, it is inevitable that SLNs will not be identified in some patients, which defeats the purpose of the SLN biopsy procedure.

REFERENCES

1. Sherman AI, Ter-Pogossian M, Tocus EC, Lymph node concentration of radioactive colloidal gold following interstitial injection. *Cancer* 1953; **6:**1238–40.
2. Fee HJ, Robinson DS, Sample WF et al, The determination of lymph shed by colloidal gold scanning in patients with malignant melanoma: a preliminary study. *Surgery* 1978; **84:**626–32.
3. Meyer CM, Lecklitner ML, Logic JR et al, Technetium-99m sulfur-colloid cutaneous lymphoscintigraphy in the management of truncal melanoma. *Radiology* 1979; **131:**205–9.
4. Sullivan DC, Croker BP, Harris CC et al, Lymphoscintigraphy in malignant melanoma: Tc-99m antimony sulfur colloid. *Am J Roentgenol* 1981; **137:**847–51.
5. Bergqvist L, Strand S, Hafstrom L, Jonsson PE, Lymphoscintigraphy in patients with malignant melanoma: a quantitative and qualitative evaluation of its usefulness. *Eur J Nucl Med* 1984; **9:**129–35.
6. Norman J, Cruse W, Espinosa C et al, Redefinition of cutaneous lymphatic drainage with the use of lymphoscintigraphy for malignant melanoma. *Am J Surg* 1991; **162:**432–7.
7. Eberbach MA, Wahl RL, Lymphatic anatomy: functional nodal basins. *Ann Plast Surg* 1989; **22:**25–31.
8. Yoffey JM, Courtice FC, *Lymphatics, Lymph and the Lymphomyeloid Complex.* Academic Press: London, 1970.
9. Casley-Smith JR, Lymph and lymphatics, In: Kaley G, Altura BM, eds, *Microcirculation,* 423–502. University Park Press: Baltimore, 1977.
10. Kaplan WD, Davis MA, Rose CM, A comparison of two technetium-99m-labeled radiopharmaceuticals for lymphoscintigraphy. *J Nucl Med* 1979; **20:**933–7.
11. Kapteijn BAE, Nieweg OE, Muller SH et al, Validation of gamma probe detection of the sentinel node in melanoma. *J Nucl Med* 1997; **38:**362–6.
12. Alazraki NP, Eshima D, Eshima LA et al, Lymphoscintigraphy, the sentinel node concept, and the intraoperative gamma probe in melanoma, breast cancer, and other potential cancers. *Semin Nucl Med* 1997; **27:**55–67.
13. Nathanson SD, Anaya P, Karvelis KC et al, Sentinel lymph node uptake of two different technetium-labeled radiocolloids. *Ann Surg Oncol* 1997; **4:**104–10.
14. Wong JH, Terada K, Ko P, Coel MN, Lack of effect of particle size on the identification of the sentinel node in cutaneous malignancies. *Ann Surg Oncol* 1998; **5:**77–80.
15. Tonakie A, Yahanda A, Sondak V, Wahl RL, Reproducibility of lymphoscintigraphic drainage patterns in sequential TC-99M HSA and TC-99M sulfur colloid studies: implications for sentinel node identification in melanoma. *J Nucl Med* 1998; **39:**25P.
16. Nathanson SD, Nelson L, Karvelis KC, Rates of flow of technetium 99m-labeled human serum albumin from peripheral injection sites to sentinel lymph nodes. *Ann Surg Oncol* 1996; **3:**329–35.
17. Uren RF, Howman-Giles RB, Thompson JF et al, Variability of cutaneous lymphatic flow rates. *Melanoma Res* 1998; **8:**279–82.
18. Jonk A, Kroon BBR, Mooi WJ, Hoefnagel CA, Contralateral inguinal lymph node metastasis in patients with melanoma of the lower extremities. *Br J Surg* 1989; **76:**1161–2.
19. Thompson JF, Saw RP, Colman MH et al, Contralateral groin node metastasis from lower limb melanoma. *Eur J Cancer* 1997; **33:**976–7.
20. Uren RF, Thompson JF, Howman-Giles RB, *Lymphatic Drainage of the Skin and Breast: Locating the Sentinel Nodes.* Harwood: Amsterdam, 1999.
21. Bergqvist L, Strand SE, Persson BRR, Particle sizing and biokinetics of interstitial lymphoscintigraphic agents. *Semin Nucl Med* 1983; **8:**9–19.
22. Nopajaroonsri C, Simon GT, Phagocytosis of colloidal carbon in a lymph node. *Am J Pathol* 1971; **65:**25–42.
23. Strand SE, Persson BRR, Quantitative lymphoscintigraphy I: basic concepts for optimal uptake of radiocolloids in the parasternal lymph nodes of rabbits. *J Nucl Med* 1979; **20:**1038–46.
24. Thompson JF, Niewind P, Uren RF et al, Single-dose isotope injection for both preoperative lymphoscintigraphy and intraoperative sentinel

lymph node identification in melanoma patients. *Melanoma Res* 1997; **6:**500–6.

25. Uren RF, Howman-Giles RB, Thompson JF, Demonstration of second tier lymph nodes during preoperative lymphoscintigraphy for melanoma: incidence varies with primary tumor site. *Ann Surg Oncol* 1998; **5:**517–21.

26. Ludwig J, Ueber kurschlusswege der lymphbahnen und ihre beziehungen zur lymphogen krebsmetastasierung. *Path Microbiol* 1962; **25:**329.

27. Bronskill MJ, Radiation dose estimates for interstitial radiocolloid lymphoscintigraphy. *Semin Nucl Med* 1983; **13:**20–5.

28. Glass EC, Essner R, Morton DL, Kinetics of three lymphoscintigraphic agents in patients with cutaneous melanoma. *J Nucl Med* 1998; **39:**1185–90.

29. Morton DL, Wen D-R, Wong JH et al, Technical details of intraoperative lymphatic mapping for early stage melanoma. *Arch Surg* 1992; **127:**392–9.

30. Uren RF, Howman-Giles RB, Thompson JF et al, Lymphoscintigraphy to identify sentinel nodes in patients with melanoma. *Melanoma Res* 1994; **4:**395–9.

31. Uren RF, Howman-Giles R, Thompson JF et al Interval nodes: the forgotten sentinel nodes in patients with melanoma. *Arch Surg* 2000; **135:**1168–72.

32. Uren RF, Howman-Giles RB, Thompson JF et al, Lymphatic drainage to triangular intermuscular space lymph nodes in melanoma on the back. *J Nucl Med* 1996; **37:**964–6.

33. Uren RF, Howman-Giles RB, Thompson JF, Lymphatic drainage from the skin of the back to intra-abdominal lymph nodes in melanoma patients. *Ann Surg Oncol* 1998; **5:**384–7.

34. Uren RF, Howman-Giles RB, Thompson JF, McCarthy WH, Exclusive lymphatic drainage from a melanoma on the back to intraabdominal lymph nodes. *Clin Nucl Med* 1998; **23:**71–3.

35. Uren RF, Howman-Giles RB, Thompson JF et al, Lymphatic drainage from peri-umbilical skin to internal mammary nodes. *Clin Nucl Med* 1995; **20:**254–5.

36. Robbins KT, Medina JE, Wolfe GT et al, Standardizing neck dissection terminology. Official report of the Academy's committee for head and neck surgery and oncology. *Arch Otolaryngol Head Surg* 1991; **117:**601–5.

37. O'Brien CJ, Petersen-Schaefer K, Ruark D et al, Radical, modified, and selective neck dissection for cutaneous malignant melanoma. *Head Neck* 1995; **17:**232–41.

38. O'Brien CJ, Uren RF, Thompson JF et al, Prediction of potential metastatic sites in cutaneous head and neck melanoma using lymphoscintigraphy. *Am J Surg* 1995; **170:**461–6.

39. Uren RF, Howman-Giles R, Thompson JF, Quinn MJ, Direct lymphatic drainage from the skin of the forearm to a supraclavicular node. *Clin Nucl Med* 1996; **21:**387–9.

40. Hunt JA, Thompson JF, Uren RF et al, Epitrochlear lymph nodes as a site of melanoma metastasis. *Ann Surg Oncol* 1998; **5:**248–52.

41. Clouse ME, Wallace S, Lymphatic Imaging. Lymphography, computed tomography and scintigraphy. In: Harris JHJ, ed, *Golden's Diagnostic Radiology,* 2nd edn, 15–21. Williams & Wilkins: Baltimore, 1985.

42. Vendrell-Torne E, Setain-Quinquer J, Domenech-Torne FM, Study of normal mammary lymphatic drainage using radioactive isotopes. *J Nucl Med* 1972; **13:**801–5.

43. Turner-Warwick RT, The lymphatics of the breast. *Br J Surg* 1959; **46:**574–82.

44. Uren RF, Thompson JF, Howman-Giles R, Shaw HM, Melanoma metastases in triangular intermuscular space lymph nodes. *Ann Surg Oncol* 1999; **6:**811.

45. Borgstein PJ, Meijer S, Pijpers R, Intradermal blue dye to identify sentinel lymph-node in breast cancer. *Lancet* 1997; **349:**1668–9.

46. Uren RF, Howman-Giles RB, Thompson JF et al, Mammary lymphoscintigraphy in breast cancer. *J Nucl Med* 1995; **36:**1775–80.

47. Vera DR, Wisner ER, Stadalnik RC, Sentinel node imaging via a nonparticulate receptor-binding radiotracer. *J Nucl Med* 1997; **38:**530–5.

48. Moghimi SM, Hawley AE, Christy NM et al, Surface engineered nanospheres with enhanced drainage into lymphatics and uptake by macrophages of the regional lymph nodes. *FEBS Lett* 1994; **344:**25–30.

4

The intraoperative gamma probe: design, operation, and safety

Pat Zanzonico

CONTENTS   Radioactivity and radiation   •   Basic conditions in radiation detection and measurement   •   Radiation detectors   •   Practical considerations   •   Dosimetry and radiation protection

Radionuclide detection of sentinel lymph nodes (SLNs) and visually occult tumors can be enhanced using small intraoperative probes in a surgical setting because of the close proximity of the detector and the elimination, through collimation, of most interfering radiation from radioactivity in surrounding tissues.[1,2] While such probes have been used almost exclusively for counting x-rays and gamma-rays (γ-rays), intraoperative beta probes have also been developed.[3–5] In addition, small field-of-view intraoperative gamma cameras, or imaging probes, have been developed.[6–8] This review, however, is limited to the technical aspects of nonimaging intraoperative gamma probes.

A compilation of the pertinent physical properties of current or potential radionuclides for use with intraoperative gamma probes is presented in Table 4.1.

RADIOACTIVITY AND RADIATION

Terminology

The terminology of radiation physics is complex, and terms such as "radioactivity" and "radia-tion" are sometimes confused. Radioactivity is a property of certain atomic nuclei: as a result of inherent structural instability, radioactive nuclei may spontaneously and randomly undergo an alteration, or "disintegration," to a different, more stable nuclear structure. This process is sometimes also known as a "transformation," "transmutation," or "decay." In the process of or immediately after such a radioactive decay, energy and matter may be emitted in the form of photon and/or particulate radiation. Photon radiations are x- or γ-rays: electromagnetic radiations having neither (rest) mass nor electric charge and similar to, but much higher in energy than, visible light. Particulate radiations have mass and charge. The most common particulate radiations are beta-rays (β-rays): high-energy positively or negatively charged electrons— positron (β$^+$) or negatrons (β$^-$), respectively. Generally, β-rays not explicitly identified as either positive or negative are assumed to be negatrons (β$^-$).

Quantities and units

The physical quantity of "activity" specifies the

Table 4.1 Physical properties of radionuclides used with intraoperative gamma probes						
	Fluorine-18	Technetium-99m	Indium-111	Iodine-123	Iodine-125	Iodine-131
Physical half-life, $T_{\frac{1}{2}}^{a}$	110 min	6.02 h	2.83 d	13.1 h	60.1 d	8.04 d
X- or γ-ray energy (keV)	511	140	171, 247	159	27	364
Half-value layer (cm)^b						
Soft tissue/water	7.1	4.6	5.1	4.7	1.7	6.3
Lead	0.46	0.017	0.09	0.05	0.005	0.024
Specific gamma ray constant, Γ (R-cm^2/mCi-h)^c	5.7	0.78	2.0	0.75	1.5	2.5

^{a} The time required for the activity to decrease by radioactive decay to 50%.
^{b} Thickness (cm) to reduce number of x- or γ-rays to 50%.
^{c} The exposure rate (in R/h) in air at 1 cm from a 1-mCi point source.

amount of radioactivity and is the number of radioactive disintegrations that occur per unit time; activity is commonly expressed in disintegrations per second (dps) or disintegrations per minute (dpm).[9] The older, or conventional, unit of activity is the curie (Ci), which represents 37 billion, or 3.7×10^{10} dps. (This somewhat odd value is the number of dps in 1 gram of radium, which was originally used as a standard relative to which the activities in radioactive materials were expressed.) Relative to the amounts of radioactivity used clinically, 1 Ci is a very large activity. Accordingly, submultiples of the curie are often used: 1 millicurie (mCi), 3.7×10^7 dps, is one-thousandth of 1 Ci and 1 microcurie (μCi), 3.7×10^4 dps, is one-millionth of 1 Ci. The newer, Système International d'Unités (SI) unit of activity is the becquerel (Bq), which corresponds to 1 dps. In contrast to 1 Ci, 1 Bq is a very small activity, and so multiples of the becquerel are often used clinically: 1 kilobecquerel (kBq), 1×10^3 dps, is one thousand Bq, and 1 megabecquerel (MBq), 1×10^6 dps, is one million Bq. Note that 1 μCi = 37 kBq, and 1 mCi = 37 MBq. For a given activity, measured count rate (such as counts per second or counts per minute) is highly dependent on the counting system and the source-detector geometry, and therefore generally is not a quantitative

measure of—and should not be mistaken for—activity.

Energies of both photon and particulate radiations are expressed in units of electron volts (eV) or multiples thereof. An electron volt is the amount of energy equal to the kinetic energy of an electron after it has been accelerated through a potential difference of 1 volt (V). Radiation energies are typically expressed as multiples of the electron volt: 1 kiloelectron volt (keV), 1×10^3 eV, is one thousand eV, and 1 megaelectron volt (MeV), 1×10^6 eV, is one million eV.

The probability and/or severity of harm from radiation is directly related to the "dose." Over the years, a seemingly bewildering array of quantities have been devised to express radiation dose, especially as related to biological effects. The oldest such quantity is "exposure" (X), the amount of electric charge produced by x- or γ-rays per unit mass of air. The conventional unit of exposure is the roentgen (R), which equals 0.000258 coulombs (C) per kilogram of air (2.58×10^{-4} C/kg), and the SI unit is 1 C/kg (=3876 R). A generally applicable and perhaps more familiar quantity is the "absorbed dose" (D), the energy deposited by any radiation per unit mass of any material. The conventional unit of absorbed dose is the rad (=100 erg/g), and the SI unit is the gray

(Gy) (=1 J/kg); 1 rad is one hundredth of a gray (or 1 cGy), and 1 Gy = 100 rad. A newer quantity, the "dose equivalent" (DE), equals the absorbed dose (D) multiplied by a dimensionless "quality factor" (QF) or "radiation weighting factor" (w_R). The quality factor is different for different types of radiations: 1 for x-, γ-, and β-rays; 10 for neutrons (n) and protons (p); and 20 for alpha-rays; it reflects the relative effectiveness of that radiation in producing biological damage. Thus, for different radiations, equal dose equivalents presumably correspond to equal biological damage. The conventional unit of dose equivalence is the rem, and the SI unit is the sievert (Sv); 1 rem is a hundredth of a sievert (or 1 cSv), and 1 Sv = 100 rem. Finally, the "effective dose equivalent" (H_E or EDE) equals the sum over all the tissues of the body of the dose equivalent (DE) to each tissue multiplied by its respective tissue weighting factor (w_T), which reflects the relative radiation sensitivity of that tissue. The effective dose equivalent is thus a single value that presumably reflects the overall biological damage (specifically, the total risk of cancer or genetic abnormality) of an irradiation regardless of how nonuniform the irradiation is among the tissues of the body. The units of effective dose equivalent are the same as those of dose equivalent: the conventional unit is the rem, and the SI unit is the sievert. In principle, a given effective dose equivalent incurs the same risk of cancer to the irradiated individual or of a genetic abnormality in that individual's subsequently conceived offspring as an equal, uniform total-body dose equivalent; for x-, γ-, and β-rays (QF = 1), this latter quantity corresponds to a uniform total-body absorbed dose. The effective dose (E) is yet another quantity to express such risk and is essentially identical to the effective dose equivalent.

Interactions of radiation with matter

Radiations emitted as a result of radioactive decay, such as x-, γ- and β-rays, are "ionizing" radiations; that is, such radiations ionize the atoms or molecules of a stopping medium and produce free negative electrons and positive

ions. Gamma rays and x-rays are far more penetrating than β-rays: in soft tissue, x- and γ-rays with energies of several hundred keV will travel 5–10 cm, while β-rays with similar energies will travel no further than approximately 1 mm (=0.1 cm). Because of their greater penetration, x- and γ-rays can be conveniently and sensitively detected, counted, and localized with intraoperative probes. At the same time, x- and γ-rays from a relatively large volume of tissue can contribute to the count rate measured with an intraoperative probe, potentially confounding the precise localization of an SLN or tumor.

Gamma- and x-rays interact with matter by the photoelectric effect or by Compton scatter (Figure 4.1). Because of their change in direction, rays that are Compton-scattered in the patient's body and detected with an intraoperative probe may misleadingly appear to originate from a direction different from that of the original ray. Compton scatter thus represents one of the major impediments to accurate spatial localization and high-contrast detection of radionuclides in situ.

BASIC CONSIDERATIONS IN RADIATION DETECTION AND MEASUREMENT

Statistics

Statistical fluctuations will occur in the measured counts or count rates arising from decay of radioactivity. Thus, if an intraoperative probe were used repeatedly to measure the counts or count rates from a given amount of radioactivity, a different value would probably be obtained for each measurement. The lower the activity and/or the shorter the counting interval, the smaller the average number of counts per measurement and the greater this statistical fluctuation will be. Such fluctuations complicate the accurate detection and measurement of radioactivity, especially if one is attempting to perform such measurements quickly, as in a surgical setting.

There is actually no way to establish with absolute certainty that the apparent target-to-background (SLN-to-adjacent normal tissue) count-rate ratio is accurate; that is, that it is *not*

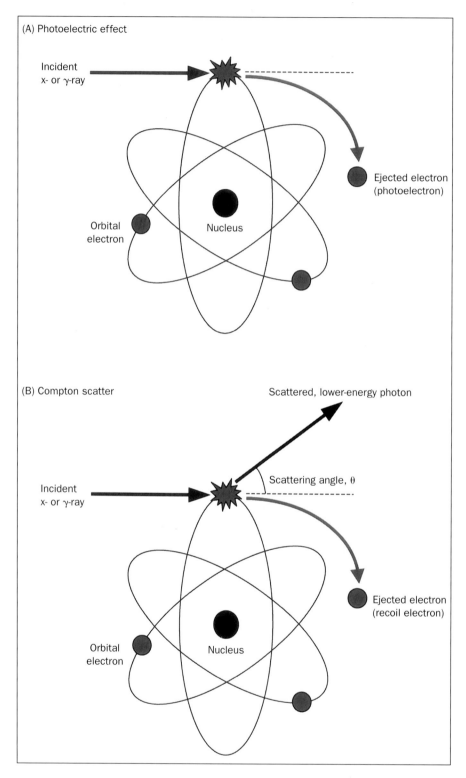

(A) Photoelectric effect

Incident
x- or γ-ray

Ejected electron
(photoelectron)

Orbital
electron

Nucleus

(B) Compton scatter

Scattered, lower-energy photon

Scattering angle, θ

Incident
x- or γ-ray

Ejected electron
(recoil electron)

Orbital
electron

Nucleus

Figure 4.1 Interactions of x- and γ-rays with matter. (A) In the photoelectric effect, an x- or γ-ray's energy is completely transferred to an orbital electron in an atom of the stopping medium, ejecting the electron from the atom as a "photoelectron." The x- or γ-ray thus disappears in the process. (B) In Compton scatter, only a portion of the incident x- or γ-ray's energy is transferred to an orbital electron, which is ejected from the atom as a "recoil electron." The scattered x- or γ-ray's energy is therefore less than that of the incident x- or γ-ray and it travels in a different direction.

caused by unavoidable random fluctuations in the measured count rates. The detection of the SLN can be made statistically reliable, however. As the lymph node-to-background count-rate ratio and/or the lymph node count-rate increase, it takes less time to acquire a sufficient number of counts to achieve a statistically significant difference between the target and the background count rates (Figure 4.2). For example, for an apparent count-rate ratio of 2 ("low contrast"), a node count rate of 25 counts per second (cps) requires a counting interval of 500 seconds to actually establish such a ratio with statistical reliability, a prohibitively long counting interval per site in a surgical setting. Even for a lymph node count rate of 250 cps, a counting interval of 50 seconds is still required for a node-to-background ratio of only 2. With clinically realistic count rates, then, low-contrast lymph nodes or tumors may be missed (i.e., not distinguished from background) with short counting intervals. On the other hand, for an apparent count-rate ratio of 10 ("high contrast"), counting intervals of only 30 seconds and 3 seconds are required for lymph-node count rates of 25 cps and 250 cps, respectively.

Shielding and collimation

The purpose of shielding and collimation is to prevent radiations from directions other than the direction of counting from striking the detector and producing counts, since such counts may confound the localization of SLNs or small tumors. Along with adequate shielding on the back and sides of the detector, such directional counting requires a collimator (Figure 4.3) to stop (or "attenuate") x- or γ-rays emitted in a direction other than the desired counting direction from striking the detector (such as Event 3 in Figure 4.4). The length and

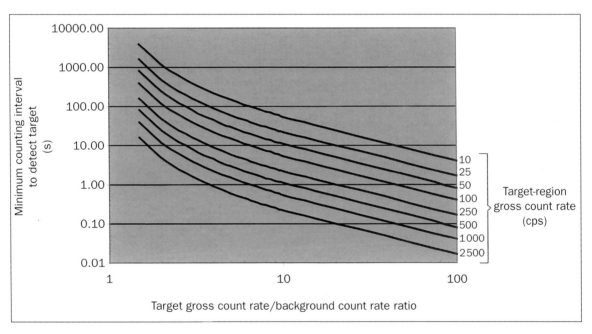

Figure 4.2 Minimum counting interval (in seconds) to "reliably" detect a target region as a function of the ratio of the target-region gross count rate to the background count rate, and of the target region gross count rate (in cps). This is based on the statistics of counting data and the "detection" criterion that the target-region net count rate is 2 standard deviations above the background count rate, yielding a 95% probability that it is actually greater than the background count rate. The net count rate is the difference between the gross (or total) and the background count rates.[10,11,34]

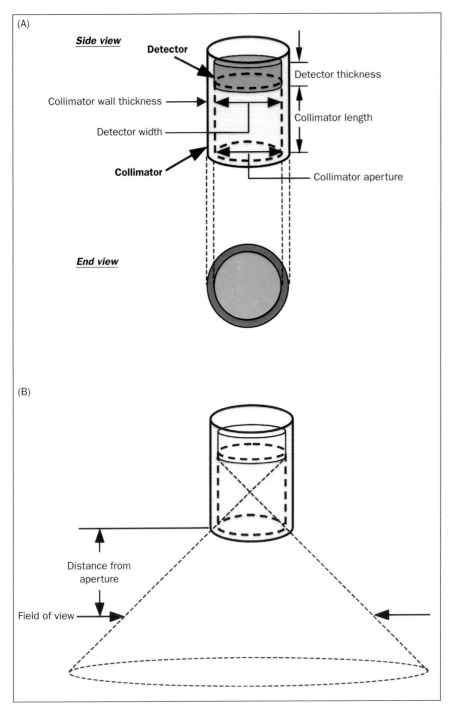

(A)

Side view

Detector

Detector thickness

Collimator wall thickness

Collimator length

Detector width

Collimator

Collimator aperture

End view

(B)

Distance from aperture

Field of view

Figure 4.3 Gamma-probe collimator. (A) Basic design. The collimator may be thought of as an extension of the detector shielding in the forward direction, that is, beyond the detector face in the desired counting direction. A collimator may be characterized by its aperture (generally, but not necessarily, equal to the width of the detector), its length, and its wall thickness. (B) The probe's field of view—the area of tissue from which unscattered x- or γ-rays may reach the detector—increases with increasing distance from the collimator aperture. The volume of tissue from which unscattered x- or γ-rays may reach the detector is thus a three-dimensional cone diverging outward from the collimator (the dotted line).

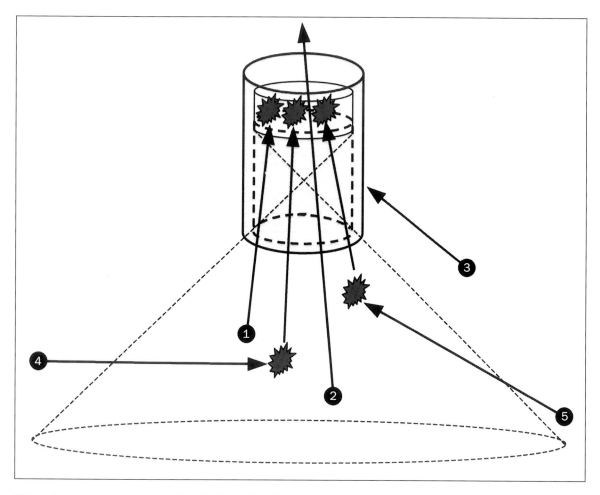

Figure 4.4 In the detection and localization of an SLN or small tumor with intraoperative gamma probes, a variety of "events" contribute to the measured counts. Events 1 and 2 represent unscattered x- or γ-rays emitted within the field of view (FOV) and traveling in the direction of the detector. The x- or γ-ray corresponding to Event 1 is then stopped within the detector and counted, and represents a correctly positioned event. The x- or γ-ray corresponding to Event 2 simply passes through the detector and is not counted. Event 3 represents an unscattered x- or γ-ray emitted outside the FOV and traveling towards the detector in a direction different from the desired counting direction. It therefore strikes the collimator and is stopped, never reaching the detector, and is, correctly, *not* counted. Event 4 represents a *sharply* Compton-scattered x- or γ-ray emitted outside the FOV. Although it is scattered in the direction of the detector, the scattering angle and therefore the energy loss are sufficiently large that the energy of the scattered photon has been reduced to a value that lies below the photopeak energy window. Event 4 is therefore correctly *not* counted. Event 5 represents a *less sharply* Compton-scattered x- or γ-ray emitted outside the FOV. It is also scattered in the direction of the detector, but the scattering angle and therefore the energy loss are small enough that the energy of the scattered photon still lies within the photopeak energy window (see text). Event 5 is therefore counted but mispositioned as having been emitted within the FOV.

aperture determine the detector's field of view: by lengthening the collimator and/or narrowing its aperture, the detector's field of view is reduced (see Figure 4.9 and text discussion).

For higher-energy and therefore more penetrating radiations, thicker shielding and thicker collimation may be required. To maximize attenuation, collimators should be fabricated out of materials with a high atomic number (the atomic number, Z, is the number of protons in the nucleus or the number of orbital electrons in the nonionized atom of the material) and a high mass density (the mass density, ρ, is the mass per unit volume, typically expressed in g/cm^3). Among such materials, lead is inexpensive, widely available, and machinable, and has long been the most commonly used shielding and collimation material. Other materials such as tungsten, gold, and platinum provide even greater attenuation than lead and are not prohibitively expensive in the small amounts needed for intraoperative probe collimators. The relative attenuation of lead, tungsten (8% copper), gold, and platinum (iridium alloy) are 1, 1.2, 1.6, and 1.7, respectively.[12]

RADIATION DETECTORS

Basic design and operating principle of radiation detectors used in intraoperative probes

Radiation detectors can generally be characterized in terms of their operation as either scintillation or ionization detectors (Figure 4.5).[10,11] In scintillation detectors, visible light is produced as radiation, excites atoms of a crystal, and is converted to an electron signal or pulse which is then amplified by a photomultiplier tube (PMT) and its high voltage (500–1500 V). In ionization detectors, free electrons produced when radiation ionizes a stopping medium are electrostatically collected by a bias voltage (10–500 V) to produce an electron signal. In both scintillation and ionization detectors, the unprocessed electron signal is then shaped and amplified and the resulting pulses sorted by their amplitude (or "pulse height"). Importantly, the pulse height is directly related to the x- or γ-ray energy absorbed in the detector. Only pulses in a preset pulse-height (or energy) range are actually counted and the number of such counts or the count rate displayed.

The high voltages used in scintillation and in semiconductor detectors are 700–1500 V and 10–500 V, respectively. The actual detector in typical intraoperative probes is 10–20 mm in diameter and approximately 10 mm thick in scintillation detectors but is only roughly 1 mm thick in semiconductor detectors.[2,10–16] Scintillators include thallium-doped sodium iodide, NaI(Tl) (effective atomic number Z = 42); thallium-doped caesium iodide, CsI(Tl) (Z = 54); and samarium-doped lutecium ortho-oxysilicate, LSO (Z = 66). Although NaI(Tl) is the most widely used clinical scintillator, among the halides CsI(Tl) has a higher effective atomic number than NaI(Tl) and, therefore, greater attenuation, especially for photons with energies greater than that of technetium-99m (Tc-99m) γ-rays (140 keV). All are hygroscopic (i.e., readily absorb moisture, including moisture in air) and must be placed in hermetically sealed as well as light-tight containers to exclude moisture and prevent yellowing and the resulting decrease in light emission and sensitivity. Semiconductors used in ionization-detector probes include cadmium telluride, CdTe (Z = 52); cadmium zinc telluride, CdZnTe (Z = 47); and mercuric iodide, HgI_2 (Z = 65).[2,10–12,14–16]

Detector parameters

Radiation detectors, including intraoperative probes, may be characterized by various performance parameters, including energy resolution, sensitivity (or efficiency), and their spatial resolution.[10,11,14,15,17,18] A general summary of performance parameters of current intraoperative gamma probes is presented in Table 4.2.

Energy resolution and energy-selective counting
An x-ray or γ-ray is emitted from a radioactively decaying atom with a single well-defined

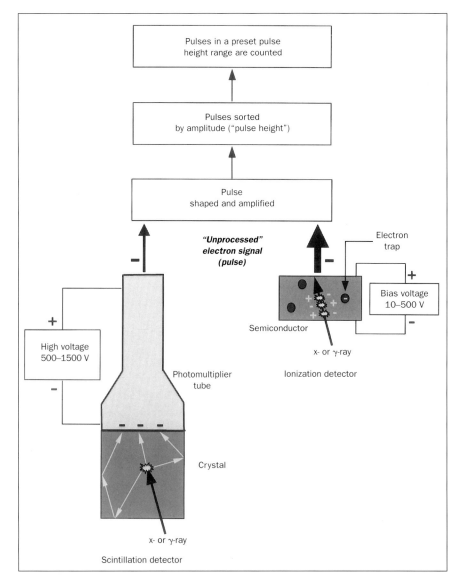

Figure 4.5 Basic design and operating principle of a scintillation detector and a semiconductor ionization detector. The heavier arrow emerging from the back of the ionization detector is meant to indicate the greater number of electrons per keV of radiation energy absorbed in its unprocessed electron signal.

energy. Even in the absence of scatter (e.g., in air), however, the *detected* energy of such radiations will not correspond precisely to this energy but will fall within a range of energies centered about this energy. A detector's "energy resolution" indicates the extent of this dispersion of detected energies about the actual energy of the x- or γ-ray (Figure 4.6). It is related to the "noise," or statistical uncertainty, inherent in the detection process and is therefore inversely related to the number of electrons comprising the "unprocessed" electron signal (see Figure 4.6). For scintillation detectors, the energy resolution is typically of the order of 10%. For ionization (i.e., semiconductor) detectors, more electrons are produced per keV of radiation energy absorbed; therefore, the energy resolution is generally better.[14,15]

The importance of energy resolution lies in elimination of scattered radiation and therefore of mispositioned events. Radiation loses energy when scattered and the lower-energy scattered

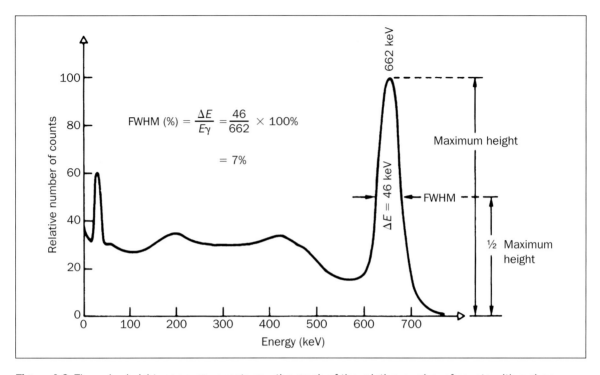

Figure 4.6 The pulse-height, or energy, spectrum—the graph of the relative number of counts with a given detected energy versus the detected energy—for the 662 keV γ-rays emitted by caesium-137. The photopeak, the prominent bell-shaped component of the spectrum at the 662-keV energy level, represents detected unscattered ^{137}Cs γ-rays. Energy resolution is defined as the full width at half-maximum height (FWHM = ΔE) of the photopeak expressed as a percentage of the photopeak energy (E_γ), FWHM (%) = $\Delta E/E_\gamma$ 100% (adapted from reference 34).

Table 4.2 Typical structural characteristics and performance parameters of current intraoperative probes

	Scintillation probes	Ionization probes
Detector materials	NaI(Tl), CsI(Tl), LSO	CdTe, CdZnTe
Detector thickness (mm, approx.)	10	1
Detector diameter (mm)	10–20	10–20
Energy resolution (%FWHM)	15–30	5–10
Tc-99m sensitivity at 1 cm in air (cps/μCi)	200–400	200–400
Tc-99m spatial resolution at 1 cm (mm FWHM)	10–20	10–20

The data in this table (taken from references 2, 10–12, 15, and 16) are intended to summarize, in a general way, the prevailing performance parameters among current intraoperative probes. Because the measured values of such parameters are highly dependent upon the measurement conditions, one should be aware of the respective conditions in comparing performance parameters among probes.

radiation may therefore be discriminated from the unscattered radiation on the basis of their respective energies. The finite energy resolution of radiation detectors means, however, that there will be overlap of scattered and unscattered radiations, as illustrated in Figure 4.7. As energy resolution improves (i.e., the FWHM decreases and the photopeak becomes narrower—see Figure 4.6), the separation of unscattered and scattered radiations increases and more counts corresponding to mispositioned, scattered radiation may be eliminated while discarding fewer counts corresponding to correctly positioned, unscattered radiation.

Because of finite energy resolution, a so-called "20% photopeak energy window" $(E_\gamma \pm 10\%)$ is commonly employed, where E_γ is the photopeak x- or γ-ray energy. For example, $(140 - 14 = 126)$ keV to $(140 + 14 = 154)$ keV represents the 20% energy window typically used to count the 140-keV γ-ray of Tc-99m (Figure 4.7A). Depending on the device, such an energy window may be set by specifying the center-line energy and the percentage width of the window (E_γ and $\Delta E = 0.2\, E_\gamma$, respectively, for a 20% window), the baseline energy and width of the window ($0.9\, E_\gamma$ and $\Delta E = 0.2\, E_\gamma$, respectively, for a 20% window), or the lower-level discriminator and upper-level discriminator energies ($0.9\, E_\gamma$ and $1.1\, E_\gamma$, respectively, for a 20% window).

The meaning of the energy window and the effect of different energy windows are illustrated in Figure 4.7. By only counting pulses with detected energies within the photopeak energy window, the most sharply Compton-scattered, and therefore the most mispositioned, x- or γ-rays (such as Event 4 in Figure 4.4) are excluded because their energies lie below the energy window. On the other hand, the energies of less sharply Compton-scattered x- or γ-rays (such as Event 5 in Figure 4.4) actually lie within the energy window, and such pulses are counted. As the energy window is narrowed, the total and the unscattered counts decrease, but the scattered counts decrease even more. Thus, sensitivity (see below) decreases, but localization of SLNs or small tumors and the count contrast (see below) between nodes

or tumors and adjacent normal tissue may improve—because scattered, misplaced events comprise a smaller fraction of the total counts. Conversely, as the energy window is widened, the total and the unscattered counts increase, but the scattered counts increase even more. Thus, sensitivity increases, but localization of SLNs or small tumors and the count contrast between nodes or tumors and adjacent normal tissue may deteriorate—because scattered, misplaced events now comprise a greater fraction of the total counts.

Sensitivity
Sensitivity (or efficiency) is the detected count rate per unit activity (expressed, for example, in cps/μCi). There are two distinct components of overall sensitivity: geometric sensitivity and intrinsic sensitivity. Geometric sensitivity is the fraction of emitted radiations that actually strike the detector. Intrinsic sensitivity is the fraction of radiations that, upon striking the detector, are then stopped within the detector and counted. As illustrated in Figures 4.8, 4.9 and 4.10, sensitivity sharply decreases with increasing distance from the collimator aperture. Geometric efficiency is also directly related to the collimator aperture and inversely related to the collimator length: as the collimator aperture is narrowed and/or lengthened, the number of radiations counted, and therefore the sensitivity, decreases markedly (Figure 4.9). Intrinsic sensitivity, on the other hand, depends only on the thickness and composition of the detector: the thicker the detector and the higher its effective atomic and mass density, the greater its intrinsic sensitivity. Since higher-energy radiations are more penetrating and are more likely to pass through a detector without being stopped and detected, intrinsic sensitivity decreases with increasing radiation energy. Detection of such radiations may therefore require detectors that are thicker and/or have a higher atomic number.

Sensitivity is an important parameter in overall SLN or tumor detectability in situations where counting intervals are limited, for example, where the surgeon's attempt to count many sites in a large surgical field is limited by the

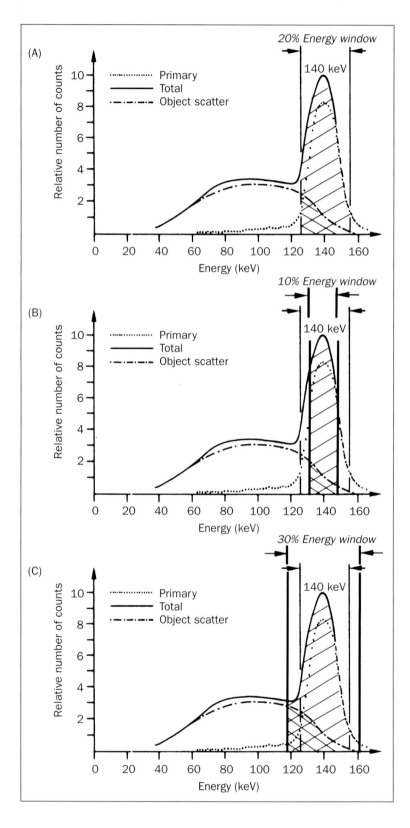

Figure 4.7 Technetium-99m energy spectra with three different energy windows. Such spectra (the solid lines) comprised at least two distinct components: the bell-shaped photopeak (the dot curves) corresponding to unscattered x- or γ-rays emitted within the probe's field of view (such as Event 1 in Figure 4.4) and the scatter curves (the dot-dash curves) corresponding to Compton-scattered x- or γ-rays (such as Events 4 and 5 in Figure 4.4). As the energy window is narrowed from the standard 20% (A) to 10% (B), the total counts (corresponding to the total hatched area) decrease, but the scattered counts (corresponding to the cross-hatched area) decrease even more. As the energy window is widened from 20% (A) to 30% (C), the total counts increase, but the scattered counts increase even more (adapted from reference 34).

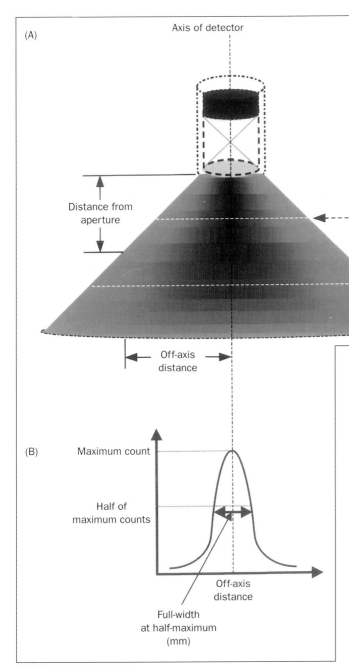

(A)

Axis of detector

Distance from
aperture

Off-axis
distance

1

2

(B)

Maximum count

Half of
maximum counts

Off-axis
distance

Full-width
at half-maximum
(mm)

Figure 4.8 The sensitivity and spatial resolution of a gamma probe as a function of the distance from the collimator aperture. (A) The intensity of the gray shading within the three-dimensional cone diverging outward from the collimator aperture is an indication of the relative counts, with black corresponding to the maximum counts and progressively lighter shades of gray corresponding to progressively fewer counts. The progressively lighter shading with increasing distance from the collimator aperture indicates that the number of radiations counted, and therefore the sensitivity, are decreasing with distance. (B) The probe's spatial resolution may be characterized in terms of its point-spread function (PSF), the graph of the detected count rate from a point source as a function of the distance of the source from the axis of the detector, and the full width at half-maximum (FWHM) of the bell-shaped PSF: the broader the PSF, the larger the FWHM of the PSF and the poorer the spatial resolution. The broader dispersion in the intensity of the gray shading with increasing distance from the aperture reflects the distance-dependent degradation of spatial resolution, that is, the distance-dependent broadening of the PSF and increase in the FWHM (as illustrated by PSFs 1 and 2 in A).

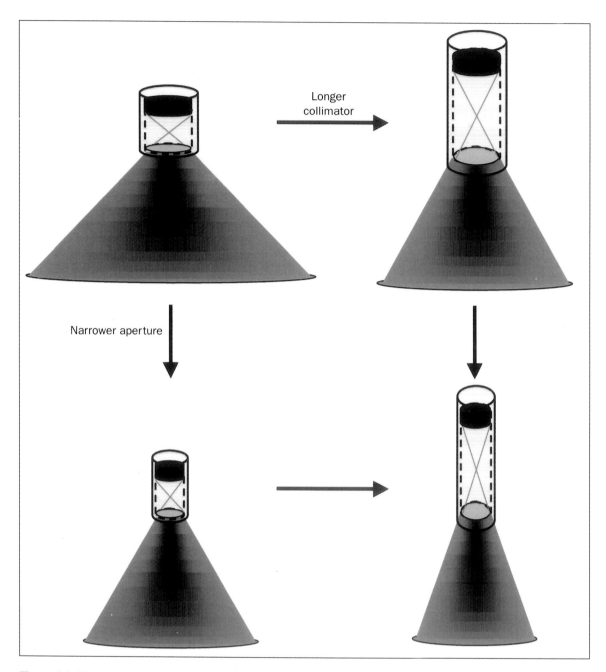

Figure 4.9 The sensitivity and spatial resolution of a gamma probe as a function of its collimator length and aperture. As in Figure 4.8, the intensity of the gray shading within the three-dimensional cone diverging outward from the collimator aperture is an indication of the relative counts, with black corresponding to the maximum counts and progressively lighter shades of gray corresponding to progressively fewer counts. As the collimator aperture is narrowed and/or as the collimator is lengthened, the three-dimensional cone of tissue from which emitted x- and γ-rays can strike the detector becomes markedly smaller; that is, the field of view becomes smaller. As a result, the number of radiations counted and the sensitivity decrease. As the collimator aperture is narrowed and/or as the collimator is lengthened, however, this dispersion (i.e., the PSF) is narrowed and the spatial resolution improves.

time available for the procedure. Sensitivity may be increased, apparently, by widening the energy window and/or by reducing collimation and shielding, but at the cost of increasing the number of scattered x- and γ-rays counted and thereby degrading the probe's ability to localize small structures such as SLNs with precision owing to the counting of more mispositioned, Compton-scattered x- and γ-rays. In comparing probes, therefore, one should check that apparently higher sensitivity is not achieved simply by using a wider energy window or a wider aperture and/or shorter collimator.

Spatial resolution

For detectors such as intraoperative probes where radiation is to be localized as well as detected and counted, spatial resolution is a critical performance parameter. It reflects the ability of the detector to determine the location of a source accurately. The probe's spatial resolution can be expressed as the full width at half-maximum height (FWHM) of the point-spread function (PSF): the narrower the PSF and the smaller the FWHM of the PSF, the better the detector's spatial resolution; that is, the more precisely a small source such as an SLN can be localized (see Figure 4.8). Narrowing the collimator aperture and/or lengthening the collimator markedly narrows the dispersion of counts about the detector axis, narrowing the PSF and improving spatial resolution (Figure 4.9). At the same time, however, the volume of tissue from which unscattered x- and γ-rays can reach the detector, and therefore the sensitivity, are also markedly reduced. This illustrates the important principle that sensitivity and spatial resolution are inversely related: sensitivity decreases as spatial resolution improves, and spatial resolution degrades as sensitivity increases.

Comparison of scintillation detectors and semiconductor ionization detectors

Scintillation-detector intraoperative probes have the advantages of reliability, relatively

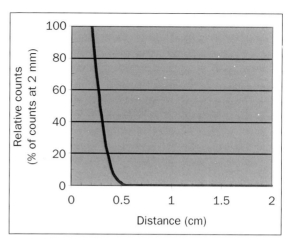

Figure 4.10 The count rate (normalized to 100% at a distance of 0.2 cm) as a function of distance from a point source. The detected count rate from a point source decreases as $1/r^2$), that is, 1 divided by the square of the distance (r) between the detector and the source; this relationship is known as the "inverse square law." It applies, exactly, only to a point source in air. In principle (i.e., ignoring scatter), a stopping medium (e.g., soft tissue) between the detector and the source attenuates some of the radiation and the detected count rate is slightly less. In reality, however, x- and γ-rays that are Compton-scattered from out of the detector's field of view towards the detector actually add counts, and the distance-dependent decrease in count rate is therefore not as pronounced as indicated in the graph.

low cost, and high sensitivity (mainly because of their greater thickness: about 10 mm versus only about 1 mm in ionization detectors), especially for medium- to high-energy photons. Disadvantages include bulkiness and relatively poor energy resolution and scatter rejection. In some scintillation-detector intraoperative probes, the light signal from the crystal is guided to a remote PMT through a flexible fiberoptic cable.[12] Thus, the probe assembly can be made lighter and more compact, and more like a surgical instrument. Up to 90% of the light produced in the scintillator may, however, be lost during transmission along the fiberoptic cable to the PMT, resulting in degraded energy resolution (38% for 140-keV Tc-99m γ-rays, versus only 10–15% for a conventional detector in which the PMT is coupled directly to the crystal in the probe housing).[12] Alternatively, electronic devices known as photodiodes have shown promise as compact replacements for PMTs without the degradation of energy resolution associated with fiberoptic light guides.[12]

Semiconductor-based probes are compact and have excellent energy resolution and scatter rejection. Defects (irregularities in the crystal lattice) can, however, trap electrons produced by radiation, thus reducing the total charge collected ("charge trapping"). As a result of such incomplete charge collection, statistical uncertainty (i.e., noise) is increased and the photopeaks in energy spectra are broadened; that is, the otherwise excellent energy resolution of semiconductors is somewhat degraded. To minimize this effect, semiconductor detectors are made relatively thin (only about 1 mm), but at the cost of lower intrinsic sensitivity.[12] Trapping can also be reduced by increasing the bias voltage across the detector (see Figure 4.5), but at the expense of greater electronic noise and poorer performance. Techniques for fabricating defect-free semiconductors and thus reducing charge trapping continue to be developed, with the potential to improve energy resolution to as low as 3%. Currently, however, the main disadvantage of semiconductor detectors remains their limited thickness and resulting lower sensitivity, especially for medium- to high-energy x- and γ-rays.[2,12,14,19] Nonetheless, while scintillation detectors can be made thicker and therefore more sensitive, semiconductor detectors do produce more electrons per x- and γ-ray stopped, and therefore have superior energy resolution.

To date, the few clinical studies directly comparing scintillation and semiconductor intraoperative probes have not provided a clear choice between the two types of probe. Harcke et al found some advantage to the compact design of the semiconductor probe but some disadvantage due to its lower sensitivity.[20] Szypryt et al found a NaI(Tl) probe to yield lower target-to-background count-rate ratios in bone lesions following administration of Tc-99m-methylene diphosphonate (Tc-99m-MDP) and to be less

reliable over time (presumably because of crystal hydration and yellowing, and consequently reduced sensitivity).[21] In surgical staging of gynecologic malignancies, Woolfenden and Barber found both types of probe performed satisfactorily,[16] and, unlike Szypryt et al,[21] found no deterioration over time of the scintillation probe. Moreover, neither the poorer energy resolution nor the better sensitivity of scintillation probes has translated into significantly different lesion detectability in phantom-based technical comparisons of scintillation and ionization probes.[12,14]

PRACTICAL CONSIDERATIONS

Probe applications, performance parameters, and design features

In practice, the most important performance characteristics of an intraoperative probe are overall sensitivity (efficiency), energy resolution, and spatial resolution.[14,15,17,18] Obviously, a probe having the highest sensitivity, the lowest energy resolution (expressed as the % FWHM of the photopeak) and therefore the best scatter rejection, and the lowest spatial resolution (expressed as the FWHM of the PSF) for all radionuclides used clinically, would be the probe of choice. Unfortunately, no single probe has, or can have, the optimum values of each of these performance parameters. In particular, sensitivity and spatial resolution are inversely related.

An intraoperative probe should be selected and its performance parameters evaluated on the basis of the specific clinical tasks for which it will be used.[11,17,22] Intraoperative probes for SLN detection require excellent spatial resolution to allow precise localization of the small target; energy resolution and sensitivity are probably somewhat less important. The relatively superficial anatomic location of SLNs, and therefore the lack of overlying scattering material, means that the contribution of scattered radiations is minimized. Since the total region to be sampled is rather limited and counting and localization can be performed prior to surgical incision, the counting interval can be made longer to compensate for lower sensitivity. The total region to be sampled for SLNs can be further restricted if the SLNs are at least approximately localized by the use of gamma-camera imaging, preferably with a cobalt-57 flood source transmission image for anatomic orientation.[23] Radioguided tumor excision, on the other hand, may require primarily high sensitivity, to allow rapid yet statistically reliable counting of many sites in large surgical fields. Finer spatial sampling within higher count-rate areas can then be used to localize the focus of activity with greater precision. Good energy resolution, to minimize the count contribution of scattered radiation, is also important, especially in the presence of variable background activity.

Among commercially available intraoperative probes, performance parameters vary widely.[11,17,18,24] For example, Tiourina et al found that sensitivity varied by a factor of 20 and energy resolution by a factor of 4 among four commercially available probes they evaluated.[18] The prospective user must be aware of the precise conditions under which performance parameters are evaluated. For example, intraoperative probes may have removable side-shielding, interchangeable collimators, interchangeable detectors, and user-selectable and/or user-adjustable energy windows. Moreover, performance parameters may be evaluated using widely varying source-detector geometries. Any or all of these variables will affect the measurements of the various performance parameters, and quoted values of such parameters should therefore be examined critically.

A basic probe consists of a control unit, a detector, and cabling (Figure 4.11). Any audible signal, the frequency or pitch of which presumably reflects the count rate, should be audible above the ambient sound level in an operating room and should have an adjustable volume. A background suppression ("squelch") feature should be available so that the audible signal is silent unless the measured count rate exceeds a user-adjusted threshold value. "Autoranging" should be included: when the detected count

rate exceeds the maximum count rate for a particular range, the system automatically switches to a higher count-rate range. A turn-key system with an integrated laptop computer, data-acquisition boards, and software for probe set-up/control and data acquisition and analysis may be desirable.

An intraoperative probe must, of course, be portable and should therefore be as light and compact as possible, especially since it is used in crowded operating rooms. The probe must be battery-operated and an on-board backup battery should be provided; battery operation virtually eliminates concerns about electrical safety. The detectors themselves should also be small, light, and compact to simulate surgical instruments to which surgeons are accustomed and to provide easier detector access to certain internal tissues. While it is common practice to improve tissue access by slight angulation of the detector head, the operator should be aware of the orientation of the probe at all times.[25,26] When used intraoperatively, the detectors must, of course, be sterile. It should therefore be possible to sterilize probes with ethylene oxide gas or glutaraldehyde. Alternatively, a removable sterile sheath may be used. A protective carrying case for the control unit, probes, removable side-shielding, collimators, cables, and check sources should be provided.

Care and routine quality control

Like electronic instruments in general, intraoperative probes are fragile and subject to mechanical damage and, of course, to water damage. Care should be taken to avoid striking or dropping the control unit and the detectors. Cables should be inserted and removed by their connectors and not by pulling the cable. Some commercial intraoperative probes have non-standard connectors for linking the detector to the control unit, and special care must be taken when using these. If applicable, only the manufacturer-provided alternating-current adapters should be used. Extremes of temperature, and rapid changes in temperature, should be avoided. Organic solvents, oils, corrosive

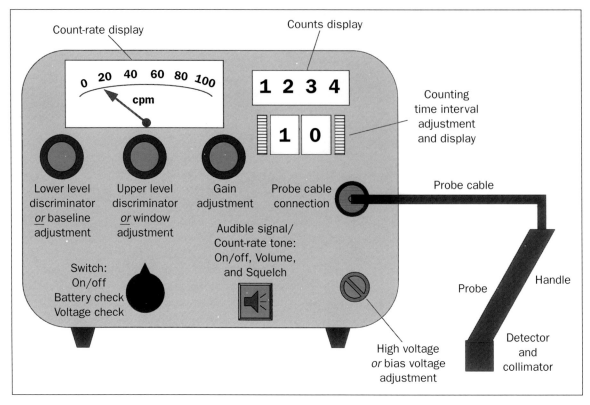

Figure 4.11 A basic intraoperative gamma probe consists of a control unit (with all displays, controls, power supplies, and electronics), a detector (generally with side-shielding and a collimator), and an electrical or fiberoptic cable. A real-time (e.g., galvanometer-type, as shown, or digital) count-rate display, audible count-rate tone ("howler"), user-selectable counting interval (with display), digital count display, and energy window settings (e.g., upper and lower level discriminators) are usually included. Battery and bias/high-voltage checks and bias/high-voltage and gain controls are also generally included. Not all features depicted are included with all probes, however.

materials such as acids and bases, and abrasive household cleaners should be avoided.

Quality control features should include a "battery check" and a "bias/high-voltage check" for both the primary and any backup battery, with a display clearly indicating that the direct current and bias/high voltages, respectively, are within the acceptable range. The battery should provide at least 8 hours of continuous operation. A visual and/or audible "low-battery" indicator, similar to those found in laptop computers, is also useful.

Unfortunately, intraoperative probes generally do not provide a display of the energy spectrum; therefore, one cannot visually check

that the probe is "peaked" (that is, that the radionuclide's photopeak actually coincides with the preset energy window), and is otherwise working properly. The lower counts or count rates resulting from an inappropriate energy window may therefore go unnoticed. Thus, a long-lived check source or set of check sources (such as cobalt-57, barium-133, and/or iodine-129) should be available for daily checks of count-rate constancy; a marked change in the count rate from one day to the next indicates an inappropriate energy-window setting or some other problem (such as a cracked crystal). Ideally, the check sources should each be incorporated into some sort of plastic cap that fits reproducibly over the probe so that spurious differences in the count rates due to variations in source-detector geometry are avoided. If the observed count rate (e.g., from a long-lived standard source in such a standardized counting geometry) deviates from that expected, the user should verify that the energy window (the lower-level discriminator, or baseline, and upper-level discriminator, or window) is set correctly. If necessary, the gain may be adjusted. Generally, however, the bias or high voltage should not be adjusted unless the count rate cannot be matched to the expected count rate by adjustment of the gain (Figure 4.11).

Daily measurements of background count rates (to check for excessive electronic noise) and standard count rates, and the results of daily battery and bias/high-voltage checks should be recorded and archived in a quality-control log book.

User training

Other than practical training in an actual surgical setting, there is generally little opportunity for a physician to learn how to use an intraoperative probe under realistic conditions, to understand in practical terms the sometimes subtle effects of scatter, background activity, and count-limited statistics, and to test one's competency in terms of node detection and localization.[11,27] A clinically relevant phantom may therefore be helpful for user training as well as for practically meaningful evaluation of the overall accuracy of probes in detecting and localizing lesions. In user training, the correct setting of energy windows must be emphasized. In particular, novice users must be trained to check that the current energy window, any removable collimation, and the probe itself match the isotope currently being counted.

DOSIMETRY AND RADIATION PROTECTION

The SLN biopsy procedure has the practical advantage of requiring the use of relatively low levels of radiopharmaceutical activity (less than 1 mCi). As discussed below, the associated radiation doses and radiogenic risks to patients and, even more so, to hospital personnel are generally quite low and compare favorably with many, more familiar, medical and non-medical exposures (Table 4.3).[26,28–31] Of course, radiation and radioactivity must always be used in the safest possible manner, with adherence to common-sense radiation protection principles and compliance with prevailing regulatory requirements. All operating-room and pathology-laboratory personnel involved in SLN biopsy procedures should attend a formal course on these topics; such a course is typically offered by a hospital's Radiation Safety Office and may total several hours in duration. Nonetheless, implementation of the SLN biopsy procedures should require only minimal modification, if any, of procedures in the surgical suite and the pathology laboratory.

Radiation dosimetry: patients

A number of analyses of the radiation doses to patients associated with SLN biopsy procedures have been performed,[26,28–31] generally based on the standard schema developed and promulgated by the Medical Internal Radionuclide Dosimetry (MIRD) Committee of the Society of Nuclear Medicine.[32] The results of these analyses for SLN biopsy procedures in breast with Tc-99m colloids are summarized in Table 4.4. Note that the doses in Table 4.4 are dose equivalents in mrem, which, for Tc-99m radiation (quality factor = 1), are numerically equal to absorbed doses in mrad; 1000 mrem = 1 rem and 1000 mrad = 1 rad. Compared with typical tissue doses associated with diagnostic nuclear medicine procedures, of the order of 1 rem (=1000 mrem), the doses to all distant tissues from an SLN biopsy procedure with 500 μCi of Tc-99m colloid are *much* less (two to three orders of magnitude less). The *mean* dose to the injected breast (1100 rem = 1.1 rem) and the *maximum* dose to regional lymph nodes (1300 rem = 1.3 rem), on the other hand, are comparable with those from routine diagnostic

Table 4.3 Radiation doses in perspective: effective dose equivalents for medical and nonmedical exposures[30]

	Effective dose equivalent (mrem)
Medical exposure	
Chest x-ray	4
SLN biopsy procedure (breast)[a]	32
Mammogram	40
Brain computed tomography (CT)	180
Tc-99m bone scan	360
Intravenous urography	460
Barium enema	500
Abdominal CT	720
Chest CT	830
Nonmedical exposure	
SLN biopsy procedure—per case[a]	
Pathologist	0.042
Surgeon	0.23
Transatlantic airline flight[b]	6
Annual maximum permissible dose for general public	100
Annual dose to nuclear medicine technologists—USA average	180
Annual natural background radiation—USA average	300
Annual natural background radiation—Denver, Colorado[b]	400
Annual maximum permissible dose for occupationally exposed individuals	5000

[a]For a procedure in which 400 μCi of Tc-99m are used.
[b]The higher doses in Denver and in a transatlantic airline flight are due to increased cosmic radiations at these higher altitudes.

nuclear medicine procedures. The doses to the injection site and to the volume of dispersion are, however, substantially greater (one to two orders of magnitude greater). The doses to these highly localized volumes of tissue, although relatively large, are probably radiobiologically insignificant because these small tissue volumes will either be excised at surgery or therapeutically irradiated to far higher doses. Consistent with its effective dose equivalent of only 32 mrem (see Tables 4.3 and 4.4), an SLN biopsy procedure with Tc-99m therefore appears to incur far less radiogenic risk overall than the already low risk associated with routine diagnostic nuclear medicine or radiological procedures (Table 4.4). For example, the effective dose equivalent associated with a Tc-99m bone scan, 360 mrem (Table 4.3),[30] is an order of magnitude greater.

Radiation dosimetry: personnel

Prevailing regulations in the United States limit the effective dose equivalent (i.e., the total-body dose equivalent and absorbed dose) to occupa-

Table 4.4 Patient dose estimates for SLN biopsy procedures (breast) with Tc-99m colloids (500 μCi)

Tissue	Dose equivalent (mrem)
Whole body (mean)	0.81–7.3
Gonads	approx. 0–8.9
Liver	1.6–24
Lung	12
Thymus	15
Lymph node	16–1300
Myocardium	
If the left breast is injected	32
If the right breast is injected	3.2
Breast	
Injection site—assuming no biological clearance	
Injection volume 0.48 ml	240 000
0.96 ml	130 000
1.92 ml	65 000
3.85 ml	34 000
5.77 ml	23 000
Injection site—with measured biological clearance	
Injection volume 0.2–0.5 ml	9700–46 000
6 ml	14 000–77 000
Volume of dispersion (measured: 2–5 ml)—assuming no biological clearance	5700–14 000
Whole injected breast (mean)—assuming no biological clearance	1100
Effective dose equivalent (mrem)	32

Data from references 28–31.

tionally exposed individuals to 5000 mrem (=5 rem) per year. For such individuals, the dose equivalent to the eye is limited to 15 rem (=15 000 mrem) per year and to the skin or any individual organ other than the eye to 50 rem (=50 000 mrem) per year. Personnel are required to be "badged" (i.e., are issued film badges) if their projected annual dose exceeds 0.5 rem (=500 mrem) to the total body, 1.5 rem (=1500 mrem) to the eye, or 50 rem (=50 000 mrem) to any other organ, that is, 10% of the respective maximum permissible doses for occupationally exposed individuals.

The hypothetical "worst-case" doses for a single SLN biopsy procedure with 500 μCi of Tc-99m are 0.23 mrem to the surgeon and 0.042 mrem to the pathologist (see Table 4.3), as well as 5.3 mrem to the surgeon's fingers and 3.5 mrem to the pathologist's fingers.[26] Thus, based on the higher finger dose, a surgeon would have to be badged if performing more than 940 such procedures per year (=[0.1 × 50 000 mrem/yr]/5.3 mrem/procedure]) and a pathologist more than 1400 procedures per year (=[0.1 × 50 000 mrem/yr]/5.3 mrem/procedure]).[26] Similarly, based on the higher finger dose, a surgeon could perform up to 9400 such procedures per year (=[50 000 mrem/yr]/5.3 mrem/procedure]) and a pathologist up to 14 000 such procedures per year

(=[50 000 mrem/yr]/3.5 mrem/procedure]) without exceeding the annual maximum permissible dose.[26]

Radiation protection

In the USA, medical use of radioactive materials (specifically, fissionable materials and fission products and their progeny) is regulated by the Nuclear Regulatory Commission (NRC). In approximately half of the 50 states, the so-called "agreement states," the NRC has agreed to transfer its regulatory authority to the state. In any medical or other facility in which radioactive materials are used, the Radiation Safety Officer (RSO), in conjunction with a Radiation Committee, is charged with ensuring that all such materials are used in a manner that is safe and compliant with all applicable regulations. Prospective users of the SLN biopsy procedure should consult with their institutional RSO for specific advice on complying with all radiation safety policies and procedures.

Owing to the relatively low activities used in SLN biopsy procedures, few radiation-safety precautions are actually required in the surgical suite or the pathology laboratory. This assumes that universal precautions are always observed. It is generally recommended that the injection of the radiopharmaceutical be performed in the nuclear medicine laboratory. Lead aprons and other shielding are generally not recommended for either the patient or for staff.[26,33] Tissue specimens sent to the pathology laboratory will contain less than 1 mCi of Tc-99m and, consistent with the applicable regulations, need not be labeled as radioactive.[26] Such labeling may be prudent, however. Normal cleaning and decontamination procedures for instruments and other nondisposable items should adequately remove any radioactive contamination.

Regulations concerning disposal of radioactively contaminated solid waste from hospitals and other institutions are especially stringent: no waste that is demonstrably radioactive (i.e., that yields a count rate significantly greater than the background count rate when surveyed with a Geiger counter) may be disposed of as nonradioactive waste. Gauze and other disposable items contaminated with tissue, blood, etc., as well as lymph nodes and other tissue specimens (including specimens sent to pathology) from the injection site *may* therefore be sufficiently radioactive to warrant decay-in-storage prior to disposal as nonradioactive medical waste.[26,30] Such items should be placed in appropriate plastic bags and the bags sealed and labeled with the date and the identity of the radionuclide (Tc-99m), then transferred to the nuclear medicine laboratory or radiation safety office for storage in a designated shielded, secure area in the institution. For radionuclides as short-lived as Tc-99m (physical half-life 6.02 hours) and for the relatively small amounts of activity used in SLN biopsy procedures (less than 1 mCi), decay-in-storage for approximately 2 days should generally be adequate. Before disposal into the nonradioactive waste stream, however, the waste must be resurveyed and shown to be no longer demonstrably radioactive. On the other hand, many hospitals have installed high-sensitivity counting systems to monitor *all* waste exiting the facility and, if necessary, to divert radioactively contaminated waste at that point for decay-in-storage. An institution's RSO may therefore decide that surgical waste from SLN biopsy procedures need not be diverted in the operating room or the pathology laboratory to decay-in-storage. Each user should consult the RSO for specific advice on waste disposal.

REFERENCES

1. Barber HB, Barrett HH, Woolfenden JM et al, Comparison of in vivo scintillation probes and gamma cameras for detection of small, deep tumours. *Phys Med Biol* 1989; **34**:727–39.
2. Woolfenden JM, Barber HB, Intraoperative probes. In: Wagner HN, Szabo Z, Buchanan JW, eds, *Principles of Nuclear Medicine*, 2nd edn, 292–297. Saunders: Philadelphia, 1995.
3. Raylman RR, Wahl RL, A fiber-optically coupled positron-sensitive surgical probe. *J Nucl Med* 1994; **35**:909–13.
4. Raylman RR, Fisher SJ, Brown RS et al, Fluorine-18-fluorodeoxyglucose-guided breast cancer

surgery with a positron-sensitive probe: validation in preclinical studies. *J Nucl Med* 1995; **36:** 1869–74.

5. Daghighian F, Mazziotta JC, Hoffman EJ et al, Intraoperative beta probe: a device for detecting tissue labeled with positron or electron emitting isotopes during surgery. *Med Phys* 1994; **21:** 153–7.

6. Barber H, Barrett H, Dereniak E et al, A gamma-ray imager with multiplexer read-out for use in ultra-high-resolution brain SPECT. *IEEE Trans Med Imaging* 1993; **40:**1140–4.

7. Hartsough N, Barber H, Woolfenden J et al, Probes containing gamma radiation detectors for in vivo tumor detection and imaging. *Proc SPIE* 1989; **1068:**184–6.

8. Moore R, Alpert N, Strauss H, A hand-held, low power gamma camera: design considerations and initial results. *J Nucl Med* 1988; **29:**832 (Abstract).

9. Zanzonico P, Internal radionuclide radiation dosimetry: a review of basic concepts and recent developments. *J Nucl Med* 2000; **41:**297–308.

10. Keshtgar M, Waddington W, Lakhani S, Ell P, Radiation detectors, In: Keshtgar M, Waddington W, Lakhani S, Ell P, eds, *The Sentinel Node in Surgical Oncology*, 19–38. Springer: Berlin, 1999.

11. Zanzonico P, Heller S, The intraoperative gamma probe: basic principles and choices available. *Semin Nucl Med* 2000; **30:**33–48.

12. Woolfenden JM, Barber HB, Design and use of radiation detector probes for intraoperative tumor detection using tumor-seeking radiotracers. In: Freeman LM, ed, *Nuclear Medicine Annual 1990*, 151–73. Raven Press: New York, 1990.

13. Attix FH, *Introduction to Radiological Physics and Radiation Dosimetry.* John Wiley: New York, 1986.

14. Barber HB, Barrett HH, Hickernell TS et al, Comparison of NaI(Tl), CdTe, and HgI2 surgical probes: physical characterization. *Med Phys* 1991; **18:**373–81.

15. Kow DP, Barber HB, Barrett HH et al, Comparison of NaI(T1), CdTe, and HgI2 surgical probes: effect of scatter compensation on probe performance. *Med Phys* 1991; **18:**382–9.

16. Woolfenden JM, Barber HB, Radiation detector probes for tumor localization using tumor-seeking radioactive tracers. *AJR Am J Roentgenol* 1989; **153:**35–9.

17. Britten AJ, A method to evaluate intra-operative gamma probes for sentinel lymph node localisation. *Eur J Nucl Med* 1999; **26:**76–83.

18. Tiourina T, Arends B, Huysmans D et al, Evaluation of surgical gamma probes for radioguided sentinel node localisation. *Eur J Nucl Med* 1998; **25:**1224–31.

19. Gulec SA, Moffat FL, Carroll RG, The expanding clinical role for intraoperative gamma probes. In: Freeman LM, ed, *Nuclear Medicine Annual 1997*, 209–37. Lippincott-Raven: Philadelphia, 1997.

20. Harcke H, Mandell G, Sharkey C, Surgical radiation probes: a comparison. *J Nucl Med* 1988; **29:**881–2 (Abstract).

21. Szypryt EP, Hardy JG, Colton CL, An improved technique of intra-operative bone scanning. *J Bone Joint Surg [Br]* 1986; **68:**643–6.

22. Britten A, How to choose a probe. In: Keshtgar M, Waddington W, Lakhani S, Ell P, eds, *The Sentinel Node in Surgical Oncology*, 39–48. Springer: Berlin, 1999.

23. Alazraki NP, Eshima D, Eshima LA et al, Lymphoscintigraphy, the sentinel node concept, and the intraoperative gamma probe in melanoma, breast cancer, and other potential cancers. *Semin Nucl Med* 1997; **27:**55–67.

24. Tiourina TB, Dries WJ, van der Linden PM, Measurements and calculations of the absorbed dose distribution around a 60Co source. *Med Phys* 1995; **22:**549–54.

25. Alex JC, Weaver DL, Fairbank JT et al, Gamma-probe-guided lymph node localization in malignant melanoma. *Surg Oncol* 1993; **2:**303–8.

26. Hillier D, Royal H, Intraoperative gamma radiation detection and radiation safety. In: Whitman E, Reintgen D, eds, *Radioguided Surgery*, 23–38. Landes Bioscience: Austin, 1999.

27. Whitman E, Training and credentialing physicians in radioguided surgery. In: Whitman E, Reintgen D, eds, *Radioguided Surgery*, 39–46. Landes Bioscience: Austin, 1999.

28. Bergqvist L, Strand S, Persson B et al, Dosimetry in lymphoscintigraphy of Tc-99m antimony sulfur colloid. *J Nucl Med* 1982; **23:**698–705.

29. Eshima D, Fauconnier T, Eshima L, Thornback J, Radiopharmaceuticals for lymphoscintigraphy: including dosimetry and radiation considerations. *Semin Nucl Med* 2000; **30:**25–32.

30. Keshtgar M, Waddington W, Lakhani S, Ell P, Dosimetry and radiation protection. In: Keshtgar M, Waddington W, Lakhani S, Ell P, eds, *The Sentinel Node in Surgical Oncology*, 91–102. Springer: Berlin, 1999.

31. Glass E, Essner R, Giuliano A, Sentinel node localization in breast cancer. *Semin Nucl Med* 1999; **29:**57–68.

32. Loevinger R, Budinger T, Watson E et al, *MIRD Primer for Absorbed Dose Calculations* (revised edition), 128. Society of Nuclear Medicine: New York, 1991.

33. Huda W, Boutcher S, Should nuclear medicine technologists wear lead aprons? *J Nucl Med Tech* 1989; **17**:6–11.

34. Sorenson JA, Phelps ME, *Physics in Nuclear Medicine*, 2nd ed. Grune & Stratton: Orlando, 1987.

Part II
Sentinel Lymph-Node Biopsy for Melanoma

5

Surgical aspects

Charles M Balch and Julie R Lange

The technique of intraoperative lymphatic mapping and sentinel lymph-node (SLN) biopsy represents a major advance in the staging and treatment of melanoma. Sentinel lymph-node biopsy is an important tool for making decisions regarding surgical management of patients with clinically negative regional lymph nodes and as an entry qualification of patients participating into melanoma clinical trials. The technique also offers new insights into the role of the lymphatics in cancer metastases.

Indeed, much of the debate and controversy about management of clinically negative lymph nodes in melanoma patients has subsided at this point for three reasons. First, the long-term results of the Intergroup Surgical Trial have demonstrated convincingly that patients who have intermediate thickness, nonulcerated melanomas have a statistically improved cure rate with elective lymph-node dissection. Second, SLN biopsy represents a technological advance that has, for the most part, supplanted the need for elective lymph-node dissection in most patients. Third, research about prognostic factors predicting the risk of nodal metastases and survival outcome has reached a point of agreement that has fostered a major revision of the melanoma staging classification.

Over the past few years, there has been a worldwide validation of the staging accuracy and reproducibility of intraoperative lymphatic mapping and SLN biopsy, pioneered by Dr Donald Morton at the John Wayne Cancer Institute in Santa Monica, California.[1] The use of SLN biopsy for melanoma is a highly significant and reproducible technical advance that has been validated and adopted by melanoma centers across the USA and around the world. This technique has provided the surgeon with a precise tool that, when properly used, can detect the presence or absence of regional metastases down to a threshold of 10^5–10^6 cells and with an accuracy of 95%.

THE IMPORTANCE OF MELANOMA NODAL METASTASES

Why are nodal metastases important in the overall clinical management of melanoma? First of all, lymph nodes are the most common sites of initial metastases. Therefore, knowledge of the presence or absence of clinically occult nodal metastases is critical for staging and treatment decisions. Regardless of whether or not it is curative, the removal of nodal metastases at the same time as removal of the primary melanoma achieves maximum disease control and spares the patient a possible second surgical treatment in the future. Second, experimental studies of metastatic patterns suggest that distant metastases (which directly cause the patient's demise) originate more often from nodal metastases than from the primary melanoma, owing to clonal selection of more inherently metastatic melanoma cells that are able to flourish despite the intense immunological defense mechanisms in the regional lymph nodes. The ability to recognize nodal metastases at the earliest possible time in the course of their progression may interrupt their inexorable pathway to distant metastases and thereby increase the probability of cure. It is known that it takes 18–24 months, on the average, for nodal metastases to grow to a size that is clinically palpable. This may be a critical window of time and may represent the difference between curative and palliative treatment for the patient. Finally, the surgical removal of nodal metastases, when done in the setting of melanoma clinical research trials, eliminates this area as a common site of relapse. The removal of these nodes is especially important in melanoma patients being followed in clinical trials of adjuvant-systemic-therapy, who otherwise would have to be taken "off study" for a relapse that could have been avoided in the first place.

Thus, the use of intraoperative lymphatic mapping and SLN biopsy has multiple advantages in the care of the melanoma patient with clinically normal-appearing lymph nodes but who may or may not have occult nodal metastases:

1. It advances the ability to accurately stage the presence of nodal metastases by 18–24 months compared with clinical or radiological assessment of the regional lymph nodes.
2. It facilitates the surgery for nodal metastases because there is no bulk disease, and the treatment can be completed at the same time as that for the primary melanoma.
3. It defines a group of "node-negative" melanoma patients who are a more homogeneous group of patients with a good prognosis and who can be spared more radical cancer treatments.
4. It improves the accuracy, interpretability, and comparability of melanoma clinical trials.
5. It may increase cure rates among some subgroups of patients with nodal metastases.
6. It provides a new and powerful tool for examining the biological role of lymphatic dissemination of metastases and the growth of metastases in regional lymph nodes as a source of distant metastases.

TECHNICAL CONSIDERATIONS IN IDENTIFYING THE SLN

It is important to emphasize that the SLN is anatomically defined as the first lymph node to receive afferent lymphatic drainage from a primary melanoma site. It would therefore be the most likely to contain micrometastases if they were present. The SLN is not a "blue node" or a "hot node," which are simply terms reflecting the technology that is applied to identify the biological event of nodal metastases. If the technique is not performed correctly, then the true SLN may not be identified, leading to a false-negative result and a clinical relapse months later. It is therefore vitally important that surgeons using SLN biopsy engage a coordinated team of surgeons, nuclear medicine physicians, and surgical pathologists.

The starting point for the SLN biopsy procedure is the cutaneous lymphoscintigram, which must be performed accurately with the correct tracer, intradermal injection, and timing of assessment with the gamma probe. The surgeon also must have experience in the selection of patients, the technique of intradermal tracer injections, and the use of the hand-held gamma probe in the operating room. Finally, the pathologist must perform serial sections and immunohistochemical (IHC) staining of the

SLN and accurately interpret the results. If the technique of intradermal injection of the tracer materials, the surgical technique, or the pathological review of the specimen is relegated to a less experienced individual, then the false-negative rate may exceed those published by experienced centers. The false-negative rate for the procedure should not exceed 5%, especially in view of the recent evidence from the Intergroup randomized surgical trial demonstrating the curative benefit of elective lymph-node dissection in nonulcerative melanomas of intermediate thickness.[2]

THE ROLE OF SLN BIOPSY IN THE SURGICAL MANAGEMENT OF MELANOMA

Surgery is the most effective and efficient method for both staging and treatment of melanoma nodal metastases. The use of SLN biopsy should be considered in clinically node-negative patients when one or a combination of the related surgical goals are beneficial: staging, local/regional disease control, and cure. For staging, SLN biopsy should be performed in all patients who are candidates for later entry into melanoma clinical trials or who have melanomas of 1.0 mm or more in thickness, or who have thinner lesions with aggressive features, such as ulceration or Level IV/V depth of invasion. Even in patients not being considered for clinical trials, the morbidity associated with SLN biopsy is so low that it may be justified in individual patients who have been informed of the procedure's benefits and risks and who would be emotionally better able to cope with their disease with knowledge of their nodal status. This approach is also justified in patients who want to be spared a later procedure excising bulk nodal metastases, especially when there are difficulties in securing reliable follow-up physical examination.

The value of SLN biopsy not only encompasses staging, but becomes even more apparent with regard to curative treatment in the context of the recently described randomized surgical trial showing improved survival rates from elective lymph-node dissection in specific groups of melanoma patients. Prospectively defined subgroups of patients with intermediate-thickness melanomas had a significant survival advantage with elective lymph-node dissection compared with patients whose initial treatment was observation of the lymph nodes.[2] This was especially true for patients who had nonulcerative, intermediate-thickness melanomas, using a Cox multifactorial regression analysis.[2] Thus, for the first time, a randomized trial has demonstrated a therapeutic benefit for elective lymph-node dissection in prospectively defined groups of clinically node-negative melanoma patients. The survival benefit of the surgical trial described above thus provides data supporting the survival advantage of early surgical intervention to remove regional micrometastases.

The use of SLN biopsy has two inherent advantages over elective lymph-node biopsy: first, in a patient who has had a SLN biopsy, the indication for a complete lymph-node dissection after SLN biopsy are based upon pathological documentation of nodal metastasis, whereas, with the elective procedure, the decision to perform a complete node dissection is based upon the mathematical probability of a patient harboring occult nodal metastases; and second, the SLN biopsy procedure provides the pathologist with a smaller, more select amount of lymph-node tissue, representing the tissue most likely to contain metastases, in which a more detailed examination with serial sectioning and IHC staining for micrometastases is better justified.

It is important for surgeons to minimize their false-negative rate when substituting SLN biopsy for elective lymph-node dissection in the patient groups defined by this randomized trial. These patients, should they later develop a recurrence, will have missed their opportunity for a curative intervention. Elective lymph-node dissection should be considered with curative intent in the subgroups described above (i.e., intermediate-thickness melanomas without ulceration) in those circumstances where SLN biopsy is not available, when a patient has already had a wide excision (which negates the accuracy of the mapping procedure), or if the mapping is not technically feasible.

Besides the staging value of SLN biopsy, will a selective approach to identifying and excising nodal micrometastases actually improve cure rates? Dr Morton and surgical colleagues from the United States, Australia, and Canada are conducting a large randomized, prospective surgical trial. In the trial, melanoma patients with tumors greater than 1.0 mm in thickness are randomly assigned to receive either observation of their clinically normal regional lymph nodes or an SLN biopsy, followed by a therapeutic radical lymphadenectomy if the SLN contains metastases. Over 1700 patients have been entered into this trial to date; the survival results, however, will not be known for some years.

As an interim approach to address the question of increasing cure rates, Dr Morton and colleagues from the John Wayne Cancer Institute performed a matched-pair statistical analysis of clinically node-negative melanoma patients, half of whom were treated by SLN biopsy followed by complete lymphadenectomy if the SLN contained metastases, and the other half by elective lymph-node dissection.[3] They found that the actuarial 5-year survival rates were essentially equivalent in both groups. In addition, the incidence of metastatic nodes in SLN biopsy specimens was twice that of elective lymph-node dissection specimens (24% vs 12%) for the 1.5–4.0 mm subgroup. The increased incidence of nodal metastases is probably due to "stage migration" because of more rigorous examination of the nodal specimens (i.e., the use of serial sectioning IHC staining).

THE ROLE OF SLN BIOPSY IN MELANOMA STAGING

Unquestionably, the SLN biopsy technique facilitates more accurate pathological staging and, as a consequence, contributes to a significant upstaging to Stage III melanoma of patients who would otherwise be designated as clinically node-negative or as having Stage I or II melanoma. The SLN biopsy technique using serial sections and IHC staining can accurately detect nodal micrometastases down to a tumor burden of 10^5 to 10^6 metastatic melanoma cells. Not surprisingly, the yield of accurately diagnosed nodal metastases with SLN biopsy is as much as 50% greater than that of conventional methods that involve examining only a single section of a bivalved lymph node solely with a hematoxylin-and-eosin stain. This staging methodology thus creates a more homogeneous group of node-negative melanoma patients for entry into clinical trials. Indeed, this advance is so profound that results from the older literature regarding the management of clinically "node-negative" patients will have to be redefined.

THE NEW MELANOMA STAGING SYSTEM

The Melanoma Staging Committee of the American Joint Committee on Cancer (AJCC) has now accepted major revisions of the melanoma TNM and stage grouping criteria for melanoma (Tables 5.1 and 5.2).[4,5] These revisions delineate those factors that, in combination, can be used accurately for predicting the risk of patients harboring clinically occult metastases at regional and distant sites that should be taken into account when making management decisions regarding regional lymph nodes. Major revisions in melanoma staging include:

1. melanoma thickness and ulceration to be used in the T classification
2. the number of metastatic lymph nodes rather than their gross dimensions and the delineation of microscopic vs macroscopic nodal metastases to be used in the N classification
3. an upstaging of all patients with Stage I, II, and III disease when a primary melanoma is ulcerated
4. a new convention for defining clinical and pathological staging so as to take into account the new staging information gained from intraoperative lymphatic mapping and SLN biopsy.

With respect to Stage III patients (i.e., those with nodal metastases), there were three prognostic factors that significantly predicted out-

Table 5.1 Melanoma TNM classifications

T classification	Thickness (mm)	Ulceration status
T1	≤1.0	a: w/o ulceration and Level II/III
		b: with ulceration or Level IV/V
T2	1.01–2.0	a: w/o ulceration
		b: with ulceration
T3	2.01–4.0	a: w/o ulceration
		b: with ulceration
T4	>4.0	a: w/o ulceration
		b: with ulceration
N classification	**No. of metastatic nodes**	**Nodal metastatic mass**
N1	One node	a: micrometastasis[a]
		b: macrometastasis[b]
N2	Two or three nodes	a: micrometastasis[a]
		b: macrometastasis[b]
		c. in-transit metastases/satellite(s) *without* metastatic nodes
N3	Four or more metastatic nodes *or* matted nodes *or* in-transit metastases/satellite(s) *and* metastatic node(s)	
M classification	**Site**	**Serum LDH**
M1a	Distant skin, subcutaneous or nodal metastases	Normal
M1b	Lung metastases	Normal
M1c	All other visceral metastases or any distant metastasis	Normal or elevated

[a]Micrometastases are diagnosed after elective or sentinel lymph-node biopsy.
[b]Macrometastases are defined as clinically detectable nodal metastases confirmed by therapeutic lymphadenectomy or when any nodal metastasis exhibits gross extracapsular extension.
LDH, lactate dehydrogenase; met, metastasis; w/o, without.

come and therefore were incorporated into the new melanoma staging system. These were the number of metastatic nodes, the tumor volume (i.e., microscopic vs macroscopic), and the presence or absence of ulceration of the primary melanoma. Their definition and stage grouping are listed in Table 5.2. The diversity of biologi-cal risk for distant metastases is evident when one compares the 5-year survival rates, which ranged from 12–24% for patients with two or more macroscopic (i.e., clinically palpable) metastatic nodes and an ulcerated primary melanoma, to about 50% for patients with one to three macroscopic nodes from a nonulcerated

Table 5.2 Stage groupings for cutaneous melanoma

Clinical staging[a]				Pathologic staging[b]			
	T	**N**	**M**		**T**	**N**	**M**
0	Tis	N0	M0	**0**	Tis	N0	M0
IA	T1a	N0	M0	**IA**	T1a	N0	M0
IB	T1b	N0	M0	**IB**	T1b	N0	M0
	T2a	N0	M0		T2a N0	M0	
IIA	T2b	N0	M0	**IIA**	T2b	N0	M0
	T3a	N0	M0		T3a	N0	M0
IIB	T3b	N0	M0	**IIB**	T3b	N0	M0
	T4a	N0	M0		T4a	N0	M0
IIC	T4b	N0	M0	**IIC**	T4b	N0	M0
III	any T	any N	M0	**IIIA**	T1–4a	N1a	M0
					T1–4a	N2a	M0
				IIIB	T1–4b	N1a	M0
					T1–4b	N2a	M0
					T1–4a	N1b	M0
					T1–4a	N2b	M0
					T1–4a/b	N2c	M0
				IIIC	T1–4b	N1b	M0
					T1–4b	N2b	M0
					T1–4b	N2c	M0
					any T	N3	M0
IV	any T	any N	any M	**IV**	any T	any N	any M

[a]Clinical staging includes microstaging of the primary melanoma and *clinical/radiological* evaluation for metastases; by convention, it should be used after complete excision of the primary melanoma with clinical assessment for regional and distant metastases.
[b]Pathological staging includes microstaging of the primary melanoma and *pathological* information about the regional lymph nodes after partial or complete lymphadenectomy. Pathological Stage 0 or Stage 1A patients do not need pathological evaluation of their lymph nodes.

primary, to about 65% for patients with up to three microscopic nodal metastases and a nonulcerated melanoma primary. The extreme diversity of metastatic risk among these patients emphasizes the importance of obtaining pathological staging via SLN technology and the critical value of accounting for these three features of Stage III melanoma when designing and interpreting melanoma clinical trials.

The AJCC Melanoma Staging Committee concluded that it is important to identify separately patients with clinically occult (microscopic) nodal metastases from those with clinically apparent (macroscopic) nodal metastases in the staging classification. Their conclusion is based on data demonstrating that patients with microscopic nodal involvement fare better than those who have a therapeutic node dissection for clinically evident nodal metastases.

THE ROLE OF THE SLN TECHNIQUE IN MELANOMA CLINICAL TRIALS

The AJCC Melanoma Committee has recommended that all patients entering into melanoma clinical trials have pathological staging of their regional lymph nodes, with either SLN biopsy or elective lymph-node dissection, to ensure accuracy of staging and comparability of trial results with those from other similarly staged melanoma patients. There is a compelling rationale for pathological staging of the regional lymph nodes for patients prior to entry into trials of adjuvant systemic therapy. Differences in 2-year and 5-year survival rates for patients with and without clinically occult nodal metastases can vary by as much as 20–25%. Indeed, one of the problems in interpreting and comparing past clinical trials involving melanoma has been the inability to account fully for the pathological differences in nodal status in a heterogeneous group of T3 and T4 patients, some of whom had pathological assessment of their regional nodes, others of whom had only clinical assessment.

THE LIMITATIONS OF SLN TECHNOLOGY

As with the transfer of any new technique, there are some limitations to the SLN technology as it is applied to melanoma patients. First, there clearly is a "learning curve" in adapting the technique by all the specialists in surgery, nuclear medicine, and pathology. Although results vary, the consensus is that an experience with this technique in about 20 patients is required before the level of false-negative rates is consistent. Second, it is unlikely that the technique is reproducible when the mapping technique is used after a wide-local excision of the primary melanoma has been performed, especially with radial margins of 1.5–2.0 cm. The resulting lymphatic flow from the skin that far from the original melanoma may not be representative of that from the skin immediately surrounding the original melanoma. Third, the injections must be precisely at the level of the dermis, not the underlying subcutaneous fat, in order to access the relevant lymphatics. Fourth, the time, additional expertise, and consumable supplies required for this procedure are still not fully reimbursable by many insurers, despite the overwhelming evidence of its value in the management of melanoma. This may act as a deterrent to its appropriate application at some centers or to the rigorous examinations of nuclear medicine and in the nodal tissues pathology necessary to interpret the results precisely.

CONCLUSION

In summary, decisions regarding node dissection for clinically occult disease are so much better today because of improved staging techniques and the technology associated with intraoperative lymphatic mapping and SLN biopsy. Biologically, the use of this technology has given new insights into lymphatic drainage patterns from the skin and revealed a much higher frequency of nodal metastases than was previously appreciated. Clinically, the improvements in melanoma staging will vastly improve both decision-making related to the selection of standard surgical treatment options and the accuracy and comparability of melanoma clinical trials. Unquestionably, the SLN biopsy technique facilitates more accurate pathological staging and, as a consequence, contributes to a significant upstaging of patients to Stage III melanoma who would previously have been designated as node-negative or Stage I or II melanoma. It thus creates a more homogeneous group of node-negative melanoma patients for entry into clinical trials and spares those with truly "node-negative" melanoma from more radical surgery or systemic therapy. At long last, extensive efforts using data from this technology in combination with other prognostic factors have achieved a reasonable consensus about the management and staging of the regional lymph nodes in melanoma patients.

REFERENCES

1. Morton DL, Wen DR, Wong JH et al, Technical details of intraoperative lymphatic mapping for early stage melanoma. *Arch Surg* 1992; **127:**392–9.
2. Balch CM, Soong S, Ross MI et al, Long-term results of a multi-institutional randomized trial comparing prognostic factors and surgical results for intermediate thickness melanomas (1.0 to 4.0 mm). *Ann Surg Oncol* 2000; **7:**87–97.
3. Essner R, Conforti A, Kelley MC et al, Efficacy of lymphatic mapping, sentinel lymphadenectomy, and selective complete lymph node dissection as a therapeutic procedure for early-stage melanoma. *Ann Surg Oncol* 1999; **6:**442–9.
4. Balch CM, Buzaid AC, Atkins MB et al, A New American Joint Committee on Cancer staging system for cutaneous melanoma. *Cancer* 2000; **88:**1484–91.
5. Balch CM, Buzaid AC, Soong SJ et al, Final version of the AJCC Staging System for cutaneous melanoma. *J Clin Oncol* 2001; in press.

6

Pathologic aspects

Alistair J Cochran and Hans Starz

Local treatment of primary melanoma is by excision with a margin of surrounding normal skin. Whether and when the regional lymph nodes should be excised in patients with metastasis-prone, thick primary melanomas is more debatable.[1] One school considers that the ipsilateral regional nodes should be dissected at the time of removal of the primary melanoma. This approach, known as elective or prophylactic lymph-node dissection,[2,3] is supported by observations that patients whose melanomas are confined to the site of origin are less likely to die of their disease than patients with tumor spread to the regional nodes. Additionally, 20–30% (the proportion varying with primary melanoma thickness) of patients with nodes that are negative on clinical assessment have nodal tumor when examined by histologic and immunohistologic methods.[4] If all individuals with high-risk melanoma are treated by elective lymph-node dissection, however, 70–80% will be subjected to an unnecessary and significantly morbid surgical operation. Alternatively, lymph-node dissection may be reserved for patients with clinically detectable nodal tumor (therapeutic lymph-node dissection).[5,6] This spares many patients an unnecessary operation, but delays definitive therapy beyond the optimum point of deployment and thus deprives these individuals of their best chance of cure.

It is reasonable to consider that a substantial minority of patients with high-risk primary melanomas would benefit from elective lymph-node dissection. Such patients are likely to have limited quantities of tumor in the nodes and absent or truly minimal systemic spread.

The authors developed techniques to identify those individuals most likely to benefit from lymph-node dissection. Identification required that we be able to identify small numbers of tumor cells in lymph nodes.[4,7] This became feasible after the development of S-100 protein as a marker for melanocytic tumors[8–10] and the emergence of antibodies to melanoma-associated epitopes, such as HMB-45,[11] NKI/C3,[12] and Melan-A.[13–15] Conventional histology underestimates the number of patients with primary melanoma ostensibly limited to the site of origin who actually have metastatic melanoma in the regional nodes by 14%.[4] Conventional histology also underestimates tumor positivity in the apparently tumor-free nodes of patients with node-spread melanoma by 30%.[7] In patients with nodal tumor identifiable only by immunohistologic examination, the number of tumor-positive nodes was small (usually one or two) and the number of tumor cells present in each node was also small. The nodes that contained occult tumor cells were located close to the primary melanoma and were selectively immune-suppressed.[16,17]

The sentinel lymph-node (SLN) biopsy technique has generated great enthusiasm among physicians and surgeons dealing with cancer patients, and there are many reports of its successful application. A prospective trial of the approach for melanoma, funded by the US National Cancer Institute (NCI), compares selective lymph-node dissection (SLN biopsy) with a "watch and wait" strategy after wide excision.

Surgical pathologists and dermatopathologists frequently receive requests to examine tissues removed by SLN biopsy. Standard hematoxylin-and-eosin (H&E) histologic evaluation of SLNs is not sufficient, since even the tiniest micrometastases must be identified. Such identification is pivotal for the success of the SLN approach.

This report is based on the extensive experience of both authors with lymphatic mapping and SLN biopsy techniques, one in the USA (AJC) and the other in Europe (HS). Alistair Cochran is one of the initiators of modern lymphatic mapping and SLN biopsy in cooperation with DL Morton and his colleagues at UCLA and at the John Wayne Cancer Institute (JWCI),[18] and Hans Starz is part of an interdisciplinary team of physicians who introduced and further developed the gamma-probe SLN biopsy technique in Germany. Both authors are main architects of the Augsburg Consensus, derived from the First International Symposium on Sentinel Lymphadenectomy in Cutaneous Malignancies, in March 1999, in Augsburg, Germany.[19] Recommendations for the evaluation of SLNs are presented here based on our productive collaboration, and represent the authors' experience with pathologic analysis of SLNs from melanoma patients treated at UCLA, the JWCI, and the Augsburg Clinic from the late 1980s to the present. We also describe approaches to the assessment of prognosis based on SLN histopathology.

IS THE NODE TRULY SENTINEL?

Since the SLN is the node most likely to contain early metastases, it is important that the node examined is truly the SLN. Determination of the SLN depends primarily on the judgment of the surgeon and the nuclear medicine specialist, who rely on localization provided by preoperative lymphoscintigraphy (LSG), observable blue coloration of the afferent lymphatics and associated lymph nodes, and enhanced radioactivity of the lymph node detected by a hand-held gamma probe.[20]

Pathologists must examine all submitted lymph nodes closely for the blue coloration that will confirm them as sentinel. In some instances, the entire node may be blue; in others, color is localized to half or less of the node. Tumor status cannot be reliably used to confirm SLN status, because not all SLNs contain tumor, and some non-SLNs contain tumor (but always in association with a tumor-positive SLN). Approaches that allow pathologists to confirm, independently, whether a node is truly sentinel are under investigation.

TISSUE PROCESSING AND SECTIONING TECHNIQUES

We developed the SLN technique on the basis of intraoperative interpretation of frozen sections.[18] Assessment of tumor status was based on scrutiny of sections stained by H&E, by anti-S-100 protein, and by HMB-45 using a 28-minute immunoperoxidase technique. We have now moved away from the use of frozen-section analysis, believing that taking material for frozen section is wasteful of the tissue most likely to contain occult tumor. Interpretation of frozen sections stained by H&E or using the rapid immunohistochemistry (IHC) approach is always more difficult and more error-prone than interpretation of well-fixed "permanent" material. Frozen-section analysis errors are usually "falsely negative": the frozen section is cleared as negative while permanent slides show the presence of tumor. Fortunately, false-positive frozen-section interpretation of SLNs is rare.

Interpretation of SLNs must be based on an adequate series of well-fixed, full-face sections. Theoretically, each SLN should be serially sectioned to extinction, but such an approach would be impossibly expensive and is clearly impractical. Any practical recommendation must compromise between the ideal and the possible. The authors have developed two different techniques of SLN processing and sectioning, both of which are practical in the daily routine and sufficiently sensitive to detect even very small micrometastases.

The Cochran method

This method involves cutting the lymph node into two equal parts through the longest circumference of the node (Figure 6.1). The two halves of the node are placed, cut face downwards, in cassettes and fixed for at least 24 hours. The technician is instructed to minimize tissue removal during the "facing-up" process. As soon as a complete cross-section can be obtained, ten serial sections are removed. Sections 1, 3, 5, and 10 are stained by H&E, section 2 by anti-S-100 protein, and section 4 by HMB-45. Section 6 and 7 are used for negative controls, and sections 8 and 9 are reserved to repeat studies that are technically unsatisfactory or for additional IHC. If suspicious or anomalous appearances are seen within the first ten sections, additional groups of ten sections can be examined.

The Starz method

The formalin-fixed SLN is cut into tissue slices about 1 mm thick, parallel to the longitudinal axis of the lymph node (Figure 6.2). Following paraffin embedding, three sections are cut from each slice, the first for H&E staining, and the second and third for IHC with anti-S-100 and HMB-45, respectively. This method is more

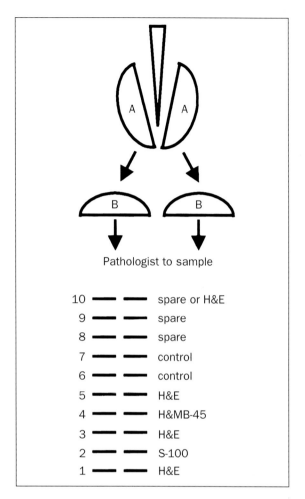

Figure 6.1 The SLN is cut into two exactly equal portions (A) through its longest circumference. The two halves of the node are placed cut face down (B), and ten serial full-face sections are cut from each. Technicians are requested to minimize tissue removal during the facing-up process. Sections 1, 3, 5, and 10 are stained by H&E. Section 2 is stained with an antibody to S-100 protein, and section 4 is stained with the antibody to HMB-45 (or Melan-A). Sections 6 and 7 are used as controls, and sections 8 and 9 are spares for any required repeats of unsatisfactory sections. If suspicious or anomalous findings are encountered, additional groups of ten sections can be prepared and stained in this way.

costly and time-consuming, but is effective for asymmetric and irregularly shaped nodes and provides an excellent basis for routine morphometric evaluations (see below).

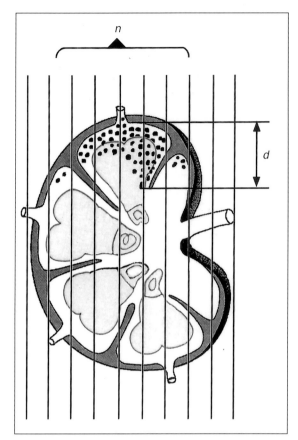

Figure 6.2 Micromorphometric evaluation of the sentinel node (S staging): the formalin-fixed SLN is cut into 1-mm slices for paraffin embedding and histologic (H&E) and immunohistochemical (S-100, HMB-45) investigation. The S classification is based on two parameters: n (number of tumor-involved tissue slices) and d (depth of tumor invasion from interior surface of the SLN capsule): S0 is defined as $n = 0$, S1 as $n = 1$ or 2 and $d \le 1$ mm, S2 as $n > 2$ and $d \le 1$ mm, S3 as $d > 1$ mm. (Reproduced from Starz et al,[21] with the generous permission of Demeter-Verlag.)

The use of immunohistochemistry

All SLNs must be examined by IHC using antibodies to S-100 protein and either HMB-45 or Melan-A (MART-1), unless the node contains overt tumor on inspection or review of H&E-stained slides. The challenge is to keep costs down by avoiding unnecessary IHC and mini-mizing report turnaround time. We order IHC (absent grossly visible tumor) at the time of gross specimen dissection.

Immunohistochemistry always increases the frequency of SLNs found to contain tumor. The proportion of SLNs in which IHC identifies occult tumor not visible in H&E sections decreases to a minimum of about 12% as (dermato) pathologists gain experience in evaluating SLNs. This is the pathologists' equivalent of the surgeons' "learning curve."

Immunohistochemistry with anti-S-100 protein

The S-100 protein is a highly robust marker for melanoma cells, detectable in virtually 100% of melanomas. We look for epithelioid, oval, or spindle-shaped cells (usually in the subcapsular sinus), which express S-100 protein epitopes in both cytoplasm and nucleus (Figure 6.3E, F). Other cells in lymph nodes express S-100 protein. The dendritic leukocytes of the paracortex are the most prominent of these potentially confounding cells. Identification of these cells is not difficult in reactive paracortices, where they are strikingly polydendritic (Figure 6.4A). In inactive lymph nodes, however, the dendritic leukocytes show either no or minimal dendrite formation (Figure 6.4B). The S-100 protein is also expressed by capsular or trabecular nevocyte collections (Figure 6.5B) and Schwann cells of node-associated nerves.

Immunohistochemistry with HMB-45

Although HMB-45 is a more specific marker for melanoma cells, the cells of up to 20% of melanomas (especially metastases) do not express this epitope. In contrast to S-100 protein, HMB-45 epitopes are confined to the cytoplasm. It does not stain dendritic leukocytes, and either does not stain capsular nevocytes or stains them at low intensity (with few exceptions) (Figure 6.5C). The antibody Melan-A (MART-1) may be used in a similar role to HMB-45, but has the same defect: a proportion

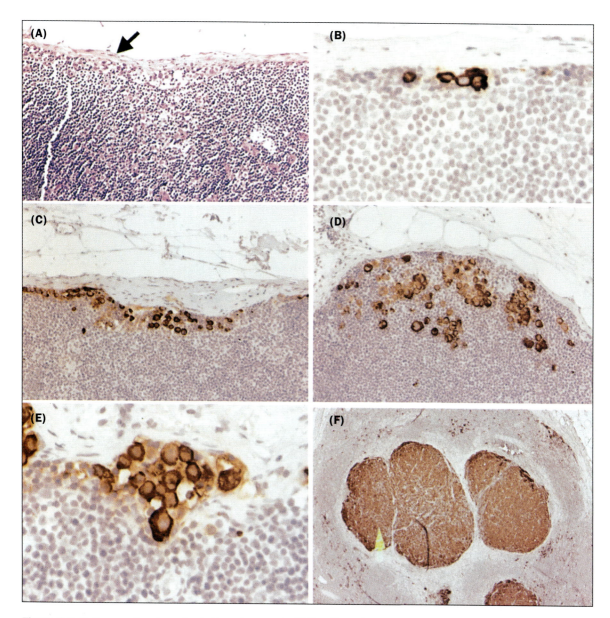

Figure 6.3 Patterns of early metastatic melanoma in SLNs. (A, B) Single subcapsular cells (H&E and HMB-45, respectively). In the H&E section, tumor cells lie in the subcapsular sinus to the right of the arrow. The presence of limited amounts of tumor is more readily appreciated in the immunohistologic preparation. (C) Increasing numbers of single melanoma cells expand the subcapsular sinus (HMB-45). (D) Melanoma cells singly and in small clusters expand into the lymphoid tissues of the node (HMB-45). (E) A microcolony of melanoma cells (HMB-45). (F) Macrocolonies of melanoma cells (yellow arrow) (S-100 protein). Illustrations (A) through (F) illustrate the sequence of colonization and expansion that characterizes the progressive involvement of an SLN by metastatic melanoma.

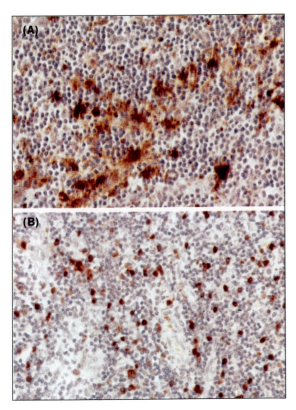

Figure 6.4 (A) Polydendritic dendritic cells in the paracortex of a non-SLN. (B) Nondendritic dendritic cells in the paracortex of an immune-suppressed SLN (an occasional cell is polydendritic) (both S-100 protein).

of melanomas does not express this epitope. Both authors have used HMB-45 as their second antibody to S-100 and have found no compelling reason to change to MART-1.

One potential source of error with HMB-45 is that in lymph nodes (mainly in the groin or iliac area) with trabecular calcification, extracellular HMB-45 reactivity may be identified.

Staging based on routine micromorphometry of the SLN

If a metastasis is identified in an SLN, a morphometrically determined stage ("S stage") is of clinical relevance.[21,22] Volumetric measurements

by Cavalieri's principle are time-consuming and require special equipment, which is not always readily available. Therefore, using standardized techniques for processing, histology, and IHC established in Augsburg, a practical staging concept was developed (see Figure 6.2). The process of S-staging requires only a few minutes and an ocular micrometer, which should be part of the standard equipment of any working laboratory.

Two parameters are recorded: the number of 1-mm slices of the SLN that contain metastatic melanoma (N) and the depth of invasion, measured as the distance of the most deeply invasive tumor cells from the interior surface of the nodal capsule (d). If several SLNs exist in one lymph node basin, n is the sum of the number of tumor-containing tissue slices in all individual tumor-positive nodes, and d is the maximum thickness of the various tumors in different SLNs.

Four S stages are distinguished (see Figure 6.2). In S0, no tumor is detected in the SLN ($n = 0$); in S1, there are circumscribed tumor deposits in the nodal periphery ($1 \leq n \leq 2$ and $d \leq 1$ mm); in S2, there are extended or multifocal peripheral nodal metastases ($n > 2$ and $d \leq 1$ mm); and in S3, there is involvement of the more central areas of the SLN ($d > 1$ mm). If SLNs coexist in different nodal basins, S stages are separately determined for each region.

At UCLA, we are evaluating the role of SLN status in the assessment of prognosis. The likelihood of there being tumor in a non-SLN and of death from melanoma is significantly increased if more than 5% of the SLN is occupied by tumor ($p < 0.0001$ in both cases). The likelihood of a tumor-positive non-SLN and of death from melanoma was also significantly higher in patients with primary tumors that were Clark's Level III and above ($p = 0.0063$ and 0.003, respectively). Indices of immune modulation, such as density of paracortical dendritic leukocytes, also correlate with the tumor status of non-SLNs ($p = 0.04$) and death from melanoma ($p = 0.0001$).[23]

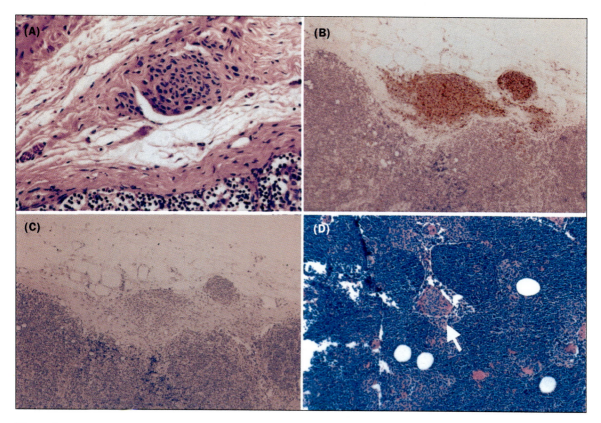

Figure 6.5 (A) Capsular nevus in an SLN (H&E). (B) Capsular nevus in an SLN (S-100 protein). (C) Capsular nevus in an SLN (HMB-45). (D) Trabecular nevus (arrow) in an SLN (H&E).

The handling of SLNs identified by radioisotope

Technetium-99m, the isotope generally used in SLN mapping, has limited tissue penetration and a short half-life (6 hours). The risk to operating room and pathology personnel from this radiation source is considered slight. According to local practices, and in line with regional regulation of radiation safety, it may be prudent to place the SLN in formalin in a safe place for 24 hours after surgical excision and prior to handling in the cutting room.[20]

PITFALLS IN THE MICROSCOPIC INTERPRETATION OF SLNs

S-100 protein staining

The major problem is the interpretation of S-100 positive dendritic leukocytes in the paracortex or sinuses. Dendritic leukocyte identification (see Figure 6.4A) is especially difficult if the "dendritic leukocytes" are nondendritic, as is often the case in immune-suppressed inactive SLNs (Figure 6.4B).[24] With good-quality IHC preparations, sinus macrophages do not stain for S-100 protein; however, if there is substantial background staining, these cells may present interpretative difficulties.

Capsular nevocytes (see Figure 6.5A) occur in about 10% of all SLNs from melanoma patients,[25] and are made more visible by the use of IHC (see

Figure 6.5B). Capsular nevocytes are confined to the capsule and trabeculae (see Figure 6.5D) of the lymph node. They are smaller than melanoma cells (with the exception of nevocytoid melanoma cells) and, while reacting strongly with S-100-protein, react with HMB-45 at a relatively weak level or not at all (see Figure 6.5C). It should be noted that blue nevi in nodes may react as strongly with HMB-45 as melanoma cells. Nevocytes often cluster around capsular vessels.

The presence of neural tissue within the lymph node may occasionally cause problems. Nerve-associated Schwann cells may strongly express S-100 protein, and if the nerve is cut transversely, an appearance suggestive of a cluster of melanoma cells positive for S-100 protein may result.

HMB-45 staining

The main problem with this method is that the tumor cells in up to 20% of melanomas are unreactive with HMB-45. In hyalinized and calcified connective tissue within lymph nodes, especially lymph nodes from the groin and internal iliac areas, extracellular HMB-45 positivity may be seen, and care is required to avoid overcalling this appearance. A similar problem occurs with MART-1 in that not all melanomas express this type.

RESULTS

Early studies from JWCI and the UCLA School of Medicine

In pilot studies prior to the multicenter trial, SLN identification and excision were followed by complete lymph-node dissection regardless of the tumor status of the SLN. A total of 259 SLNs were removed from 223 patients (i.e., an average of 1.2 SLN per individual). Tumor was identified in 47 of these 259 SLNs (18%). Tumor cells were identified by H&E in 83% of patients and in the remaining 17% by immunohistology alone (see Figure 6.3). The tumor cells occurred as single cells (see Figure 6.3A), small clumps of tumor cells (see Figure 6.3C), microcolonies (see Figure 6.3D, E), and larger colonies (see Figure 6.3F). We identified tumor in a non-SLN in the absence of tumor in the SLN in only two patients very early in our experience. Since this situation has not been encountered subsequently, it is likely that in these two patients the true SLN was not correctly identified.

Overall, including SLN-negative patients who did not have a completion lymph-node dissection, we have examined 1837 SLNs from 1006 patients, and identified SLN metastases in 188 of them (18.7%). One-third of SLN-positive patients also had non-SLN metastases. Among SLN-positive patients, 70% had a single positive node, 25% had two, and the remaining 5% had three. Most often, the melanoma cells were dispersed singly or as small microcolonies, and almost always in the subcapsular sinus. All patients in the pretrial group, regardless of the tumor status of their SLNs, received a completion lymph-node dissection.

The multicenter selective lymphadenectomy trial

These patients represent early accruals into a trial that will eventually comprise 1600 patients (see Chapter 14). Altogether, 860 SLNs were removed from 512 lymph-node basins in 446 patients. Ninety-nine SLNs contained tumor (19% positive, analyzed by lymph-node basin). Tumor was identified in 85 SLNs by H&E (86%) and in the remaining 14 nodes by IHC (14%).

Studies from the Augsburg Clinic

At the Augsburg Clinic 718 SLNs from 337 melanoma patients have been evaluated, including 54 patients with melanomas thinner than 0.76 mm. All SLNs from low-risk patients (Stage T1) were tumor-free (Stage S0), and the thinnest melanoma with a tumor-positive SLN was 0.8 mm thick. From the data, we determined 0.76 mm as the lower limit of tumor thickness at which SLN biopsy is useful. Sixty-two of the remaining 283 patients (22%) had at least one positive SLN. The distribution of S stages was 25 S1, 22 S2, and 17 S3. One patient had a tumor-positive SLN in each axilla, each Staged as S1.

There is a highly significant relationship between S stage and T stage. The S3 metastases occurred only with primary melanomas thicker than 1.5 mm. The presence of S3 metastases was associated with a 60% chance of finding non-SLN metastases at the completion lymph-node dissection. The risk of non-SLN metastases in stages S2 and S1 was 18% and 0%, respectively.

The risk of eventual development of distant metastases also correlates with S stage, with a high level of significance comparable to T stage. The best prediction of distant spread of melanoma is achieved by an additive score combining T and S stages with equal weighting. Only one of 275 patients staged S0 has subsequently developed regional lymph-node metastases, nearly 3 years after SLN biopsy.

DISCUSSION

The combination of preoperative lymphoscintigraphy and intraoperative gamma-probe mapping assisted by blue dye permits a nearly 100% rate of SLN identification in melanoma patients.[19,26,27] Sentinel lymph-node biopsy spares node-negative patients the morbidity of a regional node dissection, and allows node-positive patients a new level of staging accuracy, enhancing prognostication and aiding in the selection of adjuvant therapy. Despite the widespread adoption of SLN technology, there is as yet no evidence that this approach is therapeutic. The multicenter trial will address this issue within 2–3 years.

Despite its apparent simplicity, SLN biopsy has its pitfalls. Those wishing to undertake the procedure must undertake a learning phase, preferably under experienced supervision. This is equally true for surgeons, pathologists, and nuclear medicine professionals, and each is likely to achieve full proficiency only after treating around 30 patients. The technique is also being investigated for its applicability to a variety of other cancers including breast cancer,

prostatic cancer, colon cancer, and endometrial, cervical and vulvar carcinomas. A somewhat similar approach was previously investigated for the treatment of salivary gland cancer[28] and penile carcinoma.[29] While the broad lessons from our extensive experience with melanoma are likely to be applicable to other tumors, caution and care are required in bringing SLN methodology to different cancer systems.

One proof of the effectiveness of SLN biopsy will be the frequency at which patients develop metastases in the ipsilateral regional nodes after removal of a negative SLN. In our experience, this is infrequent; we have seen eight patients in whom ipsilateral regional failure occurred despite an allegedly "negative" SLN. Detailed re-examination of the pathologic material and clinical records of these individuals indicated that in half (4 of 8) a positive SLN had been incorrectly interpreted as negative. In two cases a few single tumor cells were missed, and in two others, the tumor cells were not visible on the original H&E preparation. Neither patient's SLN had been initially examined by IHC. In the remaining four patients, despite extensive additional sampling of the SLN by H&E and IHC, no evidence of tumor was identified. It is likely that the surgeons did not correctly identify the SLN in these cases.

It is thus essential to identify the SLN with complete accuracy. For the moment, this remains primarily the responsibility of the surgeon and the nuclear medicine specialist. Techniques are being developed to allow independent confirmation by the pathologist that a submitted lymph node is truly a "sentinel" node.

Correct determination of the tumor status of the SLN is of the utmost importance. This depends on careful sampling of the node and the routine use and accurate interpretation of IHC preparations. Both of the techniques presented here have served the authors well, and both identify similar percentages of melanoma-positive SLNs. While Cochran's technique (see Figure 6.1) is sparing of time, material, and costs, Starz's method (see Figure 6.2), morphometric study and routine S staging, is an ingenious new approach that requires in return only a small increment in expense and professional time.[20,21] The S stage is an important and accurate prognosticator of the status of the non-SLNs and the likelihood of distant metastases. Combined with T staging, it permits high precision in risk assessment for individual melanoma patients, and better selection or stratification of patient subgroups for adjuvant and other therapeutic studies. Whether it is possible to dispense with completion lymph-node dissection for patients with early stages of SLN involvement (Stage S1, perhaps even S2) will require a further prospective randomized, multicenter trial to answer.

Molecular biological techniques may provide information additional to that provided by conventional pathology and IHC in evaluating nodes for the presence of tumor.[30–32] Conventional pathology and IHC identify tumor in about 20% of SLNs, and regional lymph-node relapse in patients treated by wide-local excision alone occurs at a similar frequency. Molecular biologists claim that by using reverse transcriptase–polymerase chain reaction (RT-PCR) technology, they can identify signals for messenger RNA species derived from metastatic melanoma cells in lymph nodes that are negative by H&E and IHC. This work was initially undertaken using primers for tyrosinase mRNA and is compromised by observations that cells including capsular nevocytes and Schwann cells in node-associated nerves other than metastatic melanoma cells contain mRNA for tyrosinase.[23,33] Therefore, a signal for tyrosinase mRNA cannot be interpreted as certainly indicating the presence of metastatic melanoma. Studies in progress, in which multiple primers (for example to mRNA for MAGE or MART-1) are used,[32] represent a scientifically more interesting approach. The need to evaluate the role and significance of molecular biology in the analysis of SLNs is clear. Pathologists should, however, be careful to avoid providing SLN tissue for scientific study in a manner that may compromise diagnosis. It is inappropriate to arbitrarily provide portions of an SLN for research. We prefer instead to provide sections cut from the lymph node in a serial fashion and interspersed with sections stained by H&E and IHC. This approach has the additional advantage that it facilitates interpretation of the RT-PCR results, by allowing close morphologic comparison.

CONCLUSION

The surgical pathologist is an essential member of the SLN team, and will continue to have a key role in the evolution of this new technology. A consistent and meticulous approach to the sampling and interpretation of the SLN is required; in melanoma patients this requires systematic serial sectioning of the SLN, routine H&E staining, and IHC stains for both S-100 and HMB-45. Melanoma cells must be distinguished from capsular and trabecular nevus cells, interdigitating dendritic leukocytes, macrophages, and intranodal neural tissues. Morphometric staging of the SLN is a new technique that allows enhanced prediction of metastases to the non-SLN and to distant sites. Ultrastaging of the SLN by RT-PCR remains investigational. The biology of melanoma is unique, and the lessons learned from SLN biopsy in this setting may not be universally applicable as SLN biopsy is extended to breast cancer and other tumor systems.

REFERENCES

1. Balch CM, Soong S-J, Bartolucci AA et al, Efficacy of an elective regional lymph node dissection of 1 to 4 mm thick melanomas for patients 60 years of age and younger. *Ann Surg* 1996; **224**:255–66.
2. Balch CM, The role of elective lymph node dissection in melanoma: rational, results and controversies. *J Clin Oncol* 1988; **6**:163–72.
3. Coats AS, Ingvar CI, Peterson-Schaefer K et al, Elective lymph node dissection in patients with primary melanoma of the trunk and limbs treated at the Sydney Melanoma Unit from 1960 to 1991. *Am Col Surg* 1995; **180**:402–9.
4. Cochran AJ, Wen D-R, Morton DL, Occult tumor cells in the lymph nodes of patients with pathological Stage I malignant melanoma: an immunohistological study. *Am J Surg Pathol* 1988; **12**:612–18.

5. Veronesi U, Adamus J, Bandiera DC et al, Inefficacy of immediate node dissection in Stage I melanoma of the skin of the lower extremities. *N Engl J Med* 1977; **297**:627–30.

6. Veronesi U, Adamus J, Bandiera DC et al, Delayed regional lymph node dissection in Stage I melanoma of the skin and lower extremities. *Cancer* 1982; **49**:2420–30.

7. Cochran AJ, Wen D-R, Herschman HR, Occult melanoma in lymph nodes detected by antiserum to S-100 protein. *Int J Cancer* 1984; **34**: 159–63.

8. Gaynor R, Herschman HR, Irie R et al, S-100 protein: a marker for human malignant melanomas? *Lancet* 1981; **1**:869–71.

9. Cochran AJ, Wen D-R, Herschman HR, Gaynor RB, Detection of S-100 protein as an aid to the identification of melanocytic tumors. *Int J Cancer* 1982; **30**:295–7.

10. Cochran AJ, Lu H-F, Li P-X, Wen D-R, S-100 remains a practical marker for melanocytic and other tumors. *Melanoma Res* 1993; **3**:325–30.

11. Gown AM, Vogel AM, Heak D et al, Monoclonal antibodies specific for melanocyte tumors distinguished subpopulations of melanocytes. *Am J Pathol* 1986; **123**:195–203.

12. Hagen EC, Vennegoor C, Schilingemann RO et al, Correlation of histopathological characteristics with staining patterns in human malignant melanoma assessed by (monoclonal) antibodies reactive on paraffin sections. *Histopathology* 1986; **10**:689–700.

13. Starz H, Suspected diagnosis: malignant melanoma. In: Starz H, ed, *Immunohistochemistry on Paraffin Sections: Technical Principles and Diagnostic Applications in Routine Pathology*, 42–43. GIT: Darmstadt, 1991.

14. Chen Y-T, Stockert E, Jungblith A et al, Serologic analysis of Melan-A (MART-1), a melanocyte-specific protein homogeneously expressed in human melanomas. *Proc Natl Acad Sci USA* 1996; **93**:5915–19.

15. Fetsch PA, Cromier J, Hijazi YM, Immunocytochemical detections of MART-1 in fresh and paraffin embedded malignant melanomas. *J Immunother* 1997; **20**:60–4.

16. Cochran AJ, Pihl E, Wen D-R et al, Zoned immune suppression of lymph nodes draining malignant melanoma: Histologic and immunohistologic studies. *J Natl Cancer Inst* 1987; **78**:399–405.

17. Hoon DSB, Korn EL, Cochran AJ, Variations in functional immunocompetence of human tumor-draining lymph nodes. *Cancer Res* 1987; **47**: 1740–4.

18. Morton DL, Wen D-R, Wong JH et al, Technical details of intraoperative lymphatic mapping for early stage melanoma. *Arch Surg* 1992; **127**:392–9.

19. Cochran AJ, Balda B-R, Starz H et al, The Augsburg Consensus. Techniques of lymphatic mapping, sentinel lymphadenectomy and completion lymphadenectomy in cutaneous malignancies. *Cancer* 2000; **89**:237–41.

20. Cochran AJ, The pathologist's role in sentinel lymph node evaluation. *Semin Nucl Med* 2000; **30**:11–17.

21. Starz H, Bachter D, Balda B-R et al, Qualitative and quantitative evaluation of sentinel lymph nodes in cutaneous malignancies. *Nuklearmediziner* 1999; **22**:253–60.

22. Starz H, Balda B-R, Sentinel lymphadenectomy and micromorphometric S-staging, a successful new strategy in the management of cutaneous malignancies. *Giorn Ital Dermatol Venereol* 2000; **135**:161–9.

23. Cochran AJ, Morton DL, Johnson TD et al, Prediction of outcome and tumor-status of the non-sentinel node in melanoma patients with a positive sentinel node. *Modern Pathol* 2000; **13**:61A.

24. Huang RR, Wen D-R, Guo J et al, Modulation of paracortical dendritic cells and T lymphocytes in breast cancer sentinel nodes. *Breast J* 2000; **6**: 228–32.

25. Carson KF, Wen D-R, Li P-X et al, Nodal nevi and cutaneous melanomas. *Am J Surg Pathol* 1996; **20**:834–40.

26. Bachter D, Balda B-R, Vogt H, Büchels H, "Sentinel" lymphadenectomy with scintillation detector. A new strategy in treatment of malignant melanoma. *Hautarzt* 1996; **47**:754–8.

27. Bachter D, Balda B-R, Vogt H, Büchels H, Primary therapy of malignant melanomas: sentinel lymphadenectomy. *Int J Dermatol* 1998; **37**:278–82.

28. Gould EA, Whiship T, Philbin PH et al, Observations on a "sentinel node" in cancer of the parotid. *Cancer* 1960; **13**:77–8.

29. Cabanas RM, An approach for the treatment of penile carcinoma. *Cancer* 1977; **39**:456–66.

30. Wang X, Heller R, Van Voorhis N et al, Detection of submicroscopic lymph node metastases with polymerase chain reaction in patients with malignant melanoma. *Ann Surg* 1994; **220**: 768–74.

31. Van der Velde Zimmermann D, Roijers JF, Bouwens Rombouts A et al, Molecular test for the detection of tumor cells in blood and sentinel

nodes of melanoma patients. *Am J Pathol* 1996; **149:**759–64.

32. Bostick PJ, Morton DL, Turner RR et al, Prognostic significance of occult metastases detected by sentinel lymphadenectomy and reverse transcriptase-polymerase chain reaction in early-stage melanoma patients. *J Clin Oncol* 1999; **17:**3238–44.

33. Starz H, Balda BR, Büchels H, Sentinel-Lymphonodektomie bei malignen Melanomen. Eine vorläufige Bilanz aus histomorphologischer Sicht. In: Garbe C, Rassner G, eds, *Dermatologie, Leitlinien und Qualitätssicherung für Diagnostik und Therapie,* 274–277. Springer: Heidelberg, 1998.

7

The blue-dye technique

Richard Essner and Donald L Morton

CONTENTS **Initial experience** • **Technique of dye-directed SLN biopsy** • **Difficulty with gamma-probe use** • **Conclusion**

The John Wayne Cancer Institute technique for SLN biopsy in melanoma

Technique	Combination	**Isotope**	*Type*: Various
Dye	*Type*: Isosulfan blue dye		*Filtered*: Yes (0.2–μm filter)
	Volume: 0.5–1.0 ml (cc)		*Dose*: 0.5–0.8 mCi (18.5–30 MBq)
			Volume: 0.5–1.0 ml (cc)
Injection site	*Isotope*: Intradermal		
	Dye: Intradermal		

The controversy surrounding the surgical management of the regional lymph nodes in early-stage melanoma began over a century ago. In 1892, Herbert L Snow,[1] in his lecture "Melanotic Cancerous Disease," advocated wide excision and elective lymph-node dissection as a method to control lymphatic permeation of metastases. His recommendation that treatment of melanoma routinely include excision of the draining lymph nodes was based upon his studies suggesting a direct connection of the primary tumor with the regional lymph nodes. Elective lymph-node dissection for patients with early-stage melanoma has remained controversial since Dr Snow first proposed this management approach. While many retrospective studies suggest a survival benefit for patients undergoing this procedure compared with those for whom initial treatment is limited to removal of the primary tumor alone, the therapeutic benefit of removing clinically normal lymph nodes has never been proved by randomized prospective studies.[2–12] Although elective lymph-node dissection is considered a valuable staging procedure, the cost, morbidity, inaccuracy of predicting patterns of metastases, and overall low yield of tumor-containing nodes with this procedure have led most surgeons to abandon it as a routine part of patient care. Yet, the tumor status of the regional lymph nodes has become exceedingly important for determining prognosis and directing the use of adjuvant therapy.[13,14]

As a result of their dissatisfaction with the elective procedure, Morton and associates developed the technique of intraoperative lymphatic mapping and sentinel lymph-node biopsy. This minimally invasive procedure allows the surgeon to map the route of lymphatic permeation from the primary to the regional lymph nodes and then selectively excise the first or "sentinel" nodes. Because the sentinel lymph node (SLN) has been shown to be the most likely site for metastases, focused pathologic examination of the SLN leads to accurate staging of the lymph-node basin. Patients with metastases undergo complete lymph-node dissection, while those without metastases are spared the expense and morbidity of complete lymph-node dissection.

INITIAL EXPERIENCE

The early development by Morton and associates of the technique of lymphatic mapping and SLN biopsy (Figure 7.1) as a minimally invasive alternative to elective lymph-node dissection for patients with clinically uninvolved regional lymph nodes has been described in Chapter 1.[15–17] After confirmation of the validity of the

surgical approach in a feline animal model (Figure 7.2),[17] lymphatic mapping and SLN biopsy were performed in a series of 223 patients by intradermal injection of a vital dye at the primary site. Patients with primary melanoma on the torso or head and neck underwent preoperative lymphoscintigraphy (LSG) to determine the directionality of lymph flow and the basin at risk for metastases. Morton et al were able to identify a blue-stained SLN in 194 (82%) of 237 regional lymphatic drainage basins. All 223 patients underwent complete lymph-node dissection, regardless of the pathology of the SLN, in order to verify the accuracy of the procedure. Of these specimens, 40 (21%) contained metastases in at least one lymph node. In only 2 of 194 complete lymph-node dissection specimens, non-SLNs were the exclusive site of regional metastases, rendering a false-negative rate of 1%. These results are quite remarkable considering that in most cases

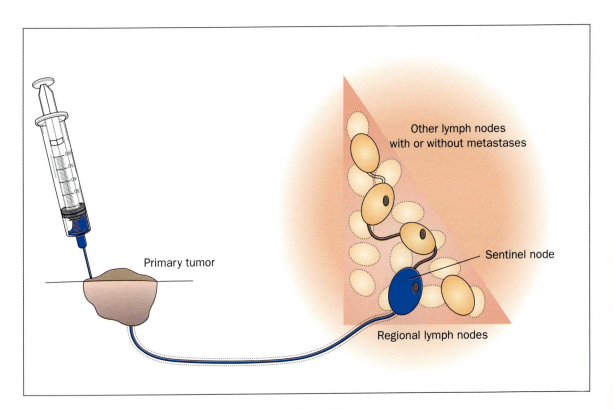

Figure 7.1 Intraoperative injection of blue dye to identify an SLN.

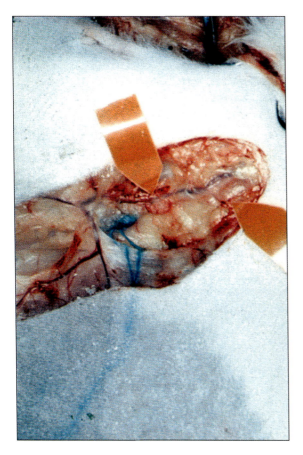

Figure 7.2 Demonstration of blue-stained SLN in feline model. Blue dye injected into the skin is visualized traveling through the subdermal lymphatics (arrows) in the regional lymph nodes. Adapted from Wong et al.[17]

preoperative LSG was not used, and the kinetics of the blue dye had not been well defined in patients.[15,17]

Occult regional metastases were identified by both standard hematoxylin-and-eosin (H&E) staining and newer immunohistochemical (IHC) techniques. Fifty-seven per cent of nodal metastases were found using conventional techniques; the remainder were identified by IHC staining alone.[18,19] Using IHC staining techniques with an antiserum to S-100 protein, Cochran and associates had previously demonstrated that 29% of lymph nodes that stained negative with H&E actually contained

metastatic melanoma.[19] The 3338 lymph nodes excised in the lymphatic mapping/SLN biopsy patients were stained with the melanoma-specific murine monoclonal antibody NKI/C3 to confirm the presence of melanoma cells. Few additional metastases were found with serial sectioning of the nodes compared with the number found by just examining the bivalved faces. The role of additional sectioning of the SLNs is unknown.[19]

The procedure of lymphatic mapping and SLN biopsy is relatively difficult, and its learning curve can be steep. During their initial 58 cases, Morton's group identified only 81% of blue-stained SLNs; however, during the next 58 cases, their rate of SLN identification increased to 96% and now approaches 100%. The surgeon with the most experience with the procedure achieved an early success rate of 96%, while the surgeon with the least experience had the lowest level of success, 72% ($p < 0.01$).[15] The gradual improvement in the rate of SLN detection is partially based on increased experience with the technique. The blue-stained afferent lymphatics and nodes can be difficult to identify: in some cases the blue-stained node may be obscured by adjacent fatty tissue, or only a small portion of the lymph node will be blue. While most surgeons have little experience dissecting the lymphatic channels prior to ever performing lymphatic mapping and SLN biopsy, careful dissection with attention to the path of the afferent channels will lead to a high degree of accuracy.

In 1993, Morton's group also reported on their experience of lymphatic mapping and SLN biopsy for head and neck melanoma draining to the cervical lymph nodes.[21] The purpose of examining this group of patients was to determine the accuracy of lymphatic mapping and SLN biopsy in a setting where the traditionally ambiguous patterns of lymphatic drainage potentially make lymphatic mapping and SLN biopsy impractical. At the time of surgery, blue dye alone was used to identify the SLN. The SLN was found in 71 (90%) of the 79 cervical drainage basins. Most of the missed SLNs were from the occipital, postauricular, or parotid basins, where the blue dye can be difficult to identify. There were no lymph-node recurrences in patients with tumor-negative dissections after a mean follow-up of 27 months. Although preoperative LSG was used in all cases, our early experience demonstrated the intrinsic difficulty with lymphatic mapping and SLN biopsy for the cervical basin. The lymphatic drainage from the head and neck is not reliably determined from anatomic location of the primary tumor.[22,23] As our own experience suggests, SLNs in the midst of the parotid gland, deep within the neck muscles, adjacent to the numerous facial veins, or in the thick soft tissue of the posterior neck can be hard to locate.

In 1993, Morton's group reported their experience with lymphatic mapping and SLN biopsy for melanoma of the lower torso and extremities draining to the groin basin.[24] The participants were 128 patients who underwent both lymphatic mapping and SLN biopsy. Preoperative LSG was used only for nonextremity primaries. Blue-stained SLNs were identified in 96% of the 51 patients who had routine selective complete lymph-node dissection and in 98% of the next 77 patients who had lymphatic mapping and SLN biopsy alone. The incidence of false-negative biopsies was less than 1%. In 12% of lymphatic mapping and SLN biopsy procedures, lymphatic drainage was to two lymph nodes. In most cases, a single SLN was identified just inferior to the inguinal ligament; however, some of the SLNs were located at the apex of the femoral triangle, and occasionally two SLNs were identified, usually on opposite sides of the femoral vein. While LSG may be considered unnecessary for some primaries on the extremities, the routine use of this procedure for all primaries helps to identify the aberrant lymph nodes in the groin, or in the popliteal or contralateral groin basins.[25]

Reintgen and associates from the H Lee Moffitt Cancer Center were the first group to confirm the original series by Morton.[26] Forty-two patients underwent lymphatic mapping and SLN biopsy, all of whom had undergone preoperative LSG. A blue-stained lymph node was found in each basin (100% accuracy). In 8 of the cases, metastases were found in the SLN, and in 7 of the 8 (88%) cases, the SLN was the exclusive site of disease. None of the remaining 34 patients had metastases either in SLNs or non-SLNs. Their initial experience re-emphasized the importance of preoperative LSG for localizing the site of the SLN. They also validated Morton's hypothesis that the blue-stained SLN reflected the tumor status of the entire regional basin.

Thompson and colleagues subsequently reported their experience with lymphatic mapping and SLN biopsy.[27] A total of 118 patients underwent preoperative LSG to identify the 120 basins at risk. At the time of surgery, blue-stained SLNs were located in 105 of the 120 (88%) basins. In 18 of the 22 (82%) basins with metastatic disease, the SLN was the exclusive site of metastases. Their rate of false-negative lymphatic mapping and SLN biopsy (1.9%) was no different from that reported in Morton's series. Thompson and colleagues confirmed the steep learning curve associated with this procedure. In the first half of their experience, SLNs were found in 74% of cases and in 92% during the second half.

A number of other investigators have also reported their experience with lymphatic mapping and SLN biopsy using blue dye alone (Table 7.1).[15,21,24,26–29] Most investigators had no prior experience with lymphatic mapping and SLN biopsy, yet achieved an accuracy rate of at least 90%. This relatively high rate of success is based on the more rapid learning of the technique through the experience gained by Morton and the other pioneers of this procedure. More importantly, complete lymph-node dissection was performed in most of the cases to evaluate the accuracy of dye-directed lymphatic mapping and SLN biopsy and to validate the technique.

In Morton's initial experience, the axilla and neck basins were the most difficult in which to identify SLNs. The anatomy of the axilla and neck prevent the nuclear medicine physician from directly marking the site of the SLN, even when the patient is positioned for surgery. We have found that the two-dimensional LSG images do not provide sufficient information about the depth of the SLN from the skin.[30] If the blue-stained afferent lymphatic is lacerated

Table 7.1 Initial experience with blue dye alone for SLN biopsy. Accuracy rates of SLN identification were based upon visual verification of blue-stained lymph nodes alone. In most of these series, complete lymph-node dissection (CLND) was performed to validate the accuracy of the procedure

Investigator (year)	N	Basins	CLND all cases	Accuracy rate (%)
Morton et al (1992)[15]	223	All	+	82
Morton et al (1993)[21]	72	Neck	+	90
Essner et al (1993)[24]	128	Groin	+	97
Reintgen et al (1994)[26]	42	All	+	100
Thompson et al (1995)[27]	118	All	+	96
Karakousis et al (1996)[28]	55	All	+	93
Belli et al (1998)[29]	74	All	−	90

during surgery as a result of not knowing the depth for dissection, the blue node is almost impossible to identify.

Several factors can lead to inaccurate identification of the SLN. Patients who have had wide excisions with margins 1.5 cm or more, or who have had rotational-flap closures, are not candidates for lymphatic mapping and SLN biopsy.[31] Similarly, any operative procedure that may have altered the lymphatic drainage patterns to the regional lymph nodes may make lymphatic mapping and SLN biopsy inaccurate. If for any reason LSG cannot be performed or is felt to be unreliable (such as in cases where the primary tumor is adjacent to the regional lymph node basin), lymphatic mapping and SLN biopsy should not be performed. Patients with clinical signs of regional lymph-node or distant disease are not candidates for lymphatic mapping and SLN biopsy, nor are patients for whom the tumor status of the regional lymph nodes will not be used to guide treatment decisions.

TECHNIQUE OF DYE–DIRECTED SLN BIOPSY

While the early success with blue dye led to the adoption of the lymphatic mapping and SLN biopsy technique by many centers, it was clear

that the learning phase was too long for most surgeons to become proficient with this technique. The smallest series we reviewed had 42 cases, which is more cases than the average surgeon is likely to see in 5 years—a fact that underscores the impracticality of a long learning phase in most centers. The routine use of cutaneous LSG has improved the accuracy rate and diminished the length of the learning curve for this technique.

The routine use of preoperative LSG in all cases has played a significant role in decreasing the incidence of missed SLN. In the United States, the most commonly employed agents for LSG are: technetium-99m-labeled human albumin colloid; Tc-99m-sulfur colloid (Tc-99m-SC), filtered (0.20 μm); or Tc-99m-human serum albumin (Tc-99m-HSA).[32–34] The agents are typically passed through a 0.2-micron filter to remove large particles. Approximately 18.5–30 MBq (0.5–0.8 mCi) of radiopharmaceutical is injected intradermally at four sites around the primary melanoma. A scintillation camera is used to document the drainage pattern from the primary via the dermal lymphatics to the regional nodes. The skin overlying the SLN is marked. Because there is some variation in the kinetics between the various pharmaceuticals, the nuclear medicine physician perform-

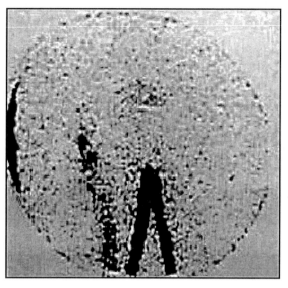 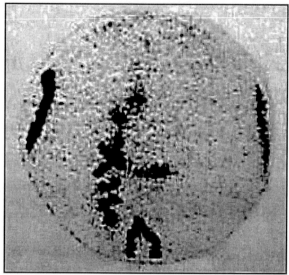

Figure 7.3 Cutaneous LSG with filtered Tc-99m-SC from a lower-extremity primary. Cutaneous LSG with filtered Tc-99m-SC injected intradermally around the calf primary site was performed with images obtained at 30 minutes and subsequently at 3 hours. The 30-minute image (left) demonstrates two inguinal lymph nodes, while more delayed images demonstrated multiple nodes. In the 3-hour image (right) the two lymph nodes seen in the earlier image are obscured by the other "hot" nodes.

ing the procedure must be careful to differentiate SLN from non-SLN. In our experience the SLN can be identified 30 minutes after injection (depending on the agent and the distance of the primary to the regional nodes); and usually by 3–4 hours after injection the SLN can no longer be differentiated from the adjacent non-SLN (Figure 7.3).[32] Lymphoscintigraphy is used to determine the regional lymph-node basin at risk for metastases, and is particularly helpful in sites on the head and neck or torso. Norman and associates demonstrated that up to 59% of primaries from the head, neck, and torso will have unexpected patterns of drainage.[33]

Glass and associates from the John Wayne Cancer Institute (JWCI) reviewed their experience with LSG using the three radiopharmaceuticals mentioned above.[32] Their studies suggested that all three agents were equally effective for LSG. A more important finding was that in over half of the cases they reviewed, more than one SLN was identified in the basin. Because the blue dye appears to travel along the same pathways as the radiopharmaceuti-

cals, LSG is critical for the accuracy of the lymphatic mapping and SLN biopsy, and is important not only for locating the site but also for assessing the number of SLNs.[35]

At surgery, 0.5–1.0 ml (cc) of isosulfan blue dye is injected intradermally around the primary site. The dye must not be injected into the biopsy cavity or incision. Gentle pressure on the injection site increases the intralymphatic pressure and decreases the transit time to the lymphatic basin.

The volume of blue dye injected is based on the site and distance of the primary from the regional lymph-node basin. Larger volumes of injection are made for tumors on the distal upper and lower extremities (about 1.0 ml) than for those on the face or proximal extremities (≤0.5 ml). The dye should be injected at four quadrants around the biopsy site, and in cases where an incisional biopsy is made, the volume of injection needs to be increased to surround the lesion. Smaller excisional biopsy wounds require a smaller volume of blue dye.

Primary lesions on the face, extremities, or

torso that are within 5–6 cm of the regional lymph node basin should have a small volume (≤0.25 ml) of blue dye injected. The blue dye can permeate through the soft tissue, resulting in the lymphatic channels being obscured by the surrounding blue coloration. In our experience, the number of blue nodes identified by the surgeon closely approximates the number seen on LSG. Typically, the portion of the node closest to the primary site will stain blue. The ability of the surgeon to adequately define the afferent lymphatic channels leading to the SLN diminishes the possibility that the blue-stained lymph node will be missed.

If the number of dye-stained lymph nodes does not equal that imaged by preoperative LSG, the surgeon must continue the surgical exploration until satisfied that all SLNs have been identified (Figure 7.4). Lengthening the surgical incision in order to gain access to the afferent lymphatics can lead to the identification of secondary and rare tertiary SLNs. Care must be taken not to transect any of the blue-stained lymphatics. The dye rapidly passes through the SLN, and the blue staining can be lost if the afferent channels are cut.

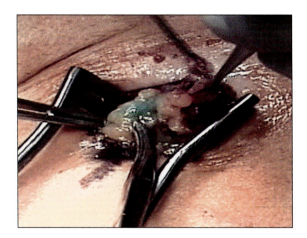

Figure 7.4 Blue-stained lymph node obtained from SLN biopsy of the groin. A blue-stained SLN is identified during lymphatic mapping and SLN biopsy approximately 10–15 minutes after intradermal injection of 1.0 ml of isosulfan blue around the primary melanoma site.

DIFFICULTY WITH GAMMA-PROBE USE

Krag and associates,[36] using the information obtained from LSG, were the first group to demonstrate a high success rate of SLN identification with the use of a radiopharmaceutical for gamma-probe direction of lymphatic mapping and SLN biopsy (radio-LSG). A group of 121 patients underwent lymphatic mapping and SLN biopsy, the majority with radiopharmaceutical alone. An SLN was defined as a node having at least 15 counts in 10 seconds and a count ratio 3 times background. Ninety-eight per cent of patients had a successful lymphatic mapping and SLN biopsy. However, the interval between injection of the radiopharmaceutical and surgery ranged from 15 minutes to 24 hours. The mean follow-up for these patients was relatively short (220 days). With this variation in technique, no clear definition of background, and short patient follow-up, we suspect that the true SLN may not always have been identified. Although Krag and associates advocated the use of the gamma probe alone, their greatest success (100% accuracy rate) was with the 44 patients who had blue dye incorporated into the technique.

In 1994, Morton and associates combined dye-directed lymphatic mapping and SLN biopsy with intraoperative injection of Tc-99m-HSA. The object of this approach was to standardize the time of injection of both blue dye and radiopharmaceutical. A radioactive SLN was defined as having an in vivo node/background count ratio of at least 2. Concurrence between blue and radioactive nodes approached 100% in their 30 cases. The logistics of the surgeon injecting radiopharmaceuticals in the operating room, however, make this technique impractical.[37]

A large number of series have since been published with radio-LSG (Table 7.2).[36,38–46] Accuracy rates in these studies range from 96% to 100%, and many investigators use these data as justification for using the probe alone (without blue dye) for lymphatic mapping and SLN biopsy. While the learning curve for radio-LSG is generally shorter than that for blue dye alone, there is no consensus about the definition of a radioactive SLN.

Table 7.2 Accuracy rates of probe-directed SLN biopsy. Accuracy rates for identification of SLNs (N = total patients in each study) were based upon the presence of blue dye in the nodes and/or demonstration of radioactivity with the use of a hand-held gamma probe. In many of these studies, the concurrent use of blue dye and radiopharmaceuticals makes it difficult to determine the true accuracy rate of either technique alone

Investigator (year)	N	Accuracy rate (%)
Krag et al (1995)[36]	121	98
Pijpers et al (1995)[38]	41	100
Mudun et al (1996)[39]	13	100
Albertini et al (1996)[40]	106	96
Thompson et al (1997)[41]	21	100
Bostick et al (1997)[42]	23	98
Leong et al (1997)[43]	163	98
Essner et al (2000)[44]	247	98
Murray et al (2000)[45]	360	99
Jansen et al (2000)[46]	200	99

Investigators have used an assortment of methods to perform radio-LSG and define a radioactive SLN (Table 7.3).[36,38–46] Our own data suggest that the in vivo count ratios for blue-stained lymph nodes can vary almost 100-fold, even when surgery is uniformly performed within 4 hours after injection of the radiopharmaceutical, and that there is no consensus on the definition of a radioactive SLN.[42,47–50] Although the use of radiopharmaceutical and the gamma probe for lymphatic mapping and SLN biopsy may improve the accuracy rate of the technique, the results from these studies suggest Tc-99m-SC is not perfect for this procedure. While larger particles such as unfiltered Tc-99m-SC and Tc-99m-labeled human albumin colloid would be expected to be trapped in the SLN, some of the particles are shunted through to adjacent lymph nodes.[51–53] Similarly, our experience with Tc-99m-HSA demonstrated that this agent passes quickly from the primary to the SLN and to adjacent non-SLNs.

Bostick and associates reviewed the JWCI experience with lymphatic mapping/SLN biopsy and radio-LSG in 100 lymph node basins from 87 patients with primary tumors in a variety of sites.[54] All patients underwent LSG with one of the three commonly used radio-

Table 7.3 Proposed "standard" definitions of radioactive SLNs. Radioactive SLNs have been defined by various methods and by a variety of investigators. The range of definitions may relate to the differences in techniques employed by each surgeon

Investigator	Definition of SLN
Krag et al (1995)[36]	15 counts/10 s plus in vivo node/background ratio ≥3
Pijpers et al (1995)[38]	Node with highest counts
Mudun et al (1996)[39]	300–3000 counts/10 s plus in vivo node/background ratio ≥3
Albertini et al (1996)[40]	In vivo node/background ratio ≥2
Thompson et al (1997)[41]	Node/residual basin background ratio ≥3
Bostick et al (1997)[42]	In vivo node/background ratio ≥2
Leong et al (1997)[43]	In vivo node/background ratio ≥3
Essner et al (2000)[44]	In vivo node/background ratio ≥2
Murray et al (2000)[45]	Node with highest counts
Jansen et al (2000)[46]	Node with highest counts

pharmaceuticals. Lymphatic mapping and SLN biopsy was performed with either concurrent injection of blue dye and Tc-99m-HSA or Tc-99m-SC injected up to 4 hours prior to the operative procedure. A total of 136 blue-stained and radioactive lymph nodes and 8 additional non-stained but hot nodes were removed in 98 lymph-node basins (success rate 98%). A hand-held gamma probe was used to determine the radioactive counts over the blue nodes, adjacent nonstained nodes, and an irrelevant background site. Ninety-two per cent of the blue-stained lymph nodes had an in vivo node/background count ratio of 2 or more, and 87% had an in vivo count ratio of 3 or more. Seventeen SLNs from 15 basins contained metastases: 16 were located with blue dye and gamma probe, and 1 was found with blue dye alone. None of the tumor-positive lymph nodes was identified with the gamma probe alone. Using the definition of a radioactive SLN as one having an in vivo count ratio of 2 or more, a success rate of 85% was achieved. When the in vivo count ratio was increased to 3 or more to improve the specificity of the technique, the success rate decreased to 78%. The concordance between the two techniques was not 100%. Not all blue-stained lymph nodes will have an elevated count ratio, and conversely, not all nodes with an elevated count ratio will be blue. In fact, the in vivo count ratios for all the blue-stained lymph nodes exhibited a wide variation, ranging from less than 1 to 100. Similar results were observed when the ex vivo count ratio of the nodes was examined, suggesting that the use of radiopharmaceuticals alone can be misleading for lymphatic mapping and SLN biopsy. Both of the radiopharmaceuticals were found to give similar count ratios for radio-LSG and led to surgical excision of a similar number of lymph nodes. At the JWCI center, we have little difficulty with performing LSG and lymphatic mapping/SLN biopsy on the same day, but logistically this approach can be difficult.

Essner and associates from the JWCI recently reviewed an expanded series of patients who underwent radio-LSG by one of three techniques:

1. intraoperative injection of blue dye and Tc-99m-HSA with LSG performed at least 24 hours earlier
2. same-day LSG combined with lymphatic mapping/SLN biopsy with a single injection of filtered Tc-99m-SC
3. prior-day LSG with filtered Tc-99m-SC.[44]

Preoperative LSG identified 299 drainage basins from the 247 patients. Sentinel lymph nodes were located using the combined technique of blue dye plus radiopharmaceuticals in 142 (97%) of 146 basins using Tc-99m-HSA, 119 (98%) of 121 basins using same-day Tc-99m-SC, and 32 (100%) of 32 basins using prior-day Tc-99m-SC. A total of 463 SLNs were identified from the 293 lymph basins (average 1.6 SLNs per basin). While there were no differences in accuracy rates among the three techniques, same-day injections of Tc-99m-SC led to the greatest in vivo node/background count ratios ($p < 0.0001$) and the greatest fall-off from in vivo node counts to the postexcision basin counts ($p < 0.0001$). Same-day LSG and lymphatic mapping and SLN biopsy with Tc-99m-SC are now our method of choice, because the high level of concurrence of blue dye and radioactivity and the large fall-off in counts reassures the surgeon that all SLNs have been removed. Yet the lack of absolute concordance between blue dye and the probe makes the combined technique less than optimum (Table 7.4).[36,38–46] The ideal radiopharmaceutical for this procedure would be one that travels quickly from the primary site to the SLN and concentrates without leakage to adjacent lymph nodes. Until the kinetics of the radiopharmaceuticals are better defined for lymphatic mapping and SLN biopsy, or better agents are developed, we recommend that these agents should not be used without blue dye.

Most investigators now employ the combination of blue dye and radiopharmaceuticals for lymphatic mapping and SLN biopsy. Preoperative LSG is performed using one of the filtered colloid radiopharmaceuticals on the same day as surgery (if not possible, the day before). At the time of surgery, the hand-held gamma probe directs the surgeon to the site of

Table 7.4 Variety of techniques used for radiolymphoscintigraphy. A variety of definitions have been employed for defining a radioactive SLN. These definitions are based on the use of different radiopharmaceuticals, injected at different times prior to surgery with or without blue dye

Investigator	Blue dye	Radiopharmaceuticals	Time postinjection
Krag et al (1995)[36]	+/−	Tc-99m-Sc, Tc-99m-HSA	15 min–24 h
Pijpers et al (1995)[38]	+	Tc-99m-colloidal albumin	2–18 h
Mudun et al (1996)[39]	−	Filtered Tc-99m-SC	≤18 h
Albertini et al (1996)[40]	+	Filtered Tc-99m-SC	≤4 h
Thompson et al (1997)[41]	+	Tc-99m-antimony colloid	20–29 h
Bostick et al (1997)[42]	+	Filtered Tc-99m-SC, Tc-99m-HSA	≤4 h
Leong et al (1997)[43]	+	Filtered Tc-99m-SC	<7 h
Essner et al (2000)[44]	+	Filtered Tc-99m-SC, Tc-99m-HSA	≤4 h
Murray et al (2000)[45]	−	Filtered Tc-99m-SC	?
Jansen et al (2000)[46]	+	Tc-99m-colloidal albumin	>12 h

the blue-stained SLN. Occasionally, the probe will lead the surgeon to an unexpected blue-stained lymph node.[55,56] We have found the concordance between the two techniques to be at least 80%. While there are a variety of methods for defining a radioactive SLN, a blue-stained lymph node remains the "gold standard" for this procedure.

The addition of the gamma probe to lymphatic mapping and SLN biopsy has generally increased the accuracy rate of SLN identification over blue dye alone. Yet the potential advantages of probe use must be considered in light of the need to standardize the technique. Some investigators have even recommended using the probe alone because of the rare allergic reactions to the blue dye.[57,58] Each center using radiopharmaceuticals must be aware of the guidelines for use of these agents, and must put into place protocols for their acquisition, preparation, distribution, monitoring, and disposal. Several studies have determined that the risk of significant radiation exposure to patients, physicians, and operating-room staff is small.[59–61] While some investigators believe that the Tc-99m-labeled tissue should be set aside for several days before it is handled by the pathologists, the 6-hour half-life of the low-energy gamma rays makes the samples relatively radiation-free in 1 day.[62]

The therapeutic value of lymphatic mapping and SLN biopsy is unknown.[63] The international Multicenter Selective Lymphadenectomy Trial (MSLT), initiated in 1994 at the John Wayne Cancer Institute, is examining as a primary end-point the survival of patients with intermediate-thickness melanoma treated by wide excision alone or in combination with lymphatic mapping and SLN biopsy. Only patients with tumor-positive SLN, or those who develop a clinical recurrence after wide excision alone, undergo selective complete lymph-node dissection. The preliminary results of this study demonstrate that the technique can be uniformly performed in a number of centers, with a high degree of accuracy for identifying SLN.[64] The addition of the gamma probe to lymphatic mapping and SLN biopsy has improved the accuracy of the procedure (95% for blue dye vs 99% for blue dye and radio-LSG) (Figure 7.5), but the success rate with blue dye was quite high from the onset of the study in 1994.

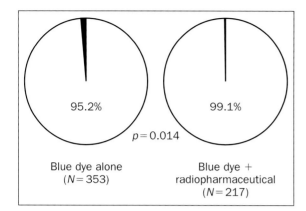

95.2%   99.1%

$p = 0.014$

Blue dye alone
($N = 353$)

Blue dye +
radiopharmaceutical
($N = 217$)

Figure 7.5 Experience of the Multicenter Selective Lymphadenectomy Trial with lymphatic mapping and SLN biopsy. The accuracy of SLN identification was significantly higher ($p = 0.014$) with blue dye and radiopharmaceuticals (99.1%) than with blue dye alone (95.2%). Adapted from Morton et al.[64]

CONCLUSION

The technique of lymphatic mapping and SLN biopsy has been shown by a number of investigators to be a reliable indicator of the tumor status of the regional lymph nodes. Based on these studies, lymphatic mapping and SLN biopsy have become a popular alternative to conventional elective lymph-node dissection and have become almost standard procedure for staging the regional lymph nodes.[65] The successful performance of lymphatic mapping and SLN biopsy, however, depends on the experience of the multidisciplinary team of surgeon, pathologist, and nuclear medicine physician. We recommend that each SLN team completes a learning phase of at least 15 cases (and perhaps up to 50) before lymphatic mapping and SLN biopsy become routine procedure at any center.[66] Our studies clearly indicate that successful mapping of the SLN is directly related to the surgeon's experience. While progressing through the learning phase, surgeons must perform complete lymph-node dissections to monitor their own false-negative rate. Although the reported rates of missed SLN are extremely low, we have observed dissected

basin recurrences as late as 5 years after negative lymphatic mapping and SLN biopsy.[67,68] The true accuracy rate of this technique has yet to be determined.[69] While this procedure has become increasingly popular, its therapeutic value is unproven.

REFERENCES

1. Snow H, Melanotic cancerous disease, *Lancet* 1892; **2:**872.
2. McCarthy WH, Shaw HM, Milton GW, Efficacy of elective lymph node dissection in 2347 patients with clinical stage I malignant melanoma. *Surg Gynecol Obstet* 1985; **161:**575–80.
3. Morton DL, Wanek L, Nizze JA et al, Improved long-term survival after lymphadenectomy of melanoma metastatic to regional nodes: analysis of prognostic factors in 1134 patients from the John Wayne Cancer Institute. *Ann Surg* 1991; **214:**491–501.
4. Balch CM, Soong S-J, Murad TM et al, A multifactorial analysis of melanoma. III. Prognostic factors in melanoma patients with lymph node metastases (stage III). *Ann Surg* 1981; **193:**377–88.
5. Callery C, Cochran AJ, Roe DJ et al, Factors prognostic in patients with malignant melanoma spread to the regional lymph nodes. *Ann Surg* 1982; **196:**69–75.
6. Balch CM, Soong S-J, Milton GW et al, A comparison of prognostic factors and surgical results in 1786 patients with localized (stage I) melanoma treated in Alabama, USA and New South Wales, Australia. *Ann Surg* 1982; **196:** 677–84.
7. Veronesi U, Adamus J, Bandiera DC et al, Inefficacy of immediate node dissection in stage I melanoma of the limbs. *N Engl J Med* 1977; **297:**627–30.
8. Veronesi U, Adamus J, Bandiera DC et al, Delayed regional lymph node dissection in stage I melanoma of the skin of the lower extremities. *Cancer* 1982; **49:**2420–30.
9. Sim FH, Taylor WF, Pritchard DJ, Soule EH, Lymphadenectomy in the management of stage I malignant melanoma: a prospective randomized study. *Proceedings of the Mayo Clinic* 1986; **61:** 697–705.
10. Balch CM, Soong S-J, Bartolucci AA et al, Efficacy of an elective regional lymph node dissection of 1 to 4 mm thick melanomas for

patients 60 years of age and younger. *Ann Surg* 1996; **224**:255–66.

11. Cascinelli N, Morabito A, Santinami M et al, Immediate or delayed dissection of regional nodes in patients with melanoma of the trunk: a randomised trial. *Lancet* 1998; **351**:793–6.

12. Rompel R, Garbe C, Buttner P et al, Elective lymph node dissection in primary malignant melanoma: a matched-pair analysis. *Melanoma Res* 1995; **5**:189–94.

13. Kirkwood JM, Strawderman MH, Ernstoff MS et al, Interferon alfa-2b adjuvant therapy of high-risk resected cutaneous melanoma: the Eastern Cooperative Group trial EST 1684. *J Clin Oncol* 1996; **14**:7–17.

14. Morton DL, Barth A, Vaccine therapy for malignant melanoma. *CA Cancer J Clin* 1996; **46**: 225–44.

15. Morton DL, Wen D-R, Wong JH et al, Technical details of intraoperative lymphatic mapping for early stage melanoma. *Arch Surg* 1992; **127**:392–9.

16. Cochran AJ, Wen DR, Morton DL, Management of the regional lymph nodes in patients with cutaneous malignant melanoma. *World J Surg* 1992; **16**:214–21.

17. Wong JH, Cagle LA, Morton DL, Lymphatic drainage of skin in a sentinel lymph node in a feline model. *Ann Surg* 1991; **214**:637–41.

18. Cochran AJ, Wen DR, Herschman HR, Occult melanoma in lymph nodes detected by antiserum to S-100 protein. *Int J Cancer* 1984; **34**:159–63.

19. Cochran AJ, Wen DR, Morton DL, Occult tumor cells in the lymph nodes of patients with pathological stage I malignant melanoma: an immunohistochemical study. *Am J Surg Path* 1988; **12**:612–18.

20. Heller R, Becker J, Wasselle J et al, Detection of submicroscopic lymph node metastases in patients with melanoma. *Arch Surg* 1991; **126**:1455–60.

21. Morton DL, Wen D-R, Foshag LJ et al, Intraoperative lymphatic mapping and selective cervical lymphadenectomy for early-stage melanomas of the head and neck. *J Clin Oncol* 1993; **11**:1751–6.

22. Shah JP, Kraus DH, Dubner S, Sarkar S, Patterns of regional lymph node metastases from cutaneous melanoma of the head and neck. *Am J Surg* 1991; **162**:320–3.

23. Wanebo HJ, Harpole D, Teates CD, Radionuclide lymphoscintigraphy with technetium 99m antimony sulfide colloid to identify lymphatic drainage of cutaneous melanoma of ambiguous sites in the head and neck and trunk. *Cancer* 1985; **55**:1403–13.

24. Essner R, Wen DR, Cochran AJ et al, Lymphatic mapping and selective lymph node biopsy: an alternative to elective lymphadenectomy for early-stage melanomas of the trunk and lower extremities. *Proc Am Soc Clin Oncol* 1993; **12**:391.

25. Thompson JF, Saw RP, Colman MH et al, Contralateral groin node metastasis from lower limb melanoma. *Eur J Cancer* 1997; **33**:976–7.

26. Reintgen D, Cruse CW, Wells K et al, The orderly progression of melanoma nodal metastases. *Ann Surg* 1994; **220**:759–67.

27. Thompson J, McCarthy WH, Bosch CMJ et al, Sentinel lymph node status as an indicator of the presence of metastatic melanoma in regional lymph nodes. *Melanoma Res* 1995; **5**:255–60.

28. Karakousis CP, Velez AF, Spellman JE, Scarozza J, The technique of sentinel node biopsy. *Eur J Surg Oncol* 1996; **22**:271–5.

29. Belli F, Lenisa L, Clemente C et al, Sentinel node biopsy and selective dissection for melanoma nodal metastases. *Tumori* 1998; **84**:24–8.

30. Robinson DS, Sample WF, Fee HJ et al, Regional lymphatic drainage in primary malignant melanoma of the trunk determined by colloidal gold scanning. *Surg Forum* 1977; **28**:147.

31. Kelemen PR, Essner R, Foshag LJ, Morton DL, Lymphatic mapping and sentinel lymphadenectomy after wide local excision of primary melanoma. *J Am Coll Surg* 1999; **189**:247–52.

32. Glass EC, Essner R, Morton DL, Kinetics of three lymphoscintigraphic agents in patients with cutaneous melanoma. *J Nucl Med* 1998; **39**: 1185–90.

33. Norman J, Cruse CW, Espinosa C et al, Redefinition of cutaneous lymphatic drainage with the use of lymphoscintigraphy for malignant melanoma. *Am J Surg* 1991; **162**:432.

34. Uren RF, Howman-Giles R, Thompson JF et al, Lymphoscintigraphy to identify sentinel lymph nodes in patients with melanoma. *Melanoma Res* 1994; **4**:395–9.

35. Essner R, The role of lymphoscintigraphy and sentinel node mapping in assessing patient risk in melanoma. *Semin Oncol* 1997; **24**:S8–10.

36. Krag DN, Meijer SJ, Weaver DL et al, Minimal-access surgery for staging of malignant melanoma. *Arch Surg* 1995; **130**:654–8.

37. Essner R, Foshag L, Morton DL, Intraoperative radiolymphoscintigraphy: a useful adjunct to intraoperative lymphatic mapping and selective

lymphadenectomy in patients with clinical stage I melanoma. Proceedings of the Society of Surgical Oncology, 47th Annual Meeting, Houston 1994 (Abstract).

38. Pijpers R, Collet GJ, Meijer S, Hoekstr OS, The impact of dynamic lymphoscintigraphy and gamma probe guidance on sentinel node biopsy in melanoma. *Eur J Nucl Med* 1995; **22:**1238–41.

39. Mudun A, Murray DR, Herda SC et al, Early stage melanoma: lymphoscintigraphy, reproducibility of sentinel node detection, and effectiveness of the intraoperative gamma probe. *Radiology* 1996; **199:**171–5.

40. Albertini JJ, Cruse CW, Rapaport D et al, Intraoperative radiolymphoscintigraphy improves sentinel lymph node identification for patients with melanoma. *Ann Surg* 1996; **223:**217–24.

41. Thompson JF, Niewind P, Uren RF et al, Single-dose isotope injection for both preoperative lymphoscintigraphy and intraoperative sentinel lymph node identification in melanoma patients. *Melanoma Res* 1997; **7:**500–6.

42. Bostick P, Essner R, Sarantou T et al, Intraoperative lymphatic mapping for early-stage melanoma of the head and neck. *Am J Surg* 1997; **174:**536–9.

43. Leong SPL, Steinmetz I, Habib FA et al, Optimal selective sentinel lymph node dissection in primary malignant melanoma. *Arch Surg* 1997; **132:**666–73.

44. Essner R, Bostick PJ, Glass EC, Standardized probe-directed sentinel node dissection in melanoma. *Surgery* 2000; **127:**26–31.

45. Murray DR, Carlson GW, Greenlee R et al, Surgical management of malignant melanoma using dynamic lymphoscintigraphy and gamma probe-guided sentinel lymph node biopsy: the Emory experience. *Am Surg* 2000; **66:**763–7.

46. Jansen L, Nieweg OE, Peterse JL et al, Reliability of sentinel lymph node biopsy for staging melanoma. *Br J Surg* 2000; **87:**484–9.

47. Lingam MK, Mackie RM, McKay AJ, Intraoperative identification of SLN in patients with malignant melanoma. *Br J Cancer* 1997; **75:**1505–8.

48. Van Der Veen H, Hoekstra OS, Cuesta MA, Meijer S, Gamma probe-guided sentinel node biopsy to select patients with melanoma for lymphadenectomy. *Br J Surg* 1994; **81:**1769–70.

49. Joseph E, Messina J, Glass FL et al, Radioguided surgery for the ultrastaging of the patient with melanoma. *Cancer J Sci Am* 1997; **3:**341–5.

50. Loggie BW, Hosseinian AA, Watson NE, Prospective evaluation of selective lymph node biopsy for cutaneous malignant melanoma. *Am Surg* 1997; **63:**1051–8.

51. Nathanson SD, Avery M, Anaya P et al, Lymphatic diameters and radionuclide clearance in a murine melanoma model. *Arch Surg* 1997; **132:**311–15.

52. Wong JH, Terada K, Ko P, Coel MN, Lack of effect of particle size on the identification of the sentinel node in cutaneous malignancies. *Ann Surg Oncol* 1997; **5:**77–80.

53. Strand SE, Persson BRR, Quantitative lymphoscintigraphy I: basic concepts for optimal uptake of radiocolloids in the parasternal lymph nodes of rabbits. *J Nucl Med* 1979; **20:**1038–46.

54. Bostick P, Essner R, Glass E et al, Comparison of intraoperative lymphatic mapping in melanoma to identify sentinel nodes in 100 lymphatic basins. *Arch Surg* 1999; **134:**43–9.

55. Nieweg OE, Kapteijn BAE, Thompson JF, Kroon BBR, Lymphatic mapping and selective lymphadenectomy for melanoma: not yet standard therapy. *Eur J Surg Oncol* 1997; **23:**397–8.

56. Nieweg OE, Jansen L, Kroon BBR, Technique of lymphatic mapping and sentinel node biopsy for melanoma. *Eur J Surg Oncol* 1998; **24:**520–4.

57. Leong SPL, Donegan E, Heffernon W et al, Adverse reactions to isosulfan blue during selective sentinel lymph node dissection in melanoma. *Ann Surg Oncol* 2000; **7:**361–6.

58. Longnecker SM, Guzzardo MM, Van Voris LP, Life-threatening anaphylaxis following subcutaneous administration of isosulfan blue 1%. *Clin Pharm* 1985; **4:**219–21.

59. Zanzonico P, Heller S, The intraoperative gamma probe: basic principles and choices available. *Semin Nucl Med* 2000; **30:**33–48.

60. Glass EC, Basinski JE, Krasne DL, Giuliano AE, Radiation safety considerations for sentinel node techniques. *Ann Surg Oncol* 1999; **6:**10–11.

61. Mincer TJ, Shriver CD, Flieck PR et al, Guidelines for the safe use of radioactive materials during localization and resection of the sentinel lymph node. *Ann Surg Oncol* 1999; **6:**75–82.

62. Eshima D, Fauconnier T, Eshima L, Thornback JR, Radiopharmaceuticals for lymphoscintigraphy: including dosimetry and radiation considerations. *Semin Nucl Med* 2000; **30:**25–32.

63. Essner R, Conforti A, Kelley MC et al, Efficacy of selective lymphadenectomy as a therapeutic procedure for early-stage melanoma, *Ann Surg Oncol* 1999; **6:**442–9.

64. Morton DL, Thompson JF, Essner R et al, Validation of the accuracy of intraoperative lymphatic mapping and sentinel lymphadenectomy for early-stage melanoma: a multicenter trial. *Ann Surg* 1999; **230:**453–65.

65. Reintgen D, Balch CM, Kirkwood J, Ross M, Recent advances in the care of the patient with malignant melanoma, *Ann Surg* 1997; **225:**1–14.

66. Morton DL, Intraoperative lymphatic mapping and sentinel lymphadenectomy: community standard care or clinical investigation? *Cancer J Sci Am* 1997; **3:**328–30.

67. Essner R, Conforti A, Kelley MC et al, Cost-conscious management of the inguinal nodes in early-stage melanoma, *Melanoma Res* 1997; **7:**S29.

68. Gershenwald JE, Colome MI, Lee JE et al, Patterns of recurrence following a negative sentinel lymph node biopsy in 243 patients with stage I or II melanoma, *J Clin Oncol* 1998; **16:** 2253–60.

69. Gershenwald JE, Thompson W, Mansfield PF et al, Multi-institutional melanoma lymphatic mapping experience: the prognostic value of sentinel lymph node status in 612 stage I or II melanoma patients. *J Clin Oncol* 1999; **17:**976–83.

8

The isotope technique

Alessandro Testori and Umberto Veronesi

The European Institute of Oncology technique for SLN biopsy in melanoma

Technique	Combination	Isotope	*Type*: Tc-99m-HSA
Dye	*Type*: Patent blue-V dye *Volume*: 1–2 ml (cc)		*Filtered*: Yes (200 –1000 nm) *Dose*: 5–10 MBq (0.135–0.27 mCi) *Volume*: 0.2–0.3 ml (cc)
Injection site	*Isotope*: Intradermal *Dye*: Intradermal		

Institutions preparing to perform sentinel lymph-node (SLN) biopsy for the treatment of patients with melanoma must first establish cooperation among clinicians from various departments. Surgeons and nuclear medicine physicians must discuss each SLN biopsy case in order to determine the preferred radiolabeled-tracer injection site. Surgeons require clear feedback concerning drainage sites and the number of SLNs detected by the labeled solution. The technique of lymphoscintigraphy (LSG) has been studied extensively during the past decades, and we now know that all cutaneous sites permit accurate mapping of the lymphatic drainage patterns.[1–4] This point is important, because some tumors may have ambiguous nodal drainage or may drain to more than one nodal basin.

Since the mid-1990s, interest in preoperative lymphatic mapping and SLN biopsy to identify the node at greatest risk for metastatic spread (the "sentinel" node) has grown rapidly. The main benefit of the SLN biopsy technique is the ability to perform accurate lymphatic staging through a minimally invasive surgical procedure. With blue dye alone, this "selective" dissection can be relatively extensive, as described in Morton's initial 1992 report.[1] With the combination of blue dye and radioisotope, however, the SLN can usually be harvested with minimal dissection, directed by the use of an intraoperative hand-held gamma probe.

Initially, the success of the SLN biopsy technique was based on the "classic" concept of individual surgical skill; in order to obtain the required result, the surgeon had to succeed in finding the SLNs using only blue dye. Subsequently, the isotope technique of SLN biopsy has been widely adopted by surgical oncologists, and the combined dye-and-isotope method of SLN biopsy represents the most modern approach available. Again, it is important to keep in mind that without the contribution of nuclear medicine and LSG, use of the SLN biopsy procedure could not have become as widespread as it is today.[5,6]

The most important benefit of preoperative radioisotope lymphatic mapping is the precise information it provides to the surgeon on the number and location of SLNs to be excised. With this information, the surgeon can decide how best to proceed, and whether to propose to the patient a procedure requiring only local anesthesia (suitable where only a single node basin is involved, particularly the groin) or to proceed with conventional general anesthesia.

During SLN surgery the radiolabeled tracer has a critical role, allowing the detection (preoperatively with LSG and intraoperatively with a gamma probe) of single or multiple radioactive, non-blue SLNs that would otherwise be missed. Several situations exist, however, in which the radioisotope can impair SLN identification. The most common is where the primary disease lies close to the lymphatic basin; the high counts at the injection site can "overshadow" the site of the SLN or even contaminate the nodal basin by direct infiltration, precluding radiolocalization. Occasionally, many nodes take up isotope, precluding a simple SLN procedure. Finally, in some cases both the deep lymphatic drainage in the pelvis and the more superficial nodes in the groin will be identified by LSG. In this setting, only a superficial groin biopsy is performed and when a negative histology is obtained, a careful ultrasound (US) follow-up at the pelvis is suggested.

Preoperative LSG, useful in mapping unexpected patterns of lymphatic drainage in the melanoma patient, is not by itself sufficient for SLN biopsy. Intraoperative use of a gamma probe is critical to the success of the procedure, and SLN biopsy should not be attempted when a gamma probe is unavailable.

Most multicenter protocols for SLN biopsy have dedicated their attention to the so-called "learning phase" of the procedure. The main reason for this is the difficulty of finding the SLN using only Patent Blue-V dye, as was commonly the case in the initial international experience of SLN biopsy. The more recent adoption of radioisotopes is likely to have reduced the importance of a formal learning phase for melanoma units starting to perform SLN biopsy.

TECHNIQUE OF SLN BIOPSY

Preoperative phase: nuclear medicine

The preoperative phase of the SLN biopsy procedure is performed by nuclear medicine 2–24 hours before surgery. Different types and doses of radiotracer can be used in LSG: the choice will depend on the local regulations in effect for the institution (or country) and on the timing of the procedure following isotope injection. The most frequently used tracers are nanocolloids of albumin, which have particles 10 nm to 100 nm in size; antimony trisulfide; and other colloids (most commonly sulfur colloid) ranging from less than 50 nm to 1000 nm in particle size.

Technetium-99m has a number of favorable characteristics that make it the isotope of choice: it reaches a distance of several centimeters from the hot area, and after 48 hours, there is no residual radioactivity.[7] We recommend the use of Tc-99m-labeled colloids of 10 nm to 200 nm particle size. Although it has been suggested that using a radiolabeled colloid with a larger particle size (e.g., sulfur colloid) would minimize the number of nodes detected and eliminate the problem of removing non-SLNs, such large particles migrate much more slowly through dermal lymphatics, thereby increasing the chance that some true SLNs are missed.

The isotope is administered as one or two intradermal injections of 0.2–0.3 ml (cc) of the agent around the scar of a previous biopsy, as described below. When LSG is performed the same day as the SLN biopsy, the amount of radiolabeled solution used should be the minimum required. In cases where the injection has delivered an excessive amount of radioactivity, the background of radioactivity can sometimes be so great as to reduce the surgeon's ability to distinguish the SLN in the basin.

The site of injection and the lymphatic basin should be visualized on the same image. If this is not possible, the lymphatic basin must be shown entirely. For melanomas of the trunk, the inguinal, axillary, and sometimes the supraclavicular or nuchal basins must be imaged. For extremity lesions, the popliteal or epitrochlear regions can be involved and should be studied. Late and static images must be obtained at least 1.5–2 hours following injection. Indeed, once the isotope has "washed out" of the lymphatic channels after an initial phase of rapid uptake, it is possible to see in-transit lymph nodes (those between the site of injection and the first regional lymph node basin). These must be considered "true" SLNs and should be localized by ultrasound prior to surgery. In these circumstances, unusual drainage is also confirmed by the dynamic images taken early in the LSG procedure.[4] For sites on the trunk or head and neck, anteroposterior, lateral, and possibly additional views may be required to localize all SLNs.[8,9]

Either the day before surgery or 2–4 hours prior to surgery, a dynamic LSG is performed following one-two intradermal injection of Tc-99m-labeled colloid particles of human serum albumin (Tc-99m-HSA) around the excision site in volumes ranging from 0.2 ml to 0.3 ml. The average injected dose can be 20–50 MBq (0.54–1.35 mCi) of Tc-99m colloids. Each patient undergoes both dynamic and static acquisitions under the gamma camera. The average acquisition time of dynamic images is 10–15 minutes postinjection, and this is followed by static evaluations at 30 minutes, 1 hour, and 2 hours (4-hour or following-day images are required in certain cases). At the end of the LSG, the most precise cutaneous projection of the sentinel node or nodes on the patient's skin is definitively marked.

Preoperative phase: ultrasonography of the SLN

Once the position of the SLN has been defined, the operation can usually begin. In some circumstances, before starting the surgical procedure, it is helpful to study the SLN with ultrasound in order to determine whether a lymph node is really present under the skin mark, whether the lymph node is superficial or deep, and to localize any in-transit SLNs. Sometimes a point of strong radioactivity in one or more unusual drainage areas can be attrib-

uted to the presence of lymphatic connections (or areas of lymphatic ectasia) in the absence of nodes, while in other situations, a radioactive node may be in the pelvis or in the retroperitoneum, in which case SLN biopsy should be avoided.

Intraoperative phase: the gamma probe and surgery

Following LSG and 10 minutes after intradermal injection of Patent Blue-V dye at the same point(s) as the colloid, the surgical procedure can begin.

Immediately prior to making the skin incision, the surgeon should check that the topographic projection of the radioactivity detected with the gamma probe corresponds with the marker on the skin. The cutaneous incision should be made based on this evaluation of the topographic projection of the radioactivity.

During the operation, the gamma probe permits a safe, minimal dissection toward the SLN. The gamma probe should be used immediately after the incision of the superficial fascia if no blue dye is visible, in order to reduce the surgical dissection required to look for the SLN. Once the SLN has been removed, it should be tested to document its isotope counts. These counts should be at least 3 times higher than the background counts in the basin, which are measured after excision of the SLN. As mentioned earlier, radiolocalization can be difficult when the melanoma site is very close to the node basin. While SLN biopsy usually precedes wide excision of the primary site, in these cases the surgeon may find it helpful to excise the primary first (thereby removing the radioactivity at the injection site) and then proceed with the SLN dissection.

While for occasional challenging cases the overall success of SLN biopsy may be determined by the surgeon's experience, with the advent of radiolocalization by the intraoperative gamma probe, SLN biopsy has become a simple and straightforward operation. A variety of centers report success rates that approach 100%.[10–22]

THE LEARNING CURVE: THE EUROPEAN INSTITUTE OF ONCOLOGY EXPERIENCE

At the European Institute of Oncology (EIO), we have analyzed our first 90 SLN biopsy procedures to determine the role of the learning curve. One surgeon (AT) performed all of the operations, all patients had preoperative LSG, and both isotope and blue-dye mapping were used in each case. Ninety consecutive patients with Stage I primary melanoma (MD Anderson classification: T1–4a, TNM) were enrolled in the study, the first of whom was the first patient to undergo SLN biopsy at the EIO in October 1994. Sentinel lymph-node biopsy was performed on all patients within 3 months of primary tumor excision. Informed consent was obtained from all patients, and the ethics committee of the EIO approved the protocol. Patient data are shown in Table 8.1.

Dynamic LSG was performed the day before surgery, following intradermal injection of Tc-99m-colloidal albumin around the excision site in individual portions ranging from 0.2 ml to 0.3 ml

each. The average injected dose in this group of patients was 37 MBq (1 mCi). Each patient underwent both dynamic and static LSG imaging under the gamma camera. The average acquisition time for dynamic images was 10–15 minutes postinjection. Static imaging followed at 30 minutes, 1 hour, 2 hours, 4 hours, and 18 hours. On the day following the LSG, and 10 minutes prior to surgery, Patent Blue-V dye was injected intradermally at the same point(s) as the colloid, and the area was gently massaged to facilitate the diffusion of the dye into the lymphatics. The amount of dye injected ranged from 1 ml to 4 ml, with a mean of 1.56 ml.

Following standard surgical preparation, the patient was anesthetized and a small incision was made over the area previously marked in the regional lymphatic drainage basin; the subcutaneous tissue was then explored in search of a blue-stained lymphatic channel. The channel was carefully dissected toward the blue-stained SLN. If no blue-stained node or vessel could be found, the SLN was traced with a hand-held gamma probe. After removal of the SLN, the gamma probe was used to confirm the radioactivity of the specimen. The resection bed and the entire nodal area were then scanned to identify any other SLNs, with further exploration (guided by the gamma probe) if the bed or basin counts remained high. Radioactivity was measured in counts per second, and a "hot" lymph node was defined as any lymph node with counts greater than 3 times the background level.

Sentinel lymph nodes were recorded as blue-stained or not, and as radioactive or not. We also noted whether the SLN was found by blue dye alone, and whether the gamma probe was essential in directing the surgeon to SLN that otherwise would have been missed. We noted the time required to identify each SLN, the number of SLNs excised, and the number of SLNs shown by the LSG.

Among the 90 patients, LSG identified a total of 135 SLNs in 105 node basins (an average of 1.2 SLN per basin). Sentinel lymph nodes could not be found in two patients, and in both the primary site was on the back, very close to the axilla. Neither patient had nodal metastases found on a Level I axillary lymph-node dissection (ALND).

Table 8.1 Description of the patients enrolled in the study ($n = 90$)	
Sex (n)	
Male	46 (51%)
Female	44 (49%)
Age (yr)	
Mean ± SE	50.5 ± 1.5
Range	18–80
Site of the primary (n)	
Trunk	44 (49%)
Head–neck	4 (4%)
Limbs	42 (47%)
Histology of the primary (n)	
Breslow value	
≤1.5 mm	35 (39%)
1.5–4.0 mm	45 (50%)
>4.0 mm	10 (11%)

To document the role of a learning curve for the SLN biopsy procedure, we compared the surgeon's ability to find the SLN using the vital dye alone, the gamma probe alone, and the two techniques in combination (Table 8.2). Of 135 SLNs identified by LSG, 133 were found at surgery; 106 (78.5%) were found by blue dye, 6 (4.4%) by blue dye alone, and 129 (95.5%) by isotope. The combination of the two techniques identified 133 of 135 SLNs overall, a success rate of 98.5%.

When the blue-dye and isotope methods are considered together, there was no "learning curve," and SLNs were identified with a high rate of success from the outset. Similarly, there was no learning curve for using isotope by itself. In contrast, blue-dye success rates improved significantly, from 57% in our early experience to 81% more recently.

The pathologic status of the SLNs harvested in our first 90 SLN biopsy cases is presented in Table 8.3. As expected, SLN status is significantly related to lesion thickness.

Table 8.2 Success rates of harvesting SLNs by method in 90 patients

Method	Total no. of SLNs (%)	14 patients	76 patients	
		Early series	Late series	p value
Preoperative LSG	135 (100%)	14 (10.4%)	121 (89.6%)	
Intraoperative gamma probe	129 (95.5%)			
Blue dye	106 (78.5%)	14 (57.1%)	121 (81.0%)	0.04
Blue dye + gamma probe	133 (98.5%)			

Table 8.3 Pathologic status of SLNs of 90 primary melanoma patients by Breslow evaluation

Primary melanoma thickness	No. of patients	SLN-negative		SLN-positive		p value
		(n)	(%)	(n)	(%)	
≤1.5	35	34	97.1	1	2.9	<0.01
>1.5	55	34	61.8	21	38.2	
≤2	47	41	87.2	6	12.8	<0.01
>2	43	27	62.8	16	37.2	
≤2.5	59	51	86.4	8	13.6	<0.01
>2.5	31	17	54.8	14	45.2	
≤3	69	57	82.6	12	17.4	<0.01
>3	21	11	52.4	10	47.6	
≤3.5	75	61	81.3	14	18.7	<0.01
>3.5	15	7	46.7	8	53.3	
≤4	80	64	80.0	16	20.0	<0.01
>4	10	4	40.0	6	60.0	
Breslow mean value 2.41 mm		1.98 mm		3.77 mm		

Table 8.4 Intraoperative time required to find stained and nonstained SLNs

Biopsy site	Mean time (min)	Stained SLN		Nonstained SLN		Student's t-test	p value
		Mean time (min)	n	Mean time (min)	n		
All SLNs	11.5	10.1	106	16.8	29	3.78	<0.01
Groin	10.3	9.4	57	15.8	10	2.26	0.03
Axilla	12.9	11.3	46	19.3	12	3.11	<0.01

Finally, we analyzed the time required to find the SLN, to test the hypothesis that the presence of blue lymphatic staining could help to reduce operative time. This hypothesis has been confirmed, as shown in Table 8.4. The time required to find stained and nonstained SLNs was analyzed for all biopsy procedures and separately for the two most frequently biopsied lymph nodal basins: the groin and the axilla. Overall, blue-stained SLNs were found significantly sooner (10.1 min) than non-stained SLNs (16.8 min), with similar findings for the separate analyses of the groin and axillary procedures.

In summary, the addition of isotope to blue dye eliminates the learning curve of SLN mapping for melanoma. We recommend the use of blue dye as an adjunct to isotope, primarily because it allows faster localization of the SLN in the 80% of patients in whom it is successful.

REFERENCES

1. Morton DL, Wen DR, Wong JH et al, Technical details of intraoperative lymphatic mapping for early stage melanoma. *Arch Surg* 1992; **127**:392–9.
2. Morton DL, Wen DR, Cochran AJ, Management of early stage melanoma by intraoperative lymphatic mapping and selective lymphadenectomy: an alternative to routine lymphadenectomy or "watch and wait". *Surg Oncol Clin N Am* 1992; **1**:247–59.
3. Wong JH, Cagle LA, Morton DL, Lymphatic drainage of shin to sentinel node in a feline model. *Ann Surg* 1991; **214**:637–41.
4. Wong JH, Truelove K, Ko P et al, Localization and resection of an in transit sentinel lymph node by use of lymphoscintigraphy, intraoperative lymphatic mapping, and a hand-held gamma probe. *Surgery* 1996; **120**:114–16.
5. Bartolomei M, Testori A, Chinol M et al, Sentinel node localization in cutaneous melanoma: lymphoscintigraphy with colloids and antibody fragments versus blue dye mapping. *Eur J Nucl Med* 1998; **25**:1489–94.
6. Testori A, Bartolomei M, Grana C et al, Sentinel node localization in primary melanoma: learning curve and results. *Melanoma Res* 1999; **9**:587–93.
7. Pijpers R, Collet JG, Meijer S et al, The impact of dynamic lymphoscintigraphy and gamma probe guidance on sentinel node biopsy in melanoma. *Eur J Nucl Med* 1995; **22**:1238–41.
8. O'Brien CJ, Uren RF, Thompson JF et al, Prediction of potential metastatic sites in cutaneous head and neck melanoma using lymphoscintigraphy. *Am J Surg* 1995; **170**:461–6.
9. Wells KE, Rapaport DP, Cruse CW et al, Sentinel lymph node biopsy in melanoma of the head and neck. *Plast Reconstr Surg* 1997; **100**:591–4.
10. Testori A, Sentinel node biopsy: letter to the editor. *Melanoma Res* 1999; **9**:619–20.
11. Leong SPL, Stenmetz I, Habib FA et al, Optimal selective sentinel lymph node dissection in primary malignant melanoma. *Arch Surg* 1997; **132**:666–73.
12. Krag DN, Meijer SJ, Weaver DL et al, Minimal-access surgery for staging of malignant melanoma. *Arch Surg* 1995; **130**:654–8.
13. Thompson JF, McCarthy WH, Bosch CMJ et al, Sentinel lymph node status as indicator of the presence of metastatic melanoma in regional lymph nodes. *Melanoma Res* 1995; **5**:255–60.
14. Godellas CV, Berman CG, Lyman G et al, The

identification and mapping of melanoma regional nodal metastases: minimally invasive surgery for the diagnosis of nodal metastases. *Am Surg* 1995; **61**:97–101.

15. Kapteijn BAE, Nieweg OE, Liem I et al, Localizing the sentinel node in cutaneous melanoma: gamma probe detection versus blue dye. *Ann Surg Oncol* 1997; **4**:156–60.

16. Testori A, Grana C, Bartolomei M et al, Lymphoscintigraphy with antimelanoma monoclonal antibody to detect micrometastases of the sentinel node in melanoma patients. *Int J Surg Science* 1998; **5**:117–18.

17. Lingam MK, Mackie RM, Mackay AJ, Intraoperative lymphatic mapping using patent blue V dye to identify nodal micrometastases in malignant melanoma. *Reg Cancer Treat* 1994; **7**:144–6.

18. Van der Veen H, Hoekstra OS, Paul MA et al, Gamma probe guided sentinel node biopsy to select patients with melanoma for lymphadenectomy. *Br J Surg* 1994; **81**:1769–70.

19. Krag D, Harlow S, Weaver D et al, Technique of sentinel node resection in melanoma and breast cancer: probe-guided surgery and lymphatic mapping. *Eur J Surg Oncol* 1998; **24**:89–93.

20. Rivers KJ, Roof MI, Sentinel lymph-node biopsy in melanoma: is less surgery better? *Lancet* 1997; **350**:1336–7.

21. Emilia JC, Lawrence WJ, Sentinel lymph node biopsy in malignant melanoma: the standard of care? *J Surg Oncol* 1997; **65**:153–4.

22. Bostick P, Essner R, Sarantou T et al, Intraoperative lymphatic mapping for early-stage melanoma of the head and neck. *Am J Surg* 1997; **174**:536–9.

9

The dye-plus-isotope technique

John F Thompson

The Sydney Melanoma Unit technique for SLN biopsy in melanoma

Technique	Combination	Isotope	*Type*: Tc-99m-ASC/Tc-99m-CA
Dye	*Type*: Patent blue-V dye		*Filtered*: N/A
	Volume: 0.5–1.5 ml (cc)		*Dose*: 5 MBq (0.135 mCi)
			Volume: 0.05 ml (cc)
Injection site	*Isotope*: Intradermal		
	Dye: Intradermal		

Reliable staging of patients with melanoma using the technique of selective sentinel lymph-node biopsy requires that each sentinel lymph node (SLN) must be correctly identified and removed.[1,2] It is not sufficient to identify and remove a single SLN in a lymph-node field if more than one SLN is present in that field. Similarly, staging may be inaccurate if an SLN is present outside a recognized lymph-node field (e.g., as an interval node between the primary melanoma site and the expected drainage field) and is not identified and removed for histologic examination.[3] It goes without saying that unless staging by selective SLN biopsy is completely accurate, the information obtained will be misleading, and inappropriate management decisions may be made as a result. The greatest risk is that a positive SLN will be missed. In this situation, one of two things will happen: either clinical evidence of melanoma recurrence will become apparent at a later time,

when the likelihood of successful curative treatment will be lower; or in the future, the indication for treatment with an adjuvant therapy of proven efficacy will not be recognized. The other important problem that will arise if SLN biopsy provides information that is incorrect or incomplete involves patients entering randomized trials of adjuvant therapy and being incorrectly staged. This situation increases the difficulty of interpreting the results of such trials.

For all of the reasons given above, techniques that provide the greatest possible accuracy when attempting to locate and remove SLNs are clearly desirable. Even after a surgeon has had experience with many hundreds of selective SLN biopsy procedures, cases sometimes occur in which confident identification of all SLNs proves difficult. It therefore seems logical to make full use of all available techniques that may assist in achieving maximum accuracy in SLN identification.

Carefully performed preoperative lymphoscintigraphy (LSG) will usually provide detailed and reliable information about the number of SLNs and their locations. This information obtained from the preoperative lymphoscintigram is the starting point for reliable selective SLN biopsy. If preoperative LSG is not performed, or is not undertaken with appropriate care and attention to detail, the chance of successfully identifying and removing every SLN will be markedly reduced.

At the time of surgery, intradermal blue-dye injection around the primary melanoma (if it remains in situ) or around the excision-biopsy wound (if the melanoma has been removed) remains the "gold standard" for SLN identification, but intraoperative use of a gamma probe is also of great value to indicate both that a node is "hot" (because it contains trapped radiolabeled tracer) and that the residual gamma count in the node field is low, with no focal hot spots, following the removal of all presumed SLNs in that field.

There is already a considerable body of evidence to indicate that use of either the blue-dye or the gamma-probe technique alone is likely to be less reliable than their use in combination. Both single-center and multicenter studies have shown that SLN identification rates are improved when the two techniques are used together. It seems that reliable SLN identification rates approaching 100% can be achieved by a surgeon with appropriate training and experience when a good-quality preoperative lymphoscintigram is available and both blue dye and a gamma probe are used at the time of surgery. Before considering details of the combined blue-dye/gamma-probe technique, however, key features of lymphatic mapping with blue dye and with a gamma probe that are relevant to the combined technique are reviewed briefly.

BLUE-DYE MAPPING

It has been known for over two centuries that various dyes and inks can be used to demonstrate lymphatic vessels and lymph nodes.

Indeed some of the earliest known descriptions of cutaneous lymphatic drainage pathways were based on dissection after the injection of substances such as Prussian Blue dye, Chinese ink, and mercury.[4] In the 1950s, blue-dye injections were used to demonstrate lymphatic channels in the hand and foot, so that the lymphatics could be cannulated for the newly introduced technique of x-ray lymphography. It was not until the mid-1980s, however, that systematic studies were initiated that used blue dye to identify those lymph nodes most likely to contain metastatic melanoma in a given individual.[5] The story of the development of intraoperative lymphatic-mapping techniques for early-stage melanoma[6] has been related in Chapter 1. Within a few years of the original description of the technique, the accuracy of SLN status as an indication of the status of the entire regional lymph-node field has been confirmed by other groups.[7–10]

Blue-dye injection technique

Blue dye is injected intradermally at several points around the melanoma or, if it has been removed, on either side of the central part of the excision-biopsy scar. Care must be taken to ensure that the injection is truly intradermal, because if a significant volume of dye is injected subcutaneously, rapid spread occurs in the subcutaneous plane, allowing the dye to enter lymphatic pathways some distance from the melanoma site and thus drain to a lymph node that is not the SLN draining the melanoma site on the skin. The situation then becomes analogous to that of attempting lymphatic mapping after a wide-local excision of the melanoma site has been performed; one or more SLNs will always be identified, but may not be the nodes that originally drained the primary melanoma site. There is now good evidence, however, that if only an excision biopsy has been performed with a clearance of no more than a few millimeters around the melanoma, lymphatic mapping will still reliably indicate the true SLN or SLNs. Accurate placement of the blue dye intradermally is more readily achieved with a very fine-bore needle (30 gauge). When such a needle is used, the pressure required to inject the dye is considerable, making the use of a Luer-Lok syringe mandatory if embarrassing blue-dye explosions are to be avoided. In most situations, only small-volume injections are required (total 0.5–1.5 ml), provided that measures to ensure rapid transit to the draining lymph-node field are employed.[11]

When to inject the blue dye

When general anesthesia is to be used, it is usually satisfactory to inject the blue dye 5–10 minutes before anesthetic induction. If local anesthesia is used, dye injection 5–10 minutes prior to injection of the anesthetic agent is desirable. In both situations, this provides sufficient time for the site of injection to be gently massaged and for the patient to exercise the appropriate body part if the anatomical location of the primary melanoma site makes this possible. These maneuvers are recommended because they make it more certain that the blue dye will have reached the regional lymph-node field by the time of surgical exploration of that field. They are particularly important if the preoperative lymphoscintigram has shown very slow movement of injected radiolabeled material from the injection site to the regional lymph nodes.[12] Under these circumstances, it can be helpful to inject the blue dye 15–20 minutes before anesthetic induction, allowing more time for massage and exercise. The other situation in which earlier injection of blue dye is desirable is if the patient has become cold in the preoperative period, a situation that frequently occurs when patients clad only in a thin operating-room gown spend time in a cool holding area or anesthetic room while awaiting their surgery. Skin temperatures can fall to levels well below body core temperatures in these situations, and lymphatic flow rates are dramatically reduced as a consequence. Although the intradermal blue-dye injection is uncomfortable for the patient, it is better to do this before the area is infiltrated with local anesthetic solution because the fluid in the dermis and subcuta-

neous tissues may alter physiological lymph drainage pathways from the melanoma site, and so cause identification of an incorrect node (a non-SLN) as the SLN.

Choice of blue dye

Worldwide, two types of blue dye are in routine use for lymphatic mapping: Patent Blue-V dye in Europe and Australia, and isosulfan blue dye in North America. Patent Blue-V dye is generally regarded as the more satisfactory agent, and if it is used, reinjection around the primary melanoma site is very rarely required. When isosulfan blue is used, however, the staining of lymphatics and SLNs is less intense, and the blue color disappears more rapidly. For this reason, it has been suggested that repeat injection may be required if SLN identification and removal has not been achieved within 20 minutes.[6] Patent Blue-V dye is not currently available for use in the United States.

Systemic complications of intradermal blue-dye injection

Following intradermal injection of blue dye, the patient's general skin color can change, to become gray and almost cadaveric. A pulse oximeter may indicate a low oxygen saturation, even when the actual arterial blood-oxygen tensions are well above normal. The patient's urine is likely to be green-blue in color for many hours postoperatively. It is important that the patient should anticipate and understand these common effects of blue-dye injection. More serious side-effects can occur, but they are fortunately rare. Potentially the most serious is the development of an anaphylactoid reaction to the blue dye, with the widespread appearance on the skin of large blisters filled with pale-blue fluid, accompanied in severe cases by bronchospasm and systemic hypotension. Standard treatment for an acute allergic reaction is required, including parenteral antihistamines and corticosteroids, with intravenous fluid and inotrope support if necessary.

The surgical procedure: tracing blue-stained lymphatics

Preoperative LSG will have indicated the site or sites of SLNs, allowing the surgical incision to be planned appropriately. Once the subcutaneous tissue plane is entered, very cautious dissection is required, with meticulous hemostasis, to enable identification of the blue-stained lymphatic channels and to avoid damage to them. When a blue-stained lymphatic is found, it can be traced as far as the lymph node to which it drains. This lymph node should itself be blue-stained if it is to be identified confidently as an SLN. If a node is clearly blue-stained, and has one or more blue-stained afferent lymphatics entering it, there can be no doubt that it is an SLN. Although the preoperative lymphoscintigram will have indicated the number of SLNs in a regional node field, as well as their location and approximate depth below the skin surface, it is still desirable to seek and trace blue-stained lymphatic channels. This is because SLNs can sometimes be difficult to locate even when their approximate position is known, and they may not be intensely stained. Indeed, an SLN may sometimes be blue-stained only on its undersurface, or at only one pole, if that is where the afferent lymphatic enters. In either of these circumstances, the fact that the node is stained blue may not be immediately apparent, and it may be overlooked unless a blue-stained afferent lymphatic is followed to its point of entry into the node.

When removing SLNs, it is important to cause as little interference as possible to surrounding tissues, particularly to non-SLNs and their afferent lymphatics. This minimizes the theoretical risk of tumor-cell spillage, and reduces to negligible levels the likelihood of causing lymphedema. Perhaps most importantly, however, it means that if an SLN is subsequently found to be positive and a full regional lymph-node clearance is required, the SLN biopsy site can be removed in its entirety without transgressing previously dissected and therefore potentially contaminated tissue planes.

USE OF A GAMMA PROBE

If SLN identification by tracing blue lymphatics and observing node staining proves difficult, a hand-held gamma probe may be used at this time to assist with SLN location. It must be borne in mind, however, that not every "hot" node is an SLN,[13] and to achieve the high degree of accuracy that is sought, a node must be both blue-stained *and* hot to be reliably characterized as an SLN.[14] The tip of the gamma probe, covered by an appropriate sterile sheath, is inserted into the wound and the angle of its tip moved around until a hot spot is located. This provides a direction in which dissection can proceed. The maneuver can be repeated, if necessary, until the hot node is found and its blue-staining status checked. When using the gamma probe in this way, it is important to ensure that "shine-through" from residual radioactivity around the primary melanoma site is not what is being recorded. This situation often arises, for example, if an axillary sentinel node is being sought, and if the primary melanoma site is on the upper back.

Sometimes the gamma probe is unable to selectively detect activity in an SLN because of proximity of the node field in which it is located to the primary melanoma site. Under these circumstances it is desirable to widely excise the primary melanoma site at this stage, thereby removing most of the radioactivity in the area and allowing much better discrimination by the gamma probe of the relatively small hot spot in the node field being explored.

Confirming SLN status with a gamma probe

Even 24 hours after intradermal isotope injection at a primary melanoma site, SLNs invariably remain the hottest nodes in the draining lymph-node field.[15,16] Radiolabeled colloid is trapped in SLNs not simply by a mechanical filtering process, but rather by active phagocytosis of colloid particles into cells lining the lymphatic sinuses within the SLN.[17] This persistent radioactivity in an SLN allows the gamma probe to be used for what is perhaps its most important function in the SLN biopsy procedure: to confirm the identity of any node thought likely to be an SLN. If the node is blue-stained, with a blue-stained afferent lymphatic, and is also found to be hot with a gamma probe, it can be concluded with complete certainty that it is indeed a true SLN. If blue staining is absent or dubious, and the node is not hot with the gamma probe, it is almost certainly not an SLN. For a variety of reasons, the SLN may not be obviously blue-stained.[14,18] It is very rare, however, for a node that is a true SLN not to contain detectable radioactive colloid for up to 30 hours following injection of radiolabeled tracer (if technetium-99m is the label used).[14] It may be 1–2 hours, however, before the intradermal isotope injected at the primary melanoma site is detectable in the SLN, making it possible for an SLN to be blue but not hot, when surgery is undertaken before 2 hours have elapsed (since the blue dye may travel to the SLN much more quickly than the radiolabeled colloid).

When use of a gamma probe in the selective SLN biopsy procedure was first introduced, it was proposed that the isotope be injected immediately preoperatively, either alone or in combination with the blue dye.[19,20] This proved, however, to be less satisfactory than injecting the isotope several hours preoperatively.[14,21] It has now become clear that a single isotope injection for both preoperative LSG and intraoperative SLN identification is not only more efficient but also cost-effective, and diminishes radiation exposure to both patient and operating-room staff by avoiding the need for a second injection of radioisotope in the immediate preoperative period, after a previous lymphoscintigram. Logistics are greatly simplified because the LSG can, if necessary, be performed on an outpatient basis the day before a planned selective SLN biopsy procedure; even after 24 hours, there will be sufficient residual radioactivity in the SLNs to allow their identification during surgery using a gamma probe. Further advantages of an interval of many hours between isotope injection and surgery are improved differentiation between SLNs and non-SLNs, and diminished residual radioactivity at the injection site. The latter is particularly

advantageous in cases involving a primary injection site that is close to the draining lymph-node field, which is often the case for head and neck melanomas. In these cases, this residual radioactivity may interfere with gamma-probe SLN identification.

One of the greatest advantages of using a gamma probe is that detection of gamma radiation, measured in counts per second, is completely objective, whereas confident detection of blue staining of a lymph node can sometimes be difficult and is thus less reliable. It is this less objective nature of lymphatic mapping and SLN identification with blue dye that has led to suggestions that its use might become unnecessary. The problem, however, is that it is readily demonstrable that second-tier nodes (i.e., nodes that are not SLNs) in a regional lymph-node field can sometimes become hot quite quickly after isotope injection.[12,13,22] A technique that relies on a gamma probe alone to identify SLNs is therefore likely to result in the removal of a number of additional, non-SLNs. This defeats the principal purpose of the SLN biopsy procedure, which is to be extremely selective and avoid unnecessary disturbance of lymphatic channels and lymph nodes in the lymph-node field.

Using the gamma probe to check for residual hot nodes

Nodes containing some radioactivity that remain after removal of the presumed SLN(s) are usually second-tier nodes.[23] In most cases, their status as second-tier nodes can be confirmed by a lack of staining when they are exposed, and the absence of any blue-stained afferent lymphatic draining directly from the primary melanoma site. The degree of residual activity in a node field must be assessed in relation to the activity that was present in the SLN, and is of course dependent upon the time that has elapsed since isotope was injected at the primary melanoma site. It is clearly important to assess the ratio of counts in a given node to the count in the remainder of the lymph-node field, rather than basing judgments on absolute levels of radioactivity. There has been considerable discussion at scientific meetings and in the literature on the subject of how to identify an SLN reliably with a gamma probe. It has been suggested, for example, that the ratio of counts in SLNs and non-SLNs after their removal should be greater than 3 : 1.[24] It is, however, undesirable to remove non-SLNs for the reasons already given, making this method of assessment inappropriate. Others have suggested comparing SLN activity with "background" activity, but without specifying how background levels are to be determined. The proposal from our own unit has been that the ratio of SLN activity ex vivo to residual activity in the node field after removal of the SLN should be greater than 3 : 1.[14] This ratio is usually greatly exceeded, but it provides a useful lower level, below which the likelihood of a node being a true SLN is very small. Thus, on checking a node field with a gamma probe after removal of all presumed SLNs, if a node with activity of more than three times the activity elsewhere in the node field is found, it is recommended that this node should be regarded as another possible SLN and removed for histologic examination, even when not apparently blue-stained.

ADVANTAGES OF A COMBINED BLUE-DYE AND GAMMA PROBE TECHNIQUE FOR SLN IDENTIFICATION

The original technique of intraoperative SLN identification developed by Morton et al involved the use of blue dye only. Influenced by Morton's work, as described in his publications, in his presentations at scientific meetings, and during his demonstrations of SLN biopsy procedures to those who visited him at the John Wayne Cancer Institute in Santa Monica, other pioneers of the technique performed their initial studies using the same blue-dye method.[8–10] It was not until some time later that the use of a gamma probe for intraoperative SLN identification was reported.[14,19,20,25]

This sequential introduction of the two techniques provided the opportunity for a number of institutions to compare their SLN biopsy experience using blue dye alone with their experience using a combined blue-dye and gamma probe technique. These institutions found that, without exception, a higher rate of confident SLN identification was achieved when the combined technique was used. Using the experiences of the Sydney Melanoma Unit as an example, in the initial series of patients in whom blue-dye mapping alone was used, successful SLN identification was achieved in 87% of patients.[9] The identification rate currently achieved using a combined blue-dye and gamma probe technique is of the order of 98% (author's unpublished data).

Bostick et al, reporting experience with melanomas of the head and neck treated at the John Wayne Cancer Institute,[26] reported an accuracy rate of 92% for SLN identification using blue dye only. The accuracy rate improved to 96% when blue dye and a gamma probe were used in combination. It is generally acknowledged that SLN identification in the neck is more difficult than in node fields elsewhere in the body, and the probe was found to be particularly useful in identifying SLNs in difficult sites such as the occipital, parotid, and postauricular regions. In a more recently reported melanoma study, Bostick et al achieved an SLN identification rate of 98% in lymphatic fields that were mapped using both blue dye and a gamma probe. These improved results were attributed mainly to use of the combined mapping modalities in a complementary fashion.[27]

Similarly, Pijpers et al[25] from the Free University Hospital in Amsterdam, Albertini et al[24] from the H Lee Moffit Cancer Center in Florida, Kapteijn et al[28] from the Netherlands Cancer Institute in Amsterdam, Leong et al[29] from the UCSF/Mount Zion Medical Center in San Francisco, and Gershenwald et al[30] from the MD Anderson Cancer Center in Houston all reported higher SLN identification rates using a gamma probe in conjunction with blue-dye mapping than had previously been achieved with blue dye only in their respective institutions.

More recently, Gennari et al[31] from the

European Institute of Oncology in Milan reported SLN identification success rates of 80% using blue dye only, but 98.7% using a combined blue-dye and gamma probe technique. Similarly, Wong et al[32] from the University of Hawaii School of Medicine reported that the use of blue dye alone gave a successful SLN identification rate of 72%, which increased to 97% with concurrent use of a gamma probe intraoperatively.

Data from two large multicenter studies are likewise convincing. In an important publication validating the accuracy of intraoperative SLN identification across multiple institutions worldwide, Morton et al reported a technical success rate of 95.2% for blue dye alone versus 99.1% for blue dye plus a gamma probe ($p = 0.014$).[33] Documenting the experience of participating World Health Organization (WHO) Melanoma Program centers, Cascinelli et al reported SLN identification rates of 78% and 91% for the axilla and groin, respectively, using blue dye only, compared with 86% and 97% respectively when blue dye plus an intraoperative gamma probe were used.[34]

Although the above results are likely to be biased because the early, learning-phase experience in most institutions was with blue dye alone, whereas the later experience was with the combined technique, the consistently better results achieved with the combined technique indicate clearly it is currently the most reliable procedure for intraoperative SLN identification.

CONCLUSION

Intraoperative SLN identification is sometimes a technically difficult procedure, and any maneuvers that allow it to be performed more efficiently and reliably should be employed whenever possible. All of the available evidence now indicates that as well as a carefully performed preoperative lymphoscintigram, the use of blue-dye mapping together with gamma probe identification ensures that the greatest possible accuracy is achieved. Even after experience with many hundreds of procedures,

cases will be encountered regularly where use of either blue dye alone or a gamma probe alone is not sufficient to identify an SLN with complete confidence. The risks of wrongly identifying a second-tier node as an SLN, or of missing a true SLN, are markedly reduced when both techniques are used, so that reliable SLN identification rates approaching 100% can be achieved by a surgeon with appropriate training and experience. Those undertaking selective SLN biopsy should never lose sight of the fundamental purpose of the procedure, which is to obtain accurate staging information. Unless the correct nodes are removed, the possibility exists that the staging will be inaccurate, and the patient's management compromised as a consequence.

REFERENCES

1. Morton DL, Bostick PJ, Will the true sentinel node please stand? *Ann Surg Oncol* 1999; **6**:12–14.
2. Thompson JF, Uren RF, What is a 'sentinel' lymph node? *Eur J Surg Oncol* 2000; **26**:103–4.
3. Uren RF, Howman-Giles R, Thompson JF et al, Interval nodes: the forgotten sentinel nodes in melanoma patients. *Arch Surg* 2000; **135**:1168–72.
4. Uren RF, Thompson JF, Howman-Giles RB, The history of lymphatic mapping. In: Uren RF, Thompson JF, Howman-Giles RB, eds, *Lymphatic Drainage of the Skin and Breast: Locating the Sentinel Nodes,* 21–28. Harwood: Amsterdam, 1999.
5. Morton DL, Chan AD, The concept of sentinel node localization: how it started. *Semin Nucl Med* 2000; **30**:4–10.
6. Morton DL, Wen DR, Wong JH et al, Technical details of intraoperative lymphatic mapping of early stage melanoma. *Arch Surg* 1992; **127**:392–9.
7. Wong JH, Cagle LA, Morton DL, Lymphatic drainage of skin to a sentinel node in a feline model. *Ann Surg* 1991; **214**: 637–41.
8. Reintgen DS, Cruse CW, Wells K et al, The orderly progression of melanoma nodal metastases. *Ann Surg* 1994; **220**:759–67.
9. Thompson JF, McCarthy WH, Bosch CMJ et al, Sentinel lymph node status as an indicator of the presence of metastatic melanoma in regional lymph nodes. *Melanoma Res* 1995; **5**:255–60.
10. Karakousis CP, Velez AF, Spellman JE, Scarozza

J, The technique of sentinel node biopsy. *Eur J Surg Oncol* 1996; **22**:271–5.

11. Thompson JF, Sentinel node biopsy. *J Surg Oncol* 1997; **66**:270–2.

12. Uren RF, Howman-Giles RB, Thompson JF et al, Variability of cutaneous lymphatic flow rates. *Melanoma Res* 1998; **8**:279–82.

13. McCarthy WH, Thompson JF, Uren RF, Invited commentary on article by Krag DN, Meijer SJ, Weaver DL et al, Minimal access surgery for staging malignant melanoma. *Arch Surg* 1995; **130**:659–60.

14. Thompson JF, Niewind P, Uren RF et al, Single dose isotope injection for both preoperative lymphoscintigraphy and intraoperative sentinel lymph node identification in melanoma patients. *Melanoma Res* 1997; **6**:500–6.

15. Uren RF, Howman-Giles RB, Shaw HM et al, Lymphoscintigraphy in high risk melanoma of the trunk; predicting draining node groups, defining lymphatic channels and locating the sentinel node. *J Nucl Med* 1993; **34**:1435–40.

16. Uren RF, Howman-Giles R, Thompson JF et al, Lymphoscintigraphy to identify sentinel lymph nodes in patients with melanoma. *Melanoma Res* 1994; **4**:395–9.

17. Uren RF, Thompson JF, Howman-Giles RB, Lymphatics. In: Uren RF, Thompson JF, Howman-Giles RB, eds, *Lymphatic Drainage of the Skin and Breast: Locating the Sentinel Nodes*, 1–20. Harwood: Amsterdam, 1999.

18. Pijpers R, Borgstein PJ, Meijer SJ et al, Sentinel node biopsy in melanoma patients: dynamic lymphoscintigraphy followed by intraoperative gamma probe and vital dye guidance. *World J Surg* 1997; **21**:788–92.

19. Essner R, Foshag L, Morton DL, Intraoperative radiolymphoscintigraphy: a useful adjuvant to intraoperative lymphatic mapping and selective lymphadenectomy in patients with clinical stage 1 melanoma. Presented at the Society of Surgical Oncology, 47th Annual Meeting, Houston, 1994.

20. Krag DN, Meijer SJ, Weaver DL et al, Minimal access surgery for staging malignant melanoma. *Arch Surg* 1995; **130**:654–8.

21. Essner R, Bostick PJ, Glass EC, Standardized probe-directed sentinel node dissection in melanoma. *Surgery* 2000; **127**:26–31.

22. Uren RF, Howman-Giles RB, Thompson JF, Variation in cutaneous lymphatic flow rates. *Ann Surg Oncol* 1997; **4**:279–80.

23. Uren RF, Howman-Giles RB, Thompson JF, Demonstration of second tier lymph nodes during preoperative lymphoscintigraphy for melanoma: incidence varies with primary tumor site. *Ann Surg Oncol* 1998; **5**:517–21.

24. Albertini JJ, Cruse CW, Rapaport D et al, Intraoperative radiolymphoscintigraphy improves sentinel lymph node identification for patients with melanoma. *Ann Surg* 1996; **223**:217–24.

25. Pijpers R, Collet GJ, Meijer S, Hoekstra OS, The impact of dynamic lymphoscintigraphy and gamma probe guidance on sentinel node biopsy in melanoma. *Eur J Nucl Med* 1995; **22**:1238–41.

26. Bostick P, Essner R, Sarantou T et al, Intraoperative lymphatic mapping for early-stage melanoma of the head and neck. *Am J Surg* 1997; **174**:536–9.

27. Bostick P, Essner R, Glass E et al, Comparison of intraoperative lymphatic mapping in melanoma to identify sentinel nodes in 100 lymphatic basins. *Arch Surg* 1999; **134**:43–9.

28. Kapteijn BA, Nieweg OE, Liem IH et al, Localizing the sentinel node in cutaneous melanoma: gamma probe detection versus blue dye. *Ann Surg Oncol* 1997; **4**:156–60.

29. Leong SPL, Steinmetz I, Habib FA et al, Optimal selective sentinel lymph node dissection in primary malignant melanoma. *Arch Surg* 1997; **132**:666–73.

30. Gershenwald JE, Tseng CH, Thompson W et al, Improved sentinel node localization in patients with primary melanoma with the use of radiolabeled colloid. *Surgery* 1998; **124**:203–10.

31. Gennari R, Stoldt HS, Bartolomei M et al, Sentinel node localisation: a new prospective in the treatment of nodal melanoma metastases. *Int J Oncol* 1999; **15**:25–32.

32. Wong JH, Steinemann S, Yonehara C et al, Sentinel node staging for cutaneous melanoma in a university-affiliated community care setting. *Ann Surg Oncol* 2000; **7**:450–5.

33. Morton DL, Thompson JF, Essner R et al, Validation of the accuracy in a multicenter trial of intraoperative lymphatic mapping and SLN lymphadenectomy for early-stage melanoma. *Ann Surg* 1999; **230**:453–65.

34. Cascinelli N, Belli F, Santinami M et al, Sentinel lymph node biopsy in cutaneous melanoma: the WHO Melanoma Program experience. *Ann Surg Oncol* 2000; **7**:469–74.

10

How we do it: the H Lee Moffitt Cancer Center approach

Douglas Reintgen and C Wayne Cruse

CONTENTS   Lymphatic mapping for melanoma   •   The H Lee Moffitt Cancer Center technique   •   Talking points from the lymphatic mapping experience of the H Lee Moffitt Cancer Center   •   Radiation exposure guidelines and policies

---

The H Lee Moffitt Cancer Center technique for SLN biopsy in melanoma

Technique	Combination	**Isotope**	*Type*: Tc-99m-SC
Dye	*Type*: Isosulfan blue dye		*Filtered*: Yes (0.2-μm filter)
	Volume: 1 ml (cc) per		*Dose*: 0.45 mCi (17 MBq)
	direction of drainage		*Volume*: 1 ml (cc)/direction of
			drainage
Injection site	*Isotope*: Intradermal		
	Dye: Intradermal		

Melanoma is a tumor that affects individuals who are young and at the most productive years of their lives, constituting a major public health problem. There is a melanoma epidemic in the United States and the rest of the world, and most physicians will continue to see more patients with melanoma as part of their practices. In the year 2000 an estimated 42 000 new melanoma cases will be diagnosed in the USA, and an estimated 7500 melanoma-related deaths will occur.[1]

The presence or absence of lymph-node metastases is the most powerful predictor of survival for patients with melanoma. Once patients develop metastatic melanoma to their regional nodes, prognostic factors based on the primary melanoma contribute very little to the prognostic model. The presence of lymph-node metastases decreases the 5-year survival rate of patients by approximately 40%, compared with those who have no evidence of nodal metastases. Much time, effort, and expense have been applied to the identification of prognostic factors based on the primary tumor. Yet, in multiple regression analysis performed on many collected populations in the literature, the lymph-node status of the patient with melanoma is by far the most powerful factor for predicting recurrence and survival. It makes sense to concentrate on obtaining an accurate nodal stage of patients with melanoma.

The standard of care for patients with melanoma has changed due to technological innovation and new research findings. These innovations include the development of new lymphatic mapping techniques to reduce the cost and morbidity of nodal staging, the emergence of more sensitive assays for occult melanoma metastases, and the identification of interferon alfa-2b as an effective adjuvant therapy for the treatment of patients with melanoma at high risk for recurrence.[2] This chapter describes the technique of lymphatic mapping as it is practiced for patients with melanoma at the H Lee Moffitt Cancer Center.

LYMPHATIC MAPPING FOR MELANOMA

A new procedure has been developed to assess the status of the regional lymph nodes more accurately and decrease the morbidity to patients of a complete elective lymph node dissection. The technique, termed "intraoperative lymphatic mapping and selective lymphadenectomy," relies on the concept that regions of the skin have specific patterns of lymphatic drainage not only to the regional lymphatic basin, but also to a specific lymph node in the basin—the sentinel lymph node (SLN). Morton pioneered the technique using vital blue dye and showed that in animals and initial human trials, the SLN is the first node in the lymphatic basin into which the primary melanoma consistently drains.[3,4] The use of the blue-dye method provides the surgeon with a visual clue to the whereabouts of these first nodes in the chain of lymphatics. David Krag was the first to report the use of an intraoperative radiocolloid method and hand-held gamma detectors to help locate the SLN.[5] The H Lee Moffitt Cancer Center (MCC) group were the first to describe the combination mapping technique,[6] a technique that uses both a vital blue dye and radiocolloid and is able to decrease the learning curve and increase the success rate of SLN localization to a level exceeding 99%. The combination mapping technique is almost universally accepted as the standard for SLN biopsy for melanoma and other solid malignancies throughout the world.

THE H LEE MOFFITT CANCER CENTER TECHNIQUE

Preoperative lymphoscintigraphy to define all regional nodal basins at risk for disease

Lymphoscintigraphy (LSG) has been shown to help predict lymphatic basins at risk for the development of metastatic disease in patients with cutaneous malignant melanoma.[7] To further establish the efficacy of this method, 212 patients presenting to the MCC with primary melanoma of the head, neck, and trunk have been studied. Drainage patterns identified by lymphoscintigraphy were compared with those predicted by historical anatomic guidelines and were found to be discordant in 63% of patients with tumors of the head and neck, and in 32% of those with primary lesions located on the trunk. Operative intervention was changed because of these findings in 47% of all patients, with 19% undergoing dissection of nonclassical lymph-node basins. An additional 28% did not have a node dissection because of failure of the scintigram to demonstrate a predominant drainage basin or the demonstration of multiple drainage sites. This series has now been updated to include over 2000 mappings, with a mean follow-up of 5 years. During this period, 85% of all the recurrence of melanoma should occur, yet there have been no recurrences in any basins not predicted to be at risk by LSG. This simple test provides an extremely accurate depiction of all basins at risk for metastatic disease. The lymphatic drainage from cutaneous melanoma of the head, neck, and trunk cannot be reliably predicted by clinical judgement or classic anatomic guidelines, and LSG is indicated in these patients prior to SLN biopsy.[8] This nuclear medicine test is also performed for patients with extremity melanoma, since approximately 5% of these patients will have an in-transit epitrochlear or popliteal node that by definition is the first node in the chain and the SLN.

The preoperative LSG serves as a "road map" for the surgeon and is used at MCC for four distinct reasons in planning the surgical procedure. These include:

- identification of all nodal basins at risk for metastatic disease
- identification of any in-transit nodes that can be tattooed by the nuclear medicine physician for later harvesting
- identification of the location of the SLN in relation to the rest of the nodes in the basin[9]
- estimation of the number of SLNs in the basin.

Choice of vital blue dye

Morton and colleagues investigated a number of dyes for their potential applicability for cutaneous lymphatic mapping. These included methylene blue, isosulfan blue (1% in aqueous solution), Patent Blue-V, cyalume, and fluorescein dye. All substances tested were known to be nontoxic in vivo and were injected intradermally as provided by the supplier. The Patent Blue-V and isosulfan blue dyes produced the best results among the substances tested for their accuracy in identifying the regional lymphatic drainage pattern in the cat.[10] Both dyes rapidly entered the lymphatics with minimal diffusion into the surrounding tissue; their bright blue color was readily visible and allowed easy identification of the exposed lymphatics. Isosulfan blue has worked extremely well for intraoperative SLN mapping and is the compound of choice at MCC. In some patients with thin skin, the afferent lymphatics can be seen through the skin after the injection of isosulfan blue. Additionally, upon entering the lymph node, the vital blue dye stains part of the node a pale blue, which is easily discernible from the surrounding non-SLNs.

In contrast, the other dyes were abandoned after proving unsatisfactory because of their rapid diffusion into surrounding tissue and insufficient retention by the lymphatic channels to stain the SLN. Morton and colleagues found that the fluorescent dyes fluorescein and cyalume required a dark room for optimal visualization. Additionally, because of their diffusion into the surrounding tissue, background

fluorescence made these agents unacceptable. Methylene blue proved to be poorly retained by the lymphatics, and thus the SLN stained lightly.

The use of the vital blue dyes has been void of any significant complications. Minor allergic reactions have been rare and consist of rashes or "blue" hives. More serious anaphylactic reactions are even less common, but have been reported.[11,12] There can be retention of the blue dye at the primary site for over a year with gradual fading of the dye with time. Patients can be left with a permanent tattoo, however, if the injected dye is not removed with the wide-local excision of the primary site. Fortunately, in the head and neck area, where a permanent tattoo would be unacceptable, the richness of the cutaneous lymphatics allows rapid clearance of the blue dye from the skin and subcutaneous tissues. A small amount of residual dye left behind after the wide-local excision has not been a problem and has rapidly disappeared.

All patients report the presence of dye in the urine during the first 24 hours, and the dye can interfere with transcutaneous oxygen monitoring during anesthesia.

Choice of radiocolloid

Little work has been performed to determine which radiocolloid is most optimally suited for either preoperative or intraoperative mapping. The ideal radiocolloid for intraoperative SLN mapping should have the characteristics of a proper particle size and stability that would readily be taken up by the cutaneous lymphatics and deposited and perhaps trapped or concentrated in the SLN. A uniform dispersion of small particles (<100 nm) is necessary for the colloid to translocate from the intradermal injection site to the lymphatic channels and the SLN. The ideal radiocolloid should also have a short half-life that would not complicate the handling of the excised specimen. Technetium-99m-labeled compounds, because they are gamma emitters, satisfy most of these requirements. In a direct comparison between filtered (0.1-μm) Tc-99m-sulfur colloid (Tc-99m-SC) and Tc-99m-antimony sulfur colloid (Tc-99m-ASC) (3–30 nm), it was found that the filtered Tc-99m-SC showed a faster transport rate to the nodal basin and a lower radiation dosimetry for liver, spleen, and whole body compared with Tc-99m-ASC. Unfiltered Tc-99m-SC has a relatively large particle size (100–1000 nm), and particle migration from the injection site in some series is slower. Other investigators have found, however, that this radiocolloid is slow to flow through the first SLN to higher secondary nodes, which is advantageous.[13]

In comparisons of the quality of the lymphoscintigrams between Tc-99m-human serum albumin (Tc-99m-HSA), Tc-99m-stannous phytate and Tc-99m-ASC, the latter colloid gave the superior images[14] for preoperative LSG. In a direct comparison between Tc-99m-HSA and filtered Tc-99m-SC in an animal model, it was found that the Tc-99m-SC was actually concentrated in the SLN over a period of 1–2 hours, while the Tc-99m-HSA rapidly passed through the SLN.[15] The ability of the SLN to concentrate the Tc-99m-SC provided better localization ratios at the time of intraoperative mapping, increased the success rate of localization, made the technique easier, and was thus a superior reagent.[15,16]

Others have used the unfiltered Tc-99m-SC. This colloid gives very good intraoperative mapping results. The planar imaging for LSG was poor, however, and investigators were unable to identify cutaneous lymphatic flow to any basin in 10% of the patients.[17]

Clinicians at MCC have recommended the use of filtered Tc-99m-SC prepared using a 0.2-μm filter. This particle size gives good images on LSG and is trapped and concentrated in the SLN over a period of time, so that the "hot spot" of activity in the SLN actually increases compared to surrounding tissue for 2–24 hours after injection, making the SLN easier to find. This particle size also has an advantage if the primary site is close to the regional basin or is located in a direct line with the basin so that "shine-through" is a problem (e.g., scapular melanomas mapping to the axilla). The use of filtered radiocolloid produces more uniform and smaller particles so that more of the radio-colloid will migrate to the SLN, theoretically reducing shine-through. One must keep in mind that only 1–5% of the injected activity from the primary site is delivered to the SLNs. Even if a wide-local excision is performed first, there may be so much shine-through activity from the primary site that finding the SLN in the basin is next to impossible with radiocolloid mapping alone. In such instances, the use of blue dye becomes more important.

Technique of intraoperative lymphatic mapping

The timing of the injection of the mapping reagents is critical to the success of the procedure. Compounds such as the vital blue dyes travel to the regional basin within a matter of minutes, while most radiocolloids are concentrated over hours in the SLN. Localization ratios for Tc-99m-SC are greatest 2–24 hours after injection, which is helpful to the surgeon in three ways. The increased ratios of radioactive counts (hot spot/background, SLN/neighboring non-SLN) allow for easier localization. The prolonged retention in the SLN permits the radiocolloid to be injected by a nuclear radiologist, hours prior to the actual operation; accordingly, the actual injection can be performed in the nuclear medicine area, and surgeons do not need to obtain special licenses for radioactivity handling. Finally, scheduling of cases becomes more convenient, as there is a long period (2–24 hours after injection of the radiocolloid) during which intraoperative mapping can be easily accomplished.

Patients at MCC come to the nuclear medicine suite early on the day of the surgery and undergo preoperative LSG with the injection of 0.45 mCi (17 MBq) of filtered Tc-99m-SC around the primary site. Dynamic scans are performed 5–10 minutes after the injection of the radiocolloid, and the location of the SLN is marked in the basin with an intradermal tattoo. All lymphatic basins at risk for metastatic spread, in-transit nodes, and SLNs in the regional basin are identified and marked for harvesting. The patient is then taken to the operating room from

2–24 hours later and 1 ml (cc) per direction of drainage of 1% isosulfan blue dye is injected around the primary site. After prepping and draping the primary site and regional basin and allowing 10 minutes for the vital blue dye to travel to the SLN, attention is directed initially to the regional basin. With the hand-held gamma probe, the hot spot in the regional basin is identified, and the hot spot/background ratio is noted. If shine-through from the primary site is a problem, the wide-local excision of the primary may be performed first. An incision is made over the hot spot, and small flaps are created in all directions to allow identification of the blue-stained afferent lymphatics. Surgical dissection is aided both by visualization of the stained afferent lymphatic down to the blue-stained node and by a directed dissection with the use of the hand-held gamma probe down to the SLN. At times, the surgeon can be confused as to what is proximal or distal on the afferent lymphatic, and the probe can be used to identify the direction of the dissection. The SLN is identified and removed with sharp or electrocautery dissection. The entire SLN is removed, and afferent and efferent lymphatics from the SLN, some of which are identified with blue staining, are controlled with hemostatic clips, since electrocautery does not seal the lymphatics. This technique decreases the chance of postoperative wound seroma.

The excised SLN is checked with the gamma probe to ascertain whether it is radioactive in order to correctly identify it as the SLN. The radioactivity in the basin is checked with the gamma probe after removal of the SLN to assure that all SLNs have been removed. If radioactivity has not decreased to background levels, use of the hand-held gamma probe to direct dissection will minimize unnecessary flap creation while looking for additional blue-stained afferent lymphatics.

A secondary benefit of radiocolloid mapping is immediate verification that all the SLNs have been removed from the basin. The radioactivity counts will return to background level once the radiolabeled lymph nodes are removed. This avoids the additional dissection necessary to verify that all SLNs have been excised when using the blue dye alone. In addition, the colloid has a much longer retention time than blue dye and may be concentrated in the SLN. Studies from MCC and Henry Ford Hospital have shown that the localization ratios double if the harvest occurs 2–6 hours after the injection of the radiocolloid compared with performing the mapping immediately after the injection of the radiocolloid.[6,15]

After harvesting, the SLN is then submitted for a detailed histologic examination that may include serial sectioning, immunohistochemical (IHC) staining, or the use of molecular biology assays for occult metastases. It cannot be emphasized enough that successful intraoperative SLN mapping requires close collaboration between the surgeon, nuclear radiologist, and pathologist. Each member of the team has a critical role. Lymphoscintigraphy is needed to provide a map for the surgeon and identify all basins at risk. The pathologist must perform a detailed examination of the SLN to take full advantage of the lymphatic mapping procedure. Attempts to perform this technique without appropriate support in place will result in lower success rates of localization and may harm the patient by providing inaccurate nodal staging. Inaccurate lymph-node staging may preclude a patient from receiving the benefit of adjuvant interferon alfa-2b therapy[2] or completion lymphadenectomy.

How does one define an SLN in terms of the amount of radioactivity accumulated? Clinicians must use ratios of activity when using radioguided surgery to find the SLN. Investigators at MCC have defined the SLN as having activity ratios of 3 : 1 (radioactivity in the SLN/background) in vivo or a ratio of 10 : 1 (activity in the SLN/neighboring non-SLN) ex vivo. Radioactivity ratios must be used since a number of variables exist with each harvest, namely, the amount of injected radioactivity at the primary site, the time interval between the injection and the harvest, the distance between the primary site and the regional basin, and the shine-through from the primary site and the regional basin.

Experience has shown that 98% of what MCC clinicians call an SLN have the above-mentioned ratios. A corollary is that when the opportunity presents itself without increasing the morbidity of the operation, the surgeon should try to remove a neighboring non-SLN as an internal control. This procedure allows the ex vivo ratio to be calculated, which is most meaningful since all shine-through is eliminated. Data generated from the Sunbelt Melanoma Trial help the surgeon to determine when the SLN dissection is complete. This trial has shown that if one removes all nodes in the basin that have activity within 10% of the hottest node, then 98% of SLNs that contain tumor will have been removed.[17]

Which patients are candidates for lymphatic mapping and SLN biopsy?

Women with melanomas less than 0.76 mm in thickness have less than a 1% chance of having nodal spread of their disease. Sentinel lymph-node biopsy is not indicated in this population. Patients with melanoma and tumor thickness between 0.76–1.0 mm have a 6% chance of having nodal metastases when lymphatic mapping is done, and a more detailed examination of the SLN with S-100 staining is performed. Patients in this subgroup can be given a choice of having their regional nodal basins sampled with this low-morbidity procedure. Prognostic factors have been identified for patients with "thin" melanomas who may be at greater risk of metastatic disease. Patients with tumors classified as Clark's Level IV or greater, patients with ulcerated primaries or regressed lesions, men, and patients who have axial melanomas have been shown to be at a greater risk of metastases and death at 5 years, approximately in the 10% range.[18] These patients should be treated as if they have thicker lesions, and their SLN should be harvested, even if the primary melanoma is less than 0.76 mm in thickness.

Patients with thick (>4.0 mm) melanomas have such a high rate of occult systemic metastases (70%) along with an increased rate of occult nodal metastases (60–70%) that procedures on the regional nodes (elective lymph-node dissection) have not been recommended

in the past because of the lack of survival benefit. Disease would frequently recur and these patients would die of systemic disease despite an elective lymph-node dissection that removed occult metastases. With the advent of effective adjuvant therapy, however, SLN procedures should be offered to these patients as a staging procedure. Patients with thick melanomas who also have documented nodal microscopic disease have a worse survival than patients with thick melanomas and no sign of nodal spread.[19] These patients (T4N1) were also in the subset of patients who benefited from adjuvant interferon alfa-2b.

Another question to be answered is what constitutes the standard of surgical care for the patient with melanomas greater than 1.0 mm in thickness. With the reported evidence that the histology of the SLN reflects the histology of the other nodes in the basin and with the consensus opinion from the World Health Organization, there is no need for elective lymph-node dissection if the surgeons has adequate support from nuclear medicine and pathology services. In communities and centers that do not have such collaboration in place, in circumstances in which intraoperative mapping cannot be performed (for example, when a previous wide-local excision of the primary melanoma has already been performed), or when the results of the mapping are equivocal, then the guidelines for elective lymph-node dissection from the Intergroup Melanoma Surgical Trial should be used.[20] If this approach is taken, however, the elective lymph-node dissection should also be directed by preoperative LSG.

TALKING POINTS FROM THE LYMPHATIC MAPPING EXPERIENCE OF THE H LEE MOFFITT CANCER CENTER

It is evident that lymphatic mapping technology has changed the standard of surgical care for melanoma. As the tumor thickness of the lesion increases, the chance of having a positive SLN also increases, so that patients with melanomas that are 0.76–1.0 mm, 1.0–1.5 mm,

1.5–4.0 mm, and greater than 4 mm, in depth will have positive SLNs with a frequency of 5.3%, 8%, 19%, and 29%, respectively, if routine histology and IHC are used to examine the SLN. We give patients with melanoma tumor thickness of 0.76–1.0 mm the choice of having the SLN harvested versus observation, and quote the 6.0% incidence of occult metastases. Invariably patients elect to have the SLN biopsy despite the relatively low risk of occult nodal metastases, since the morbidity of the procedure is low and the treatment recommendations are radically different if occult metastases are found.

Patients with a positive SLN are recommended to undergo a complete lymph-node dissection. When using only the vital blue dye for the harvesting process, the mean number of SLNs removed per basin dissected was 1.3, and the proportion of patients with positive nodes on the complete lymph-node dissection after a positive SLN biopsy was 22%. With the incorporation of radiocolloid mapping, the mean number of SLNs removed was 1.8 per basin dissected, but the number of patients with more nodes positive on complete lymph-node dissection after a positive SLN decreased to 6%. If metastatic disease exists in the regional basin, it is confined to the SLN 94% of the time. Evidently, the use of a combination mapping technique removes more SLNs, some of which are important since they contain metastatic disease. In fact, the MCC experience shows that no patient with a melanoma less than 2.8 mm in thickness has more than the SLN involved with disease. It is suggested that a melanoma has to reach a certain thickness before it sheds off enough cells to involve more than the SLN with disease. This hypothesis was recently supported by data from the MD Anderson Cancer Center and the Sydney Melanoma Unit, showing no positive higher nodes after a positive SLN biopsy for patients with melanomas less than 2.5 mm in thickness.

Clinicians at MCC are convinced that the blue dye, the radiocolloid, and the metastatic cells are trapped and concentrated in the SLN for a period of time. The finding of one side of the SLN being blue, or one side being hot, compared with the opposite side of the same node, argues for a confinement of the migrating mapping agents. The finding that one or more SLNs are the only sites of metastatic disease in 94% of the cases suggests that the metastatic cells are also trapped in the SLN for a period of time. Pass-through of the blue dye and the radiocolloid does occur, but not to the extent that it will make another higher node blue or another node hot with a 3 : 1 background ratio or a 10 : 1 ex vivo ratio of activity (SLN vs neighboring non-SLN). Again, these ratios would be necessary to define the higher node as an SLN. Pass-through of the radiocolloid does occur to a small degree, but as the mapping agent moves through the SLNs, it is distributed to multiple higher nodes. These will contribute to a higher background, but will not accumulate in a higher node to fulfill the criteria of an SLN.

The timing of the procedure in relation to the wide-local excision is critical to the success of the procedure. A series from MCC has compared the accuracy of the technique prior to and after wide-local excision, and it is apparent that the number of SLNs removed and the number of basins dissected are higher if mapping is performed after a wide-local excision compared to doing the SLN harvest at the same time as the wide-local excision. In addition, the "skip" metastases rate is thought to be increased. Trying to perform lymphatic mapping after a wide-local excision results in more extensive dissections than would have been necessary if the procedure was performed at the time of the wide-local excision. Patients with rotational flap closure and Z-plasty reconstruction are not considered candidates for mapping because of the extensive primary-site surgery. Physicians who perform the biopsies of suspicious pigmented lesions and who may be tempted to perform the wide-local excision as well must keep these facts in mind. With lymphatic mapping and SLN biopsy becoming the standard of care in the USA for the nodal staging of the melanoma, patient care cannot be compromised by primary-site surgery that is too extensive before lymphatic mapping.

Complications of the procedure are rare. All the SLN harvests are performed without any drainage, contributing to the lower morbidity of the procedure. Ten per cent of the patients will develop a seroma, but this is easily handled with percutaneous aspiration. Wound infections are rare, and wound healing is better compared with incisions made for elective lymph-node dissection, since large flaps are not created.

RADIATION EXPOSURE GUIDELINES AND POLICIES

The amount of injected radioactivity is minimal in comparison to the amount of radioactivity injected to perform a typical bone scan, and averages approximately 0.45 mCi. The radioactivity required for a bone scan is 20 mCi (740 MBq), or 44 times the dose for lymphatic mapping. For the first 100 cases, surgeons and pathologists at MCC wore radiation detection badges and rings during all parts of the procedure, and technicians from nuclear medicine swiped the areas in the operating room and pathology laboratory after each case. No significant exposure could be documented. Nuclear medicine technicians routinely enter the operating room to calibrate and run the gamma probes, and after removal of the specimen and processing by the surgeon, they handle the specimen and monitor its radioactivity as it is transported from the operating room to the pathology department. A separate room has been allocated for the intraoperative handling of the specimens. Sentinel lymph-node biopsies and primary sites are placed in formalin for 48 hours (eight half-lives of Tc-99m), stored in a refrigerator dedicated to this procedure, and removed later for routine processing.

Despite the experience at MCC in the handling of specimens, as investigators go back to their institutions to begin a program of lymphatic mapping, State regulatory policies must be checked and procedures put into place to meet each individual State's requirements. Clinicians may have to "reinvent the wheel" to convince the hospital and their colleagues that the SLN biopsy can be performed safely and does not result in any radioactivity exposure or health risk.

REFERENCES

1. Greenlee RT, Murray T, Bolden S, Wingo PA, Cancer statistics, 2000. *CA Cancer J Clin* 2000; **50**:7–33.
2. Kirkwood JM, Strawderman MH, Ernstoff MS et al, Interferon alfa-2b adjuvant therapy of high-risk resected cutaneous melanoma: the Eastern Cooperative Oncology Group Trial EST 1684. *J Clin Oncol* 1996; **14**:7–17.
3. Morton DL, Wen DR, Wong JH et al, Technical details of intraoperative lymphatic mapping for early stage melanoma. *Arch Surg* 1992; **127**:392–9.
4. Morton DL, Wen DR, Cochran AJ, Management of early-stage melanoma by intraoperative lymphatic mapping and selective lymphadenectomy or "watch and wait." *Surg Oncol Clin N Am* 1992; **1**:247–59.
5. Alex JC, Weaver DL, Fairbank JT et al, Gamma-probe-guided lymph node localization in malignant melanoma. *Surg Oncol* 1993; **2**:303–8.
6. Albertini J, Cruse CW, Rapaport D et al, Intraoperative radiolymphoscintigraphy improves sentinel lymph node identification in melanoma patients. *Ann Surg* 1996; **223**:217–24.
7. Norman J, Cruse CW, Wells K et al, A re-definition of skin lymphatic drainage by lymphoscintigraphy for malignant melanoma. *Am J Surg* 1991; **162**:432–7.
8. Meyer CM, Lecklitner ML, Logie JR et al, Technetium-99m sulfur-colloid cutaneous lymphoscintigraphy in the management of truncal melanoma. *Radiology* 1979; **131**:205–9.
9. Godellas CV, Berman C, Lyman G et al, The identification and mapping of melanoma regional nodal metastases: minimally invasive surgery for the diagnosis of nodal metastases. *Am Surg* 1995; **61**:97–101.
10. Wong JH, Cagle LA, Morton D, Lymphatic drainage of skin to a sentinel lymph node in a feline model. *Ann Surg* 1991; **214**:637–41,
11. Reintgen DS, Cruse CW, Berman C et al, An orderly progression of melanoma nodal metastases. *Ann Surg* 1994; **220**:759–67.
12. Ross M, Reintgen DS, Balch C. Selective lymphadenectomy: emerging role of lymphatic mapping and sentinel node biopsy in the management of early stage melanoma. *Semin Surg Oncol* 1993; **9**:219–23.
13. Tanabe KK, Lymphatic mapping and epitrochlear node dissection for melanoma. *Surgery* 1997; **121**:102–4.
14. Hung JC, Wiseman GA, Wahner HW et al,

Filtered technetium-99m-sulfur colloid evaluated for lymphoscintigraphy. *J Nucl Med* 1995; **36:**1895–900.

15. Nathanson SD, Anaya P, Eck L, Sentinel lymph node uptake of two different radio nuclides. Proceedings of The Society of Surgical Oncology, 49th Cancer Symposium, Atlanta 1996 (Abstract P64, page 53).

16. Krag DN, Meijer SJ, Weaver DL et al, Minimal-access surgery for staging of melanoma. *Arch Surg* 1995; **130:**654–60.

17. McMasters KM, Ross M, Edwards M et al, Sunbelt Melanoma Trial: How many radioactive sentinel lymph nodes (SLN) should be removed. Proceedings of The Society of Surgical Oncology, 52nd Annual Symposium, Orlando 1999 (Abstract P6, page 10).

18. Slingluff C, Vollmer R, Reintgen D, Seigler HF, Lethal thin malignant melanoma. *Ann Surg* 1988; **208:**150–61.

19. Heaton KM, Sussman JJ, Gershenwald JB et al, Surgical margins and prognostic factors in patients with thick (>4.0 mm) melanoma. *Ann Surg Oncol* 1998; **5:**322–8.

20. Balch CM, Soong S-J, Ross M et al, Long-term results of a multi institutional randomized trial comparing prognostic factors and surgical results for intermediate thickness melanomas (1.0–4 mm): Intergroup Melanoma Surgical Trial. *Ann Surg Oncol* 2000; **7:**87–97.

11

How we do it: The Netherlands Cancer Institute/Antoni van Leeuwenhoek Hospital approach

Omgo E Nieweg and Bin BR Kroon

CONTENTS   Patient selection • Lymphoscintigraphy • Surgical technique • Pathology • Results • Conclusion

The Netherlands Cancer Institute/Antoni van Leeuwenhoek Hospital technique for SLN biopsy in melanoma

Technique	Combination	Isotope	*Type*: Tc-99m-labeled human albumin colloid
Dye	*Type*: Patent Blue-V dye *Volume*: 1.0 ml (cc)		*Filtered*: No *Dose*: 60 MBq (1.6 mCi)
Injection site	*Isotope*: Intradermal *Dye*: Intradermal		*Volume*: 0.3 ml (cc)

Our interest in lymphatic mapping was raised when one of us witnessed the first sentinel lymph-node (SLN) biopsy outside the John Wayne Cancer Institute performed by Merrick I Ross at the MD Anderson Cancer Center in 1991. With interest and, admittedly, a fair dose of skepticism, the novel approach was introduced in Europe in 1993. At The Netherlands Cancer Institute, we believed that nuclear medicine had an important role in lymphatic mapping. The cooperation of the nuclear medicine physicians was solicited from the outset, and the gamma probe, then gathering dust, was given new purpose.

The aim of this chapter is to share the perti-

nent features of lymphatic mapping and SLN biopsy as it is performed at The Netherlands Cancer Institute. Various aspects of the technique are described and illustrated by our experience in over 200 such procedures in melanoma patients over a 7-year period.

PATIENT SELECTION

Lymphatic mapping provides important prognostic information. The 3-year survival rate in our patients is 93% when the SLN is tumor-negative and a mere 67% when it is tumor-positive.[1] Any benefit from early regional lymph-node dissection, however, is not apparent at this stage. Improvement in survival and regional tumor control have not been shown. These crucial issues are being addressed in clinical trials, but a potential survival benefit can be calculated to be small at best. What one can say is that the procedure is probably not worthwhile in patients with a thin melanoma because the risk of dissemination from such a lesion is small.

Conflicting data on the use of lymphatic mapping in the selection of patients for adjuvant systemic treatment have emerged, and adjuvant systemic treatment is not generally recommended at this time. Lymphatic mapping should be required in future studies of adjuvant treatment because of its value in staging melanoma patients. Accordingly, it is impossible to describe sound indications for lymphatic mapping in melanoma as yet. The procedure is still restricted to the context of clinical trials and is not part of standard care in Europe.[2]

LYMPHOSCINTIGRAPHY

Lymphatic mapping with selective lymphadenectomy requires a concerted effort from nuclear medicine physicians and surgeons. Lymphoscintigraphy is an essential first step and serves four purposes: it points out the draining lymph-node field; it indicates the number of SLNs and distinguishes them from secondary nodes; it enables the nuclear medicine physician to mark the location of the SLN on the skin; and, further, it identifies interval SLNs outside a lymph-node field (such aberrant SLNs occur in some 5% of patients and would escape our attention without preoperative imaging).[3]

The radioactive tracer used in Europe is technetium-99m-labeled human albumin colloid. A dose of 60 MBq (1.6 mCi) in a mean volume of 0.3 ml (cc) is injected intradermally around the tumor or biopsy site. It is important to disperse the tracer around the *entire* biopsy scar because its opposite ends may drain to different lymph nodes. Immediately after injection, dynamic scintigraphy is performed for 20 minutes.

Subsequent anterior and lateral static images are made 30 minutes and 2 hours after injection.

Although scintigraphy never fails to show an SLN, we have learned to interpret the images with caution. A study of the reproducibility demonstrated that a different drainage pattern is depicted in 12% of the patients when scintigraphy is repeated.[4] Lymphatic drainage is a variable physiologic process. In another study, we found that the number of SLNs visualized on the scintigraphy images did not always agree with the number of SLNs identified with intraoperative mapping using a vital dye and a gamma probe.[5] Such discrepancies occurred in 19% of patients.

It is important for the surgeon to review the images in collaboration with the nuclear medicine physician before the operation. It is rewarding for both parties when the surgeon reports the operative findings back to the nuclear medicine physician or, preferably, when the nuclear medicine physician comes to the operating room.

SURGICAL TECHNIQUE

After a wide excision, the wound edges do not necessarily drain to the same lymph node that the original lesion drained to. Because the risk of altered drainage is smaller after diagnostic excision with a narrow margin, preferably SLN biopsy should precede therapeutic excision with a wide margin.

A single-day admission is adequate for this procedure. Scintigraphy can be performed either on the day of the operation or on the day before. Depending on the circumstances, the operation can be done with general, regional or local anesthesia.

Immediately prior to commencement of the operation, 1.0 ml Patent Blue-V dye is injected intradermally as close as possible to the original melanoma site. It is wise to outline the margin for the wide-local re-excision with a marking pen before the injection because a small biopsy scar tends to become obscured by the blue dye. The dye is taken up by the lymphatic system and stains the lymphatic channel within a few minutes. There is no need to elevate the injection site.

The incision is made some 10 minutes after administration of the blue dye. The skin mark placed by the nuclear medicine physician and the transcutaneous probe reading suggest where to make the incision. When deciding on the location and the direction of the incision, bear in mind that a regional lymph-node dissection may have to follow. In that subsequent completion lymph-node dissection, the SLN biopsy scar is removed in continuity with the definitive surgical specimen.

When the number of SLNs is unclear, we start by exploring the node furthest from the primary melanoma site in order to limit the risk of damaging the lymphatic channel to another node. An incision a few centimeters in length is sufficient. The subcutaneous tissue underneath Scarpa's fascia is explored in search of the blue-stained lymphatic channel. We try to find the lymphatic channel upstream from the first-tier node. The dynamic scintigraphy images usually give us a sense of where the lymphatic channel can be found. When the lymphatic channel is not immediately apparent, we massage the injection site and the skin upstream to encourage the lymph flow. A lymphatic channel may contain just a minute quantity of blue dye so that it is barely visible. The operative field must be kept absolutely dry because a small amount of blood may obscure a blue duct.

The lymphatic duct is dissected downstream until it enters a lymph node. The operation can be done by either sharp or blunt dissection depending on personal preference. A subtle surgical technique is mandatory because lymphatic channels are fragile. Damaging the lymphatic channel deprives the remaining stretch of its supply of blue dye. It then quickly loses its color and cannot be traced any further. Finding a blue node without an afferent blue lymphatic channel requires considerable luck.

Once identified, the node is dissected and freed from the surrounding fatty tissue. Afferent and efferent lymphatic channels are ligated, and the subcutaneous cavity is obliterated to prevent postoperative lymph fistula and seroma. A drain is not necessary.

A gamma probe that can be fitted out with a collimator and a shield is also needed. The probe is used to confirm that the blue node is indeed the radioactive node that was seen on the scintigraphy images. The probe is essential in the rare case that the SLN cannot be found with the blue-dye technique. After removal of the SLN(s) that we were looking for, the probe is used to scan the wound for unexpected additional "hot" SLNs.

Most SLNs are easily detectable with the probe because their radioactivity content exceeds that of the surrounding subcutaneous fat by a factor of 600 on average.[6] The probe should not be used in lieu of the blue dye, however, for two reasons, the first being that an SLN may be blue but not radioactive. Therefore, its lymphatic channel should not be damaged prematurely. The second reason is that the patient may have many radioactive nodes that might not all be SLNs. In a review of 150 patients, we found that scintigraphy did not indicate the correct number of SLNs in 23% of cases.[5] The blue-dye approach enables the surgeon to map the drainage pattern and identify the lymphatic channels that determine whether a lymph node is a first-tier node receiving drainage directly from the primary lesion site or a second-tier node receiving drainage from a first-tier node. This mapping cannot be accomplished with the probe, since the probe lacks the capability to identify lymphatic channels. If it remains unclear whether a particular lymph node is a first-tier or a second-tier node, it is best to err on the side of aggressiveness and remove it.

Clearly, the blue-dye technique and the gamma probe both have a role in the operation. Surgeons should have both techniques in their repertoire, on the one hand to find all the SLNs, and on the other to avoid removing non-SLNs unnecessarily.

PATHOLOGY

Frozen-section microscopy and immediate formal regional node dissection in the event of a tumor-positive outcome appear attractive because the patient is spared a possible second operation. Our experience with frozen-section microscopy was unfavorable, however, in a series of 101 patients: false-negative results were encountered in 8 of 17 patients with dissemination to the SLN.[7] Making SLN biopsy and formal node dissection a two-stage procedure has the advantage that it eliminates the need to reserve operating-room time that would be wasted in 9 out of 10 patients.

All SLNs are completely embedded for microscopic evaluation. Nodes up to 1 cm in size are processed bisected in one block, larger nodes in parallel slices of 0.2 cm in more blocks. All blocks are cut at three levels at 100-μm intervals and stained with hematoxylin–eosin and immunohistochemistry (S-100 and HMB-45).

RESULTS

At The Netherlands Cancer Institute, we recently analyzed the results from the first 200 melanoma patients who underwent an SLN biopsy starting in 1993.[1] An SLN was visualized on the lymphoscintigrams in all patients, and it was identified intraoperatively in 199 of 200 patients. On average, an SLN can be identified within 10 minutes.[8]

Forty-eight patients (24%) had metastases in their SLN. Six of our patients went on to develop palpable metastatic disease in a lymph-node field from which a tumor-free SLN had been removed earlier (sensitivity 89%). Four of these patients were among the first 41 patients in whom we did the procedure. Minor complications were seen in 18 patients. Thus, the detection rate with the careful approach described in this chapter is virtually 100%. The sensitivity is a somewhat disappointing 89%.

CONCLUSION

Lymphatic mapping with SLN biopsy is a staging procedure waiting for clinical relevance.[9] Surgeons embarking upon this approach should solicit expert assistance from their nuclear medicine physician and their pathologist, and should participate in a trial. Surgeons should acquire proficiency in both intraoperative detection techniques in order to obtain the best possible results. Although the procedure is usually remarkably simple, it can be challenging at times. One must be wary of false-negative results.

REFERENCES

1. Jansen L, Nieweg OE, Peterse JL et al, Reliability of sentinel lymph node biopsy for staging melanoma. *Br J Surg* 2000; **87**:484–9.
2. Kroon BBR, Nieweg OE, Hoekstra HJ et al, Principles and guidelines for surgeons: management of cutaneous malignant melanoma. *Eur J Surg Oncol* 1998; **23**:550–8.
3. Roozendaal GK, Dr Vries JDH, Van Poll D et al, Sentinel nodes outside lymph node basins in melanoma patients. Proceedings of The Society of Surgical Oncology, 53rd Annual Meeting, New Orleans 2000 (Abstract P59, page 49).
4. Kapteijn BAE, Nieweg OE, Valdés Olmos RA et al, Reproducibility of lymphoscintigraphy for lymphatic mapping in patients with cutaneous melanoma. *J Nucl Med* 1996; **37**:972–5.
5. Jansen L, *Sentinel node biopsy: evolving from melanoma to breast cancer.* Thesis, University of Amsterdam, 2000.
6. Kapteijn BAE, Nieweg OE, Muller SH et al, Validation of gamma probe detection of the sentinel node in melanoma. *J Nucl Med* 1997; **38**: 362–6.
7. Schraffordt Koops H, Nieweg OE, Tiebosch ATMG et al, Is intraoperative evaluation of frozen sections a reliable method for sentinel nodes in malignant melanoma? *Melanoma Res* 1997; **7**:S106 (Abstract).
8. Kapteijn BAE, Nieweg OE, Liem IH et al, Localizing the sentinel node in cutaneous melanoma: gamma probe detection versus blue dye. *Ann Surg Oncol* 1997; **4**:156–60.
9. Nieweg OE, Kapteijn BAE, Thompson JF, Kroon BBR, Lymphatic mapping and selective lymphadenectomy for melanoma: not yet standard therapy. *Eur J Surg Oncol* 1997; **23**:397–8.

12

How we do it: the Memorial Sloan-Kettering Cancer Center approach

Daniel G Coit

The Memorial Sloan-Kettering Cancer Center technique for SLN biopsy in melanoma			
Technique	Combination	**Isotope**	*Type*: Tc-99m-SC
Dye	*Type*: Isosulfan blue dye		*Filtered*: Yes (0.2-μm filter)
	Volume: 0.6–1.0 ml (cc)		*Dose*: 0.2–0.4 mCi (7.4–15 MBq)
			Volume: 1.0–2.0 ml (cc)
Injection site	*Isotope*: Intradermal	**Gamma probe**	*Detection threshold*: 120–130 keV
	Dye: Intradermal		*Window*: 40 keV

The following is a description of the technique of lymphatic mapping with sentinel lymph-node biopsy in patients with melanoma used at the Memorial Sloan-Kettering Cancer Center, based on our experience with over 600 patients. We initiated this experience using blue dye alone, but have used a combination of blue dye and radioisotope for the last 270 patients; in our experience and in the experience reported in the literature, that technique yields the highest rate of sentinel lymph node (SLN) localization. The technique is fairly robust, with innumerable subtle working variations of the described procedure. Nonetheless, it does have many pitfalls, and one must be absolutely meticulous in order to maximize diagnostic accuracy.

PATIENT SELECTION

Clinical nodal status

The only patients eligible for this technique are those with clinically negative nodes. Most patients undergoing biopsy of cutaneous melanoma, in the absence of infection, develop very little in the way of reactive inflammatory nodes. As such, if enlarged regional draining nodes are found, they must be viewed as suspicious for harboring metastatic disease. Biopsy of these nodes, either by fine-needle aspiration or excision, is appropriate.

Melanoma thickness

The incidence of positive regional lymph nodes clearly increases with increasing tumor thickness. We currently offer SLN biopsy to patients with melanomas 1 mm thick or more, or Clark's Level IV (any thickness). Other centers have used ulceration as another criterion for SLN biopsy, regardless of thickness. In our experience, and in that of others, the incidence of positive regional lymph nodes in patients with melanomas less than 1 mm thick is extremely low.[1]

Prior biopsy or wide excision

We prefer to perform this procedure on patients with intact primary lesions, or on those who have undergone local excisional biopsy only. It is only in this group that the technique has been validated, either in a large series of confirmatory completion elective lymph-node dissections, or in a large series with adequate follow-up to document incidence of nodal failure in negative SLN basins.[2] These are the patients who should have had minimal disturbance of their regional draining lymphatics. Few data exist to address the appropriate procedure for patients who have undergone prior wide excision. Our feeling, consistent with that of others, is that the technique would probably work if the axis of the wide excision is parallel to the axis of the expected draining lymphatics. We discourage the performance of this procedure in patients in whom the axis of wide excision is at right angles to the draining lymphatics, and in patients who have undergone split-thickness skin grafting or where local rotation flaps have been used for coverage. In such cases one would expect the regional lymphatics to be disturbed to the extent that one could not be confident of identifying the appropriate afferent lymphatic channel with either the radioisotope or blue-dye injections.[2,3]

Head and neck

As experience accrues in this anatomic region, increasing success in staging of patients with melanoma of the head and neck has been reported (see Chapter 29).[4-7] Controversy continues regarding the appropriate management of an intraparotid SLN. Sentinel lymph nodes in other areas of the head and neck are more easily located and dealt with.[8]

In-transit disease

Although few data address the unique situation of patients with a solitary in-transit lesion in the setting of an intact regional nodal basin, our limited experience has revealed a high incidence of positive SLNs in this group. Thus, this technique may have some use in staging regional lymphatics of patients with in-transit metastases, especially those being considered for either resection or regional chemotherapy treatment.

NUCLEAR MEDICINE

Radioisotope

Technetium-99m-antimony sulfur colloid, with its highly uniform particle size, is probably the best isotope for use with lymphoscintigraphy (LSG); unfortunately, however, it is unavailable in the United States. The majority of the experience has been accrued there by using Tc-99m-sulfur colloid (Tc-99m-SC), a heterogeneous colloid with particles ranging from less than 10 nm to greater than 250 nm in size. Larger particles tend to be retained at the primary site, while smaller particles migrate quite quickly, often through the SLN into secondary-echelon nodes. In treating cutaneous melanoma, we have obtained optimal results using this colloid after passage through a 0.2-μm filter prior to injection into the patient. This results in migration of an adequate fraction of injected isotope to the regional node or nodes. We prefer a total dose of 0.2–0.4 mCi (7.4–15 MBq), in 1–2 ml (cc) of isotonic saline, injected at four equal sites intradermally around the primary site. Intradermal as opposed to subcutaneous injection is important, as interstitial pressure appears to facilitate access of the colloid into regional lymphatics.

Because of the weekly variability of the isotope, on rare occasions we see a total failure of the isotope to migrate from the primary site. This is best managed by having the patient return for another attempt at LSG a week or two later.

Lymphoscintigraphy

In contrast to the experience in breast cancer, we have found that routine LSG is extremely helpful in localizing SLNs in patients with melanoma. Usually within minutes, the radioisotope migrates to regional lymph nodes. Anatomic detail is provided by boron-transmission scans to help locate aberrant in-transit lymph nodes and multiple parallel channels to synchronous SLNs, detail secondary-echelon lymph nodes, and demonstrate drainage or lack of drainage to multiple basins predicted by anatomic considerations. We find LSG helpful in over 80% of patients, with unexpected findings discovered in at least 20% of patients. This is consistent with the observations of other investigators.[9]

We prefer to perform LSG on the morning of surgery and then take the patient to the operating room 1–4 hours later. This is convenient for the patient, avoiding the need to return on a second day. Other techniques have been reported, varying from injection of radioisotope intraoperatively, to injection of isotope 24 hours or more prior to surgery. We have little experience with either of those variants.

Radiation precautions

The total dose of Tc-99m used is quite low and its half-life is about 6 hours. No special radiation precautions are required for the patient, operating-room staff, or pathologists handling the SLNs.[10]

SURGERY

Anesthesia and patient positioning

One to four hours following LSG, the patient is taken to the operating room for the procedure of lymphatic mapping and SLN biopsy with appropriate treatment of the primary lesion. We have found that the SLNs in the groin are usually easier to find, and that, if appropriate for treatment of the primary, the procedure may be done under local anesthesia with monitored sedation. In the neck and axilla, our preference is for general anesthesia. The patient is usually supine, except in the instance of back primaries where the patient is placed in the lateral decubitus position, with the draining nodal basin up. If the back lesion reveals bilateral drainage, we start with the patient supine and perform the bilateral SLN biopsies. If a frozen-section analysis is done and found to be negative, the biopsy incisions are closed, and the patient is turned appropriately to manage the primary. If a frozen-section analysis is done and found to be positive, we proceed to completion lymph-node dissection in that basin, then turn the patient to manage the primary tumor.

Dye injection

After induction of satisfactory general anesthesia or sedation, prior to prepping and draping the patient, isosulfan blue dye is injected intradermally at the site of the primary tumor. For patients with melanoma, we use 0.6–1.0 ml intradermally, injected on the side of the primary or biopsy site closest to the draining lymph-node basin indicated by LSG. The amount of dye injected is limited such that the blue stain caused by the injection will be totally encompassed by the subsequent wide excision, a particularly important consideration for lesions of the face. If a prior wide excision has been performed, and the LSG is straightforward, we omit the dye totally, as residual retained dye may persist for weeks or even many months.

It is important that the dye injection be intradermal, as, similar to the radioisotope, interstitial pressure will facilitate entry of the dye into lymphatics. Generally, dye migrates to lymphatics within minutes and is nearly always in the SLN by the time surgeons have scrubbed and the patient is prepped and draped. Local massage or elevation is probably unnecessary.

Gamma probe

On probes where settings can be adjusted manually, we recommend using a detection threshold of 120–130 keV with a window of 40 keV, to center on the 140-keV photopeak of Tc-99m. If no counts are appreciated in the draining lymph-node basin, lowering the threshold slightly may produce successful SLN localization. In most current devices, no manual adjustment is necessary.

Transcutaneous counts are extremely helpful in the "planar" regions of the neck and groin, enabling precise transcutaneous localization of the SLN and permitting accurate positioning of a smaller incision. In the axilla, transcutaneous counting is less helpful, as the incision is usually standard, positioned as part of a planned axillary dissection incision if necessary (see below).

Probes are variably shielded and/or collimated, thus more or less directional. More directional probes are usually more helpful in locating SLNs, but are often more difficult to use to assess background nodal basin radioactivity following removal of the SLN. In general, smaller probes are easier to use, although the smaller crystals generally pick up fewer radioactive counts for the same amount of SLN radioactivity. Whether to use the straight or gently angled probe is a matter of personal preference.

In every case, the following counts must be meticulously recorded in the operative note: primary site, each SLN ex vivo, and residual background nodal-basin radioactivity following removal of the SLN(s). We prefer to record 10-second counts for each site, to minimize the variation inherent when only 1-second counts are recorded. We also record the blue-dye status of each SLN (blue, faint blue, not blue),

and whether or not there is a distinct afferent blue lymphatic channel. These data are imperative in order to understand the phenomenon of subsequent nodal-basin failure.

If the primary site is close to the SLN, or if the SLN is located between the probe and the primary, the radioactivity of the SLN may be overshadowed by the "blast zone" of radioactivity at the primary site. Radioactivity at the primary site may be 10–20 times higher than that in the SLN. If so, we have found it helpful to remove the primary site first, then proceed to lymphatic mapping with SLN localization. If this is necessary, one must be certain to allow adequate time for migration of the blue dye to regional lymph nodes prior to the wide excision.

Operation

After the patient is prepped and draped, the gamma probe is draped into the field, and transcutaneous counts are recorded at the primary site and over the nodal basin (or basins), indicated by LSG. The incision in the lymphatic drainage basin is located over the site of maximal transcutaneous counts, *taking care to plan the incision in such a way as to be able to incorporate it into the incision of a complete lymph-node dissection if the SLN is positive.* The SLN is almost always just deep to Scarpa's fascia and is generally easily located in the groin and neck. In the axilla, it is often deeper, in Level I. Usually a very delicate blue-stained afferent lymphatic channel can be found and traced to the node. It is important not to disrupt this lymphatic prior to locating the SLN.

The SLN is best defined operationally as the lymph node with an identified afferent blue lymphatic that stains the lymph-node hilus, a node that is usually "hotter" than adjacent nodes by gamma counting. While isotope may pass through the SLN to secondary echelon non-SLNs, this is rarely seen with the blue dye. The SLN is almost always blue, and is usually, but not always, the hottest node. We remove additional hot nodes from the lymphatic basin until the background radioactivity is less than 10% that of the hottest node removed, counted ex vivo. *Again, it is essential to record the ex vivo counts and color of all nodes removed, and to record the final nodal basin background ex vivo counts in the operative note, in order to provide a detailed record of the surgical procedure.*

In our early experience, we sent the SLN for frozen-section evaluation, so that if it is positive, a completion lymph-node dissection may be performed at the same session. While the frozen-section analysis was being done, we widely excised and closed the primary site. If the frozen section was negative, the SLN biopsy site was closed without a drain. If the frozen section was positive, we would proceed immediately to regional lymphatic dissection, *completely excising the lymph node biopsy cavity with a small ellipse of overlying skin.*

More recently, we have found that frozen-section evaluation detects only 50% of all positive SLNs.[11] We therefore now defer histologic evaluation of the SLN to permanent section, to include serial sectioning and immunohisto-chemistry (IHC) (see below). We have found this approach to have several advantages.

First, we now prepare only those patients with known positive SLNs for the potential morbidity of completion lymph-node dissection. Second, we avoid "misleading" the 10% of patients with negative frozen sections who will ultimately be found to have positive nodes on final review. Finally, segregating the procedures leads to more efficient use of the operating-room schedule.

The morbidity of the SLN biopsy procedure is quite low. Minor discomfort at the surgical site is anticipated and treated with local infiltration of 0.5% bupivacaine, and parenteral ketorolac injection. We rarely see persistent, mild incisional pain, seroma, hematoma, or wound infection. Extremity edema is exceedingly uncommon after an SLN biopsy. Complications related to the dye injection include minor local dye retention; all patients note a slight greenish tinge to their urine for a few hours. We have seen no allergic reactions to the low doses of isosulfan blue dye used in melanoma, although such reactions have been reported in breast-cancer patients, where substantially more dye is injected.

Failed procedures

Although failures are quite unusual, patients need to be informed preoperatively that this is a procedure that is not always successful. If no isotope migrates, because of either subcutaneous injection or an excess of large colloid particles, it is best to have the patient return for another attempt in 1–2 weeks. If the SLN cannot be located in a "reasonable" amount of time, surgery should revert to accepted clinical practice. In most instances, for patients with melanoma, this consists of a wide excision alone. *Again, all of this must be discussed with the patient preoperatively.*

PATHOLOGY

In our current practice, routine examination of the SLN no longer includes a frozen-section analysis. An exception to this approach would be the use of frozen-section analysis to assess an intraparotid node in order to avoid risk to the facial-nerve branches during delayed superficial parotidectomy in a previously operated field, if permanent section subsequently revealed metastatic disease.

Permanent paraffin section should consist of a single hematoxylin-and-eosin (H&E) section through the equator of the lymph node to include the hilus. If this is negative, we strongly recommend that at least three additional paraffin sections be taken through the node, for H&E as well as IHC evaluation with S-100 and HMB-45. In our experience, 10–40% of patients initially negative on frozen-section analysis will prove to be positive with more intensive pathologic evaluation of the SLN.[11] If the frozen-section analysis is performed and is positive, we proceed directly to immediate completion or "selective" regional lymph-node dissection; if the SLN is positive on subsequent evaluation, the patient is brought back to the operating room for a delayed "selective" lymph-node dissection. In our experience, about 10% of patients with a positive SLN will have additional positive lymph nodes at completion lymph-node dissection. This is consistent with the observations of others.[12] Although this raises the possibility that we may be able to identify subsets of patients who do not require further surgery after discovery of a positive SLN, at present there is no clear agreement on parameters that predict additional positive non-SLNs. Completion lymph-node dissection in the setting of a positive SLN therefore remains standard practice. We, as well as others, are currently investigating the use of reverse tran-scriptase–polymerase chain reaction (RT-PCR) to evaluate the SLN for submicroscopic metastatic melanoma.[13] Recognizing that some SLNs will harbor subcapsular nevi that will share messenger RNA profiles with melanoma, the clinical significance of detecting one or more mRNA transcripts characteristic of melanoma remains to be defined.[14–16]

FOLLOW-UP

Early collective experience with large follow-up series of melanoma patients has revealed that 2–5% of patients with negative SLNs will fail, with recurrence in the undissected nodal basin. Most, but not all of these "failures" have been traced back to incomplete pathologic evaluation of the SLN.[17] Review of the SLNs by serial sec-tioning and IHC has revealed a small volume of micrometastatic disease in most cases of nodal-basin relapse. It is imperative that melanoma patients undergoing intraoperative lymphatic mapping with SLN biopsy should be examined every 3–4 months for at least 3 years, to detect treatable local-regional relapse. Follow-up after that should be at 6- to 12-month intervals as clinically indicated.

VALIDATION OF THE TECHNIQUE

In order to feel comfortable with this technique, most surgeons experienced with intraoperative lymphatic mapping and SLN biopsy initially learned the procedure by validation with com-pletion lymph-node dissection, comparing stag-ing by SLN status to staging after completion lymph-node dissection. If this is not feasible, at

least someone with experience in the technique should supervise the first few procedures. Finally, if the yield of positive SLNs is less than expected, *and in every patient with nodal basin failure after a negative SLN*, every component of the procedure (LSG, surgery, and pathology) needs to be carefully reviewed.

SUMMARY

Lymphatic mapping with SLN biopsy is a tech-nique used to facilitate the accurate pathologic staging of melanoma patients at risk for regional lymph-node metastases. While, at pre-sent, information derived from the SLN biopsy will affect the choice of treatment (completion lymph-node dissection, adjuvant immunother-apy), the impact of this technique on long-term outcome in these patients remains the subject of ongoing clinical trials.[18]

REFERENCES

1. Bedrosian I, Faries MB, Guerry D et al, Incidence of sentinel node metastasis in patients with thin primary melanoma (< or = 1 mm) with vertical growth phase. *Ann Surg Oncol* 2000; **7**:262–7.
2. Kelemen PR, Essner R, Foshag LJ, Morton DL, Lymphatic mapping and sentinel lymphadenec-tomy after wide local excision of primary melanoma. *J Am Coll Surg* 1999; **189**:247–52.
3. Karakousis CP, Grigoropoulos P, Sentinel node biopsy before and after wide excision of the pri-mary melanoma. *Ann Surg Oncol* 1999; **6**:785–9.
4. Bostick P, Essner R, Sarantou T et al, Intraoperative lymphatic mapping for early-stage melanoma of the head and neck. *Am J Surg* 1997; **174**:536–9.
5. Morton DL, Wen DR, Foshag LJ et al, Intraoperative lymphatic mapping and selective cervical lymphadenectomy for early-stage melanomas of the head and neck. *J Clin Oncol* 1993; **11**:1751–6.
6. Carlson GW, Murray DR, Greenlee R et al, Management of malignant melanoma of the head and neck using dynamic lymphoscintigra-phy and gamma probe-guided sentinel lymph node biopsy. *Arch Otolaryngol Head Neck Surg* 2000; **126**:433–7.

7. Wagner JD, Park HM, Coleman JJ et al, Cervical sentinel lymph node biopsy for melanomas of the head and neck and upper thorax. *Arch Otolaryngol Head Neck Surg* 2000; **126:**313–21.

8. O'Brien CJ, Uren RF, Thompson JF et al, Prediction of potential metastatic sites in cutaneous head and neck melanoma using lymphoscintigraphy. *Am J Surg* 1995; **170:**461–6.

9. Uren RF, Howman-Giles R, Thompson JF et al, Interval nodes: the forgotten sentinel nodes in patients with melanoma. *Arch Surg* 2000; **135:**1168–72.

10. Miner TJ, Shriver CD, Flicek PR et al, Guidelines for the safe use of radioactive materials during localization and resection of the sentinel lymph node. *Ann Surg Oncol* 1999; **6:** 75–82.

11. Clary BM, Brady MS, Lewis JJ et al, Should frozen section analysis of the sentinel node be performed in patients with melanoma? First International Congress on the Sentinel Node and Treatment of Cancer, Amsterdam April, 1999. *Eur J Nucl Med* 1999; **26**(suppl):S68.

12. Wagner JD, Gordon MS, Chuang TY et al, Predicting sentinel and residual lymph node basin disease after sentinel lymph node biopsy for melanoma. *Cancer* 2000; **89:**453–62.

13. Bieligk SC, Ghossein R, Bhattacharya S, Coit DG, Detection of tyrosinase mRNA by reverse transcription-polymerase chain reaction in melanoma sentinel nodes [see comments]. *Ann Surg Oncol* 1999; **6:**232–40.

14. van der Velde-Zimmerman D, Schipper ME, de Weger RA et al, Sentinel node biopsies in melanoma patients: a protocol for accurate, efficient, and cost-effective analysis by preselection for immunohistochemistry on the basis of Tyr-PCR. *Ann Surg Oncol* 2000; **7:**51–4.

15. Goydos JS, Ravikumar TS, Germino FJ et al, Minimally invasive staging of patients with melanoma: sentinel lymphadenectomy and detection of the melanoma-specific proteins MART-1 and tyrosinase by reverse transcriptase polymerase chain reaction. *J Am Coll Surg* 1998; **187:**182–8.

16. Shivers SC, Wang X, Li W et al, Molecular staging of malignant melanoma: correlation with clinical outcome. *JAMA* 1998; **280:**1410–15.

17. Gershenwald JE, Colome MI, Lee JE et al, Patterns of recurrence following a negative sentinel lymph node biopsy in 243 patients with stage I or II melanoma. *J Clin Oncol* 1998; **16:**2253–60.

18. Morton DL, Thompson JF, Essner R et al, Validation of the accuracy of intraoperative lymphatic mapping and sentinel lymphadenectomy for early-stage melanoma: a multicenter trial. Multicenter Selective Lymphadenectomy Trial Group. *Ann Surg* 1999; **230:**453–63.

13

How we do it: the MD Anderson Cancer Center approach

Merrick I Ross and Jeffrey E Gershenwald

CONTENTS Case selection • Preoperative lymphoscintigraphy • Surgery • Pathology
• Conclusion

The MD Anderson Cancer Center technique for SLN biopsy in melanoma

Technique	Combination	Isotope	(i) *Preoperative LSG*:
Dye	*Type*: Isosulfan blue dye		*Type*: Tc-99m-SC
	Volume: 2–3 ml (cc)		*Filtered*: Yes
			Dose: 0.5–1.0 mCi (18.5–37 MBq)
Injection site	*Isotope*: Intradermal		*Volume*: 0.5 ml (cc)
	Dye: Intradermal		
			(ii) *Day of surgery (1–4 hours prior)*:
			Type: Tc-99m-SC
			Filtered: No
			Dose: 0.5–1.0 mCi (18.5–37 MBq)
			Volume: 0.5 ml (cc)

The objective of lymphatic mapping and sentinel lymph-node biopsy is to determine the histologic status of the regional lymph-node basin or basins. Through the injection of radiolabeled colloid or lymphatic blue dyes around the primary melanoma site, the first draining lymph node, the sentinel lymph node (SLN), can be identified. Published reports from several institutions including our own support the SLN concept: the first lymph nodes of drainage are the most likely to contain micrometastatic disease.[1–4] Because the biology of melanoma lymphatic metastases follows lymphatic anatomy, the accuracy of SLN biopsy relies on accurate descriptions of lymphatic drainage patterns. Therefore, the success of any lymphatic mapping program is dependent on the integration of three technical components: (a) preoperative determination of regional lymph-node basins at risk and predicted number and location of SLNs within these basins (preoperative cutaneous lymphoscintigraphy); (b) intraoperative localization and biopsy of the SLN; and (c) careful pathologic evaluation of the SLN. This minimally invasive approach for the staging of regional lymph-node basins promotes the selective and early application of therapeutic lymph-node dissections, durable regional control of disease in patients proven to have occult metastases, and finally, valuable staging information above and beyond what could be accomplished by elective lymph node dissection.[5]

CASE SELECTION

Candidates for SLN biopsy are patients with newly diagnosed primary, clinically node-negative melanoma (Stages I and II) predicted to be at intermediate or high risk of harboring occult nodal disease. Patients with one of the following primary tumor criteria are normally offered this approach:

- tumor thickness ≥1 mm
- Clark's Level greater than III (regardless of tumor thickness)
- primary tumor ulceration
- histologic evidence of extensive regression.

Other clinical scenarios where this technique may be useful include the following:

- local recurrence *subsequent to* a relatively narrow excision of a primary melanoma
- indeterminate tumor thickness, due either to tangential sectioning of a specimen improperly embedded in paraffin, or to tumor present at the deep margin of a superficial shave biopsy
- an atypical melanocytic lesion in which the differential diagnosis includes a primary melanoma more than 1 mm in thickness
- following a formal wide excision (with or without a skin graft) in patients who then wish to have accurate nodal staging.

In this last situation, the accuracy of SLN biopsy is unknown; the lymphatic drainage of the remaining skin may be different from that of the skin adjacent to the original primary melanoma; here we offer SLN biopsy selectively to patients who understand that the true false-negative rate has not been established.

PREOPERATIVE LYMPHOSCINTIGRAPHY

The technique of cutaneous lymphoscintigraphy (LSG) includes a four-point intradermal injection of 0.5–1.0 mCi (18.7–37 MBq) of *filtered* technetium-99m-sulfur colloid (Tc-99m-SC). An external gamma camera images the isotope migration to the nodal basin in real time and then in static images at various time intervals. The goals of LSG include the identification of nodal basins at risk in patients with melanomas at sites of ambiguous lymphatic drainage (especially truncal and head and neck locations); defining the number and relative location of SLNs within the basin; and identifying SLNs at either interval (in-transit) sites between the primary injection site and the regional nodal basin (Figure 13.1), or, in the case of ectopic SLNs, in completely unpredicted locations (Figure 13.2).

For primary injection sites distant from the potential draining nodal basins, the information obtained from the LSG is generally straightforward. For injection sites that overlie a nodal basin, however, clear SLN mapping may be difficult and at times impossible. In this setting, anterior/posterior, perpendicular/lateral, or other views may unveil an SLN obscured by the shine-through of the injection site. We generally obtain a formal lymphoscintigram remote from the day of surgery to allow appropriate and unambiguous surgical planning and consent. When this is logistically difficult, LSG can be performed on the morning of the surgery. Here, a single radiocolloid injection allows both preoperative LSG and intraoperative SLN mapping with a hand-held gamma probe, obviating the need for two injections. Occasionally the injected colloid will not migrate from the injection site when LSG is done too soon after a diagnostic excisional biopsy, and a repeat study should be done 7–10 days later when the surrounding inflammation has resolved.

On the day of surgery, the patient receives a four-point intradermal injection of 0.5–1.0 mCi of *unfiltered* Tc-99m-SC in the nuclear medicine department. This takes place 1–4 hours prior to the initiation of the planned surgical procedure. Performing surgery too quickly may not allow sufficient migration of the radiocolloid to the

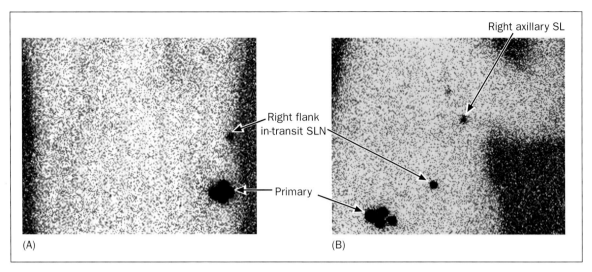

Figure 13.1 Identification of SLNs at interval (in-transit) sites between the primary injection site and the regional nodal basin. (A), Posterior flank; (B), Right lateral chest.

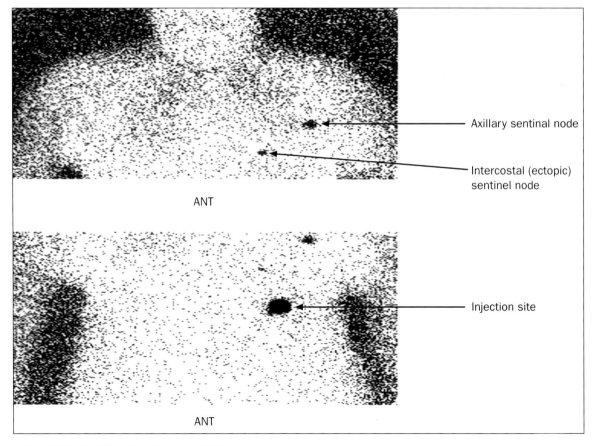

Figure 13.2 Identification of ectopic SLNs.

SLN, compromising the success of SLN localization. The minimum time required for adequate migration can be obtained by examining the preoperative LSG. Occasionally, delays between isotope injection and surgery will allow colloid (especially if filtered to select for a smaller particle size) to pass on to second-echelon nodes, leading to the unnecessary removal of multiple lymph nodes. By using an unfiltered isotope preparation (consisting of larger particles) the intent is to minimize uptake by these second-echelon (or nonsentinel) nodes.

SURGERY

Our experience with SLN biopsy for melanoma began in late 1991. We initially relied solely on intradermal injections of isosulfan blue dye to identify the SLN. Preoperative LSG was used to determine nodal basins at risk, number and location of the SLNs, and placement of the surgical incision. In 1994, we began in addition to use a hand-held gamma probe[6] at surgery to target SLNs identified by the injection, preoperatively, of a radiolabeled colloid, and since then have used a combination of dye and isotope. This evolution of techniques has improved our identification rates from 87% using blue dye alone to 99% for the combined technique.[7,8]

On arriving in the operating room from the nuclear medicine department, the patient can be scanned with the hand-held gamma probe in the holding area to make sure sufficient colloid has migrated. In the operating room, the hand-held gamma probe is used for transcutaneous scanning of the primary injection site, the intervening lymphatics, and the nodal basin proper. As the gamma probe is transcutaneously passed from the injection site to the nodal basin, the counts will diminish in proportion to the distance from the injection site. Near the SLN site, the radioactive counts will increase despite the probe being moved further away from the injection site. Beyond the SLN site, the counts decrease again. These areas are marked on the skin for surgical incision planning. We require that the actual LSG films be seen in the operating room, rather than depending on the report.

Intravenous sedation or general anesthesia is then administered followed by appropriate positioning of the patient to optimize SLN localization and minimize position changes. The type of anesthesia used is determined more by the required extent of the primary excision than by the SLN biopsy.

The primary site is then identified and approximately 2–3 ml (cc) of isosulfan blue dye is injected intradermally with the use of a tuberculin syringe and a 25-gauge needle. The patient is then prepped and draped; this allows adequate time for the blue dye to travel through the lymphatics to the SLN. The nodal basin is approached first with a small biopsy incision directed by the hand-held gamma probe. We make sure that this biopsy incision can be easily incorporated into a formal lymphadenectomy incision if that is required. A small incision is made over the "X." Once the nodal basin is entered, localization of the SLN is achieved either by following a blue channel towards the blue node or by direct visualization of the blue lymph node. The visualization of the blue dye is helpful in rapidly identifying which lymph node has accumulated the radioactive colloid. This node is then elevated from the surrounding tissues. Intervening lymphatic channels can be identified because of the blue dye, and are tied to avoid seroma formation. Ex vivo counts of the SLN are then documented with a hand-held gamma probe and recorded in the chart, on a data form, and on the pathology sheet. The lymph node is visually inspected for the presence of macroscopic metastasis or pigment. If the node is clinically normal on macroscopic examination by the pathologist, no frozen sections are performed. After removal of the initial node, the nodal basin is then scanned for residual radioactive counts with the hand-held gamma probe pointed away from the injection site. If the background activity in the nodal basin remains high because of the proximity of the injection site to the nodal basin, we widely excise the primary site, thereby removing this background activity ("shine-through") and allowing a more accurate evaluation of residual counts in the nodal basin and intervening tissues. Additional nodes identified by the presence of high radioactivity are then removed and labeled as SLNs, with numbers assigned sequentially in the order of identification. Nodes are defined as sentinel if they are blue and/or contain radioactivity significantly above background levels. Nodes are removed and labeled as "sentinel" until no focal basin count exceeds 10% of the radioactivity of the "hottest" SLN.

The SLN biopsy cavity is then irrigated, checked for meticulous hemostasis, and closed. In general, this combined dye–isotope technique entails little disruption of the lymphatic tissues, and no drain is required.

When the primary injection is remote from the nodal basin the procedure is relatively straightforward, and what is seen at the time of surgery using the blue dye should closely mimic the findings of the preoperative LSG. This is not always the case, particularly in the following situations.

Injection site close to the nodal basin

Most of the injected isotope remains at the injection site and only a small fraction actually migrates to the SLN. When the injection site is close to the nodal basin, the counts from the injection can mask or obscure the SLN. If we cannot localize the SLN transcutaneously prior to making an incision, we rely primarily on the

blue dye to visually identify the SLN. If this proves difficult, we then excise the primary melanoma site together with its injected isotope. This maneuver may unveil the counts in the SLN, allowing detection with the gamma probe.

Head and neck locations

The excision margins of head and neck melanomas may be limited by the proximity of important anatomic structures. Here we will not inject blue dye if it cannot be completely removed with the excision of the primary tumor; blue dye injected intradermally and left behind at the primary site can tattoo the skin for a long time. We avoid this problem by marking the excision margins prior to the blue-dye injection and limiting injection (by adjusting volume) to the skin that will be excised.

Identification of in-transit SLNs

In specific anatomic locations such as the trunk, LSG may identify lymph nodes outside the formal node basin, or between the primary injection site and the node basin, in 5–10% of cases.[9] These nodes, as the first to receive drainage from certain areas of the skin, are SLNs (Figure 13.3). A similar situation occurs in the

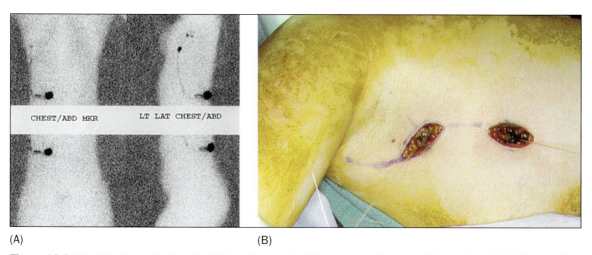

(A)   (B)

Figure 13.3 Identification of in-transit SLNs in the trunk: (A) lymphoscintigraphy; (B) location of SLN biopsy sites – axilla (left incision) and in-transit site on chest wall (right incision).

extremities distal to either the elbow or the knee, where the SLN might be an epitrochlear or popliteal node, respectively. Sometimes a single lymphatic vessel will drain from the injection site to this in-transit SLN node before traveling on, "in series," to the formal nodal basin. Alternatively, separate lymphatic channels may drain to an in-transit SLN and, "in parallel," directly to an SLN in the regional nodal basin; each of these must be considered an SLN and must be identified and removed (Figure 13.4). These nodes are best identified in advance on preoperative LSG, or at surgery by identifying an SLN in the nodal basin, removing the injection site, and then scanning the intervening tissues with the gamma probe.

While the SLN is defined as the first node of drainage from a primary injection site or afferent lymphatic channel, it is important to remember that the first node that is encountered and visualized by the blue dye may not necessarily be the first node of drainage. The dye and radiocolloid can travel through the SLN into second-echelon nodes, and the first node encountered may actually be one of these, draining "in series" from a deeper or more proximal SLN (Figure 13.5). The true SLN may be difficult to identify by visual inspection alone, and the gamma probe can be used to ensure that SLNs are not left behind after removal of the first blue node encountered. Significant residual radioactivity in the nodal basin after removal of the first blue or "hot" node found should alert the surgeon to seek others.

PATHOLOGY

The final component ensuring accurate nodal staging is a careful pathologic evaluation of the SLN; since only a few nodes are removed, they can be examined by the pathologist more carefully. We generally do not perform frozen-section evaluation of the SLN if it appears uninvolved on gross inspection. Sentinel lymph nodes are at minimum serially sectioned, stained routinely with hematoxylin-and-eosin (H&E), and immunostained with HMB-45 and S-100 antibodies. Serial sectioning allows greater tissue sampling and is therefore more likely to detect micrometastases.[10] Immunostaining reveals tumor cells among a much larger volume of normal histiocytes and lymphocytes. In prospective studies, we are evaluating the degree to which enhanced pathologic techniques—such as reverse transcriptase–

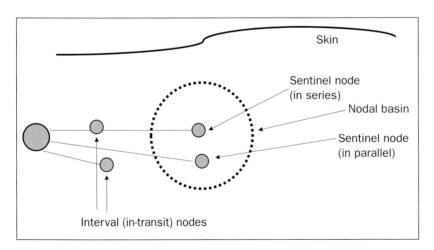

Figure 13.4 Diagram of lymphatic drainage patterns in the extremities, distal to either the elbow or the knee, involving "in series" and "in parallel" drainage. All nodes involved in these drainage patterns must be considered SLNs and must be identified and removed.

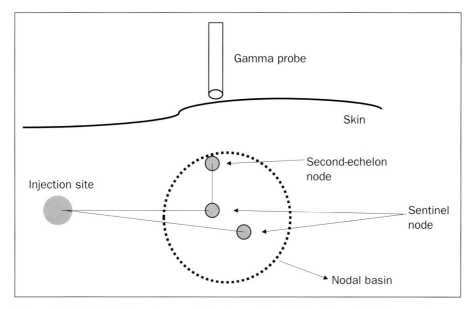

Figure 13.5 Identification of second-echelon nodes draining "in series" from a deeper or more proximal SLN.

polymerase chain reaction (RT-PCR) for tyrosinase messenger RNA—are able to detect metastases missed by routine histology. At our institution RT-PCR remains investigational and is only in use as part of a clinical trial.

CONCLUSION

Successful lymphatic mapping and SLN biopsy is not a simple undertaking and requires the integration of a sophisticated multidisciplinary team. The information obtained from this technique is extremely valuable, and therefore improper implementation is a disservice to the patient.

REFERENCES

1. Morton D, Wen D, Wong J et al, Technical details of intraoperative lymphatic mapping for early stage melanoma. *Arch Surg* 1992; **127**:392–8.
2. Ross M, Reintgen D, Balch C, Selective lymphadenectomy: emerging role for lymphatic mapping and sentinel node biopsy in the management of early stage melanoma. *Semin Surg Oncol* 1993; **9**:219–23.
3. Reintgen D, Cruse C, Wells K et al, The orderly progression of melanoma nodal metastases. *Ann Surg* 1994; **220**:759–67.
4. Thompson J, McCarthy W, Bosch C et al, Sentinel lymph node status as an indicator of the presence of metastatic melanoma in regional lymph nodes. *Melanoma Res* 1995; **5**:255–60.
5. Ross MI, Surgical management of stage I and II melanoma patients: approach to the regional lymph node basin. *Semin Surg Oncol* 1996; **12**:394–401.
6. Krag DN, Meijer SJ, Weaver DL et al, Minimal-access surgery for staging of malignant melanoma. *Arch Surg* 1995; **130**:654–8.
7. Gershenwald JE, Tseng C-H, Thompson W et al, Improved sentinel lymph node localization in patients with primary melanoma with the use of radiolabeled colloid. *Surgery* 1998; **124**:203–10.
8. Albertini J, Cruse C, Rapaport D et al, Intraoperative radiolymphoscintigraphy improves sentinel lymph node identification for patients with melanoma. *Ann Surg* 1996; **223**:217–24.
9. Thompson JF, Uren RF, Shaw HM et al, Location of sentinel lymph nodes in patients with cutaneous melanoma: new insights into lymphatic anatomy. *J Am Coll Surg* 1999; **189**:195–204.
10. Gershenwald JE, Colome MI, Lee JE et al, Patterns of recurrence following a negative sentinel lymph node biopsy in 243 patients with stage I or II melanoma. *J Clin Oncol* 1998; **16**:2253–60.

14

Clinical trials

Kelly M McMasters, Sandra L Wong and William R Wrightson

CONTENTS   Why perform SLN biopsy?   •   The Multicenter Selective Lymphadenectomy Trial   •   The Sunbelt Melanoma Trial   •   Conclusion

There has been some controversy regarding the validity and utility of sentinel lymph-node (SLN) biopsy for melanoma;[1,2] however, SLN biopsy has been adopted as the standard method of nodal staging for melanoma at nearly every major medical center in the United States. Furthermore, the World Health Organization (WHO) has issued a statement indicating that SLN biopsy should be considered the standard of care for patients with melanoma.[3] This chapter outlines the rationale for this procedure and discusses two important ongoing multicenter trials of SLN biopsy for melanoma.

WHY PERFORM SLN BIOPSY?

There are four major reasons to perform SLN biopsy. All of them involve the critically important issue of accurate staging. First, SLN biopsy improves the accuracy of staging and provides valuable prognostic information for patients and physicians to guide subsequent treatment decisions. Second, SLN biopsy facilitates early therapeutic lymph-node dissection for patients with nodal metastases. Third, SLN biopsy iden-tifies patients who are candidates for adjuvant therapy with interferon alfa-2b. Fourth, SLN biopsy identifies homogeneous patient populations for entry into clinical trials of novel adjuvant-therapy agents.

Prognostic information for patients and physicians

Sentinel lymph-node status is the most important predictor of survival for patients with melanoma. In fact, in the report by Gershenwald et al,[4] the hazard ratio for survival associated with a positive SLN was 6.43, much greater than that for any other prognostic factor. No combination of characteristics of the primary tumor can provide this prognostic information.

This nodal staging serves two purposes. First, it identifies a population of patients with a relatively favorable prognosis in whom adjuvant therapy may not be necessary. Second, it identifies a high-risk population of patients who have a poor prognosis. Therefore, SLN biopsy is a minimally invasive procedure with very little morbidity that provides important prognostic information for both patients and physicians. This information is immediately worthwhile in guiding patients to make appropriate choices regarding additional treatment and has important implications for patient follow-up.

Identification of patients who may benefit from early therapeutic lymph-node dissection

Prior to the advent of SLN biopsy, the pathologic nodal status of patients with melanoma was known only after elective lymph-node dissection. Four prospective randomized trials, however, have failed to demonstrate an overall survival benefit for patients who undergo elective lymph-node dissection,[5-9] and this conclusion has led to the common misconception that lymphadenectomy offers no therapeutic benefit for patients with melanoma. Accordingly, the important distinction between elective and therapeutic lymph-node dissection is often overlooked or obscured.

Lymph-node dissection is curative for some patients with nodal metastases. A substantial and reproducible percentage of Stage III melanoma patients are cured by lymphadenectomy, and this was true long before any adjuvant therapy was available. Furthermore, in patients with positive nodes, tumor burden as measured by the number of positive nodes has consistently been the best predictor of outcome. Therefore, it seems intuitive that early removal of lymph nodes is better than waiting until the patient develops multiple positive nodes with bulky, palpable disease. The question then arises why there has been no overall survival benefit in the trials of elective lymph-node dissection.

The answer lies in the fact that most of the patients undergoing this procedure do not have cancer in the lymph nodes. Therefore, any potential therapeutic impact of early lymph-node dissection for occult nodal metastases is diluted by the majority of patients (75–80%) who have negative lymph nodes. Even under the best circumstances, we could not expect to

see more than a 5–10% overall survival benefit in trials of elective lymph-node dissection. None of these studies was designed with adequate statistical power to detect such small differences in survival.

Two sources of data help support the notion that early removal of occult nodal metastases is better than waiting until the patient develops palpable nodal disease to perform regional lymphadenectomy. Although the 10-year follow-up results from the Intergroup Melanoma Trial demonstrated a 4% overall survival advantage in favor of elective lymph-node dissection, this conclusion did not reach statistical significance.[8,9] Certain prospectively stratified subgroups of the patients, however, specifically those who had nonulcerated melanomas, extremity melanomas, and melanomas between 1 mm and 2 mm thick, did benefit from elective lymph-node dissection. Although retrospective subgroup analysis of clinical trials is always subject to criticism, it is important to point out that patients in this study were prospectively stratified by tumor thickness, anatomic site, and ulceration, and these analyses were planned during the design of the trial.

The second crucial piece of evidence regarding the value of early lymph-node dissection is derived from the WHO Program 14 Trial of elective lymph-node dissection for patients with truncal melanomas.[7] Overall, there was no difference in survival for the two randomized arms (nodal observation versus elective lymph-node dissection). However, when the survival of the patients with positive lymph nodes, detected either histologically at elective lymph-node dissection or by palpation in the observation arm, was evaluated, quite a different picture emerged. The overall survival of patients with nodal micrometastases removed at elective lymph-node dissection was significantly greater than that of patients who underwent lymphadenectomy for palpable lymph nodes in the observation arm (48% vs 27% 5-year survival, $p = 0.04$).[7]

Therefore, if occult micrometastatic disease can be accurately identified, the data from the Intergroup Melanoma Trial and the WHO Programme 14 Trial suggest that early therapeutic lymph-node dissection may improve survival. Certainly, there is no evidence that patients who undergo delayed lymph-node dissection at the time of palpable recurrence have a better prognosis than those who undergo lymphadenectomy when they have microscopic nodal metastases. Therefore, the available evidence suggests that early therapeutic lymph-node dissection for microscopic nodal disease may be superior to delayed lymph-node dissection performed once the patient develops palpable nodal disease.[10,11]

The problem with elective lymph-node dissection, of course, is that the procedure is applied indiscriminately to all patients who have clinically negative lymph nodes. Therefore, the majority of patients (without nodal metastases) are subjected to the morbidity of lymphadenectomy without any therapeutic benefit. In the ideal situation, the patients with positive lymph nodes would be identified, and the rest would be spared the need for complete lymph-node dissection.

This is the advantage of SLN biopsy. When SLN biopsy is performed for patients with melanomas greater than or equal to 1.0 mm Breslow thickness, 20% or more will be found to have positive SLNs when careful pathologic analysis is performed.[4,12–21] Therefore, at least 20% of patients are identified as candidates for additional therapy, which includes therapeutic lymph-node dissection. Importantly, patients harboring occult metastatic disease are offered an early *therapeutic* lymph-node dissection, not an *elective* lymph-node dissection. The 80% of patients who have negative SLNs are spared the need for lymph-node dissection and have undergone a procedure that amounts to little more than a lymph-node biopsy performed on an outpatient basis at the time of the wide-local excision of the melanoma. Moreover, SLN biopsy has been shown to be cost-effective compared with elective lymph-node dissection.[22]

Identification of patients who are candidates for adjuvant interferon alfa-2b therapy

Interferon alfa-2b therapy has been approved in the United States by the Food and Drug Administration (FDA) for adjuvant therapy of high-risk melanoma patients. The vast majority of these high-risk melanoma patients are those with positive lymph nodes. This indication for interferon alfa-2b is based on the Eastern Cooperative Oncology Group (ECOG) Trial E1684, which demonstrated a disease-free and overall survival benefit for treatment with interferon.[23] A follow-up study, E1690, confirmed a disease-free survival benefit but did not demonstrate an overall survival benefit for patients treated with high-dose interferon alfa-2b.[24] This finding generated controversy about the overall benefit of interferon alfa-2b therapy for adjuvant treatment of high-risk melanoma.

The results of another important study regarding the role of high-dose interferon alfa-2b therapy, ECOG study E1694, have been presented (J Kirkwood, unpublished data). In this study, 774 high-risk melanoma patients were randomized to receive adjuvant high-dose interferon alfa-2b versus a GM2 ganglioside vaccine. The study was opened early by the data monitoring committee because of the clear superiority of interferon alfa-2b in terms of both disease-free and overall survival. Taken together, these studies indicate that high-dose interferon alfa-2b is an effective adjuvant therapy and should be offered to patients with high-risk melanoma, most notably those with nodal metastases. This conclusion provides an important rationale for performing SLN biopsy for nodal staging.

The identification of patient populations that benefit most from this therapy is the remaining goal.

Identification of homogeneous patient populations for clinical trials of adjuvant therapy

A significant concern regarding the E1684 and E1690 studies has been the heterogeneous nature of the patient populations studied. The vast majority of patients had palpable nodal disease, either synchronous with the primary tumor or recurrent at some time after the primary tumor had been excised. Very few patients (12% in E1684 and 11% in E1690) had microscopically positive lymph nodes. These studies were performed prior to the widespread acceptance of SLN biopsy for nodal staging.

At centers that perform SLN biopsy routinely, however, few patients with bulky palpable nodal disease are now seen, suggesting that the spectrum of Stage III melanoma has changed. The vast majority of Stage III patients are now those who have microscopically positive nodes detected at SLN biopsy (most frequently a single positive SLN). Therefore, the patients with Stage III disease currently identified by SLN biopsy differ significantly from populations studied in previous trials of adjuvant therapy.

The heterogeneity of the patients entered into these two studies certainly confounds the interpretation of the results. Therefore, one of the major goals of SLN biopsy is to identify homogeneously staged patient populations for entry into clinical trials. Only by entry of patients with similar prognoses will meaningful interpretation of adjuvant therapy results be possible. As a result of a major effort on the part of the American Joint Committee on Cancer (AJCC) Melanoma Task Force, major changes in the staging system for melanoma have been proposed.[25,26] These new changes incorporate several important independent prognostic factors that were not taken into account in these two trials. For instance, the number of positive lymph nodes was not a stratification criterion in E1684, although it is now known to be an important prognostic factor.[25,26] Furthermore, it is now known that tumor ulceration is such an important independent prognostic factor that it may be used to upstage patients in each T category of the new AJCC staging system.[25,26] Not only is ulceration an important prognostic factor for patients with node-negative melanoma, but it retains its prognostic significance for patients with positive lymph nodes. Therefore, a relatively minor imbalance in ulceration between treatment arms could result in significant differences in survival. Ulceration was not a stratification factor in either E1684 or E1690. This fact underscores the importance of stratifying patients in clinical trials not only by Breslow thickness, but also by the number of positive lymph nodes and the presence of ulceration.

What if SLN biopsy does not improve survival?

Sentinel lymph-node biopsy is a diagnostic staging test to determine the status of the regional lymph nodes. It has been suggested that if SLN biopsy cannot be shown to improve overall survival for patients with melanoma, there is no value in this procedure.[1,2] The value of SLN biopsy, however, is in accurate nodal staging. We do not impose the burden of therapeutic efficacy on other diagnostic staging tests in oncology, such as computed tomography scans, magnetic resonance imaging, positron emission tomography scans, or for that matter axillary lymph-node dissection (ALND) for breast cancer. Sentinel lymph-node biopsy is a minimally invasive procedure performed at the same time as the wide-local excision of the primary melanoma. It carries with it the morbidity of a lymph-node biopsy. It is certainly cost-effective and less morbid than elective lymph-node dissection. Evidence from several centers documents the accuracy of this technique for nodal staging—patients with positive SLNs unequivocally have a much worse prognosis than those patients who have negative SLNs.

THE MULTICENTER SELECTIVE LYMPHADENECTOMY TRIAL

Some have argued that SLN biopsy should be considered strictly investigational because there is no randomized, prospective study that indicates that SLN biopsy is associated with improved survival.[1,2] In fact, such a study, the Multicenter Selective Lymphadenectomy Trial (MSLT) by Dr Donald Morton and colleagues (Figure 14.1),[21] is in progress. In the MSLT trial, melanoma patients with clinically negative regional lymph nodes are randomized to one of two treatment arms: wide-local excision of the primary melanoma alone, versus wide-local excision in combination with SLN biopsy. The primary goal is to determine whether SLN biopsy with completion lymphadenectomy for patients with positive SLNs improves disease-free and overall survival rates compared with wide-local excision alone and clinical observation of the regional lymph nodes. This study will assess whether the status of the SLN can be used as a prognostic factor to identify patients who could benefit from completion nodal dissection. This study will provide definitive evidence to evaluate the role of therapeutic lymph-node dissection for patients with positive SLNs.

The National Cancer Institute-sponsored MSLT is an extension of the original studies performed by Morton and colleagues at the John Wayne Cancer Institute. The logic of the trial runs thus: while the techniques of lymphatic mapping and SLN biopsy have been widely adopted and studied in several large single-institution trials, no multicenter validation trial has taken place. Some concern existed about the ability to transfer this new technology to other surgeons while maintaining a high degree of accuracy. Because of potential technical difficulties of lymphatic mapping and SLN biopsy, its role outside of high-volume melanoma centers was questioned as well.

The MSLT is a 16-center international study that has enrolled over 1100 patients since 1995.[21] Eligible patients have invasive primary cutaneous melanoma of the head and neck, trunk, extremities, sole of the foot, palm of the hand,

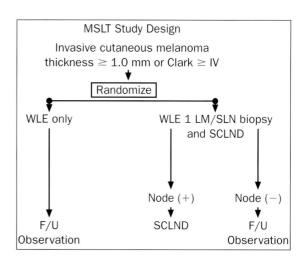

Figure 14.1 The Multicenter Selective Lymphadenectomy Trial (primary end-point overall survival). WLE: wide-local excision; LM/SLN biopsy: lymphatic mapping and sentinel lymph-node biopsy; SCLND: selective complete lymph-node dissection; F/U: follow-up. After Morton et al,[21] with permission.

or at a subungual site. Patients are included if they have primary melanomas with Breslow thickness greater than or equal to 1 mm, or Clark's Level IV/V with any Breslow thickness. Patients must be between the ages of 18 years and 75 years.

Patients are randomly assigned to either wide-local excision of the primary melanoma with nodal observation, or wide-local excision with intraoperative lymphatic mapping, SLN biopsy, and selective complete lymph-node dissection in a 40 : 60 distribution. The patients in the SLN biopsy arm all undergo lymphatic mapping with a combination of vital blue dye and radioactive colloid using a standardized technique. Strict guidelines based upon the technique originally described are followed. Participating centers have to demonstrate 85% or greater accuracy in SLN identification in at least 30 cases. All SLNs are examined in a similar manner, including serial sectioning and immunohistochemistry (IHC). The completion lymph-node dissection specimen (non-SLN) is examined by routine histologic methods only.

Patients with positive SLNs undergo completion lymph-node dissection; patients who have SLNs without evidence of metastatic disease undergo no further surgery. Adjuvant therapy is not standardized. Recent results have validated the accuracy and transferability of standardized SLN biopsy techniques in a multicenter setting.[21] It appears that successful lymphatic mapping is directly related to surgeon experience and that such experience can indeed be acquired expeditiously. This study should be closed to accrual shortly and will provide definitive data on the therapeutic impact of SLN biopsy in determining the need for completion lymph-node dissection.

What if SLN biopsy does not improve survival?

While we anxiously await the results of the MSLT study, we believe that even if SLN biopsy in and of itself does not improve survival, it has inherent value and should be continued for nodal staging until or unless another less-invasive staging test with similar predictive value is developed. This prognostic information is extremely valuable to patients and to physicians treating this disease and is vital to our efforts to find new and less toxic adjuvant therapies for melanoma. The heterogeneity of patients in clinical Stages I–III is simply too great to continue to enter patients in randomized trials based upon clinical staging of regional lymph nodes. Elective lymph-node dissection results in far too much morbidity for the vast majority of patients who have negative lymph nodes. Sentinel lymph-node biopsy therefore is appropriate for patients with a significant risk of nodal metastasis, including those with melanomas equal to or greater than 1.0 mm Breslow thickness.[4,12–22] Sentinel lymph-node biopsy for melanomas less than 1.0 mm Breslow thickness with poor prognostic features (e.g., ulceration, Clark's Level IV) is also appropriate in some cases and requires further investigation.

THE SUNBELT MELANOMA TRIAL

The Sunbelt Melanoma Trial is a multi-institutional, prospective, randomized trial that integrates the advances in melanoma staging and adjuvant therapy. The principal goal is to use ultrastaging to identify those patients who will benefit most from adjuvant therapy. The central hypothesis is that adjuvant interferon alfa-2b therapy plus regional lymph-node dissection is more effective than lymph-node dissection alone at prolonging disease-free and overall survival times for patients with early nodal metastasis.

Reverse transcriptase–polymerase chain reaction (RT-PCR) analysis of lymph nodes is a very sensitive test that can detect one melanoma cell in 1 000 000 normal cells; RT-PCR detects specific messenger RNA expressed by melanoma cells.[27] It has been reported that RT-PCR detection of tyrosinase mRNA in histologically negative SLNs correlates with decreased disease-free and overall survival.[28] Routine RT-PCR analysis of SLNs may improve our ability to identify the highest-risk groups of Stage I and II melanoma patients, who may be appropriate candidates for adjuvant therapy.

It also has been demonstrated that RT-PCR analysis of tyrosinase mRNA in peripheral blood correlates with prognosis from melanoma.[29] Although there are conflicting reports in the literature, RT-PCR analysis of peripheral blood samples may prove to be an important molecular staging test to determine the need for and effectiveness of adjuvant therapy, and for follow-up.

All patients younger than 71 years old with melanoma greater than or equal to 1.0 mm Breslow thickness, no palpable lymph nodes, no evidence of distant metastasis, and who are otherwise fit to receive interferon alfa-2b therapy, are eligible for the Sunbelt Melanoma Trial (Figure 14.2). At the time of lymphatic mapping and SLN biopsy, a portion of each SLN is frozen and stored at −70 °C for possible RT-PCR analysis at a later time. The remaining lymph is examined by routine histology, serial sectioning, and IHC staining for S-100 protein. With a median Breslow thickness of 2.3 mm,

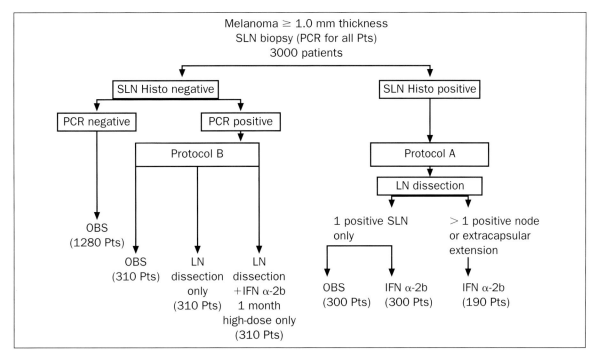

Figure 14.2 The Sunbelt Melanoma Trial. Histo, histologically; IFN, interferon; LN, lymph node; OBS, observation; PCR, polymerase chain reaction; Pts, patients.

24% of patients have had a positive SLN identified by histology or IHC. This attests to the sensitivity of the pathologic analysis of the SLNs.

Patients with histologically or IHC-positive SLNs are eligible for Protocol A (Figure 14.2). All patients undergo regional lymph-node dissection. Patients with one histologically positive or IHC-positive SLN as the only nodal metastasis are randomized to either observation or high-dose adjuvant interferon alfa-2b therapy, with stratification by Breslow thickness (1.0 mm to 2.0 mm; >2.0 mm to 4.0 mm; or >4.0 mm) and ulceration.

Patients with more than one histologically or IHC-positive SLN, any evidence of extracapsular extension of the tumor, or any non-SLN that contains metastatic melanoma are not randomized, but are treated with standard high-dose interferon alfa-2b. These patients are followed to determine the predictive value of prospective peripheral blood PCR analysis for survival and

recurrence. In this way, valuable molecular staging information will be obtained from this group of patients who receive standard adjuvant therapy.

Patients with histologically negative and IHC-negative SLNs are eligible for Protocol B (Figure 14.2). The stored portion of the SLN is evaluated by RT-PCR analysis. Markers analyzed include tyrosinase, MART-1, Mage-3, and gp100. A positive PCR test is defined as detection of tyrosinase, plus at least one other marker. If the SLN is negative by RT-PCR analysis, the patient is observed. The patients with SLNs positive by RT-PCR are stratified by tumor thickness and ulceration, and randomized to three arms: observation, lymph-node dissection, or lymph-node dissection plus interferon alfa-2b. In Protocol B, interferon alfa-2b therapy is given for 1 month only as the high-dose induction phase. Protocol B will not only define in a prospective fashion the natural history of patients with PCR-only positive SLNs but will also determine if adjuvant interferon alfa-2b therapy plus lymphadenectomy is superior to lymphadenectomy alone in terms of disease-free and overall survival. All patients will also undergo prospective analysis of peripheral blood by RT-PCR to determine the value of this molecular staging test.

The Sunbelt Melanoma Trial involves over 60 centers nationwide; over 1600 patients have been enrolled at the time of writing this chapter. This ongoing study offers a unique opportunity to use the advances in melanoma staging to determine the need for adjuvant therapy; it promises to yield important information that will be helpful in the treatment of melanoma patients in years to come.

CONCLUSION

Sentinel lymph-node biopsy, a diagnostic staging test to determine the pathologic status of the regional lymph nodes, accurately identifies the presence of nodal metastasis. The presence of a positive SLN is the single most important prognostic factor in determining the likelihood of survival. This being the case, patients should be offered the option of SLN biopsy, when appropriate, to determine the status of the regional lymph nodes. This provides the opportunity for early therapeutic lymph-node dissection, for which there is evidence of benefit in node-positive patients. Furthermore, patients in whom a positive SLN is identified are then eligible for adjuvant therapy with interferon alfa-2b, which is still the only FDA-approved adjuvant therapy for melanoma and is considered by many to be the standard of care and the reference treatment against which all other adjuvant therapies should be compared. The value of SLN biopsy for identifying homogeneous patient populations for entry into clinical trials of novel adjuvant agents cannot be underestimated. Only by identifying populations of patients with similar prognoses will we be likely to develop more effective adjuvant therapies.

Advances in the staging of melanoma will focus adjuvant therapies on patients who are most likely to benefit from them. Sentinel lymph-node biopsy has made accurate nodal staging possible with a minimally invasive procedure. The addition of RT-PCR detects "submicroscopic" disease and may identify Stage I and II patients at higher risk for recurrence, who may benefit from more aggressive treatment. Results from large prospective trials of SLN biopsy for melanoma, including the Multicenter Selective Lymphadenectomy Trial and the Sunbelt Melanoma Trial, will answer many of the remaining questions.

REFERENCES

1. Lamberg L, Dermatologists debate sentinel node biopsy, safety of liposuction, and antibiotic prophylaxis. *JAMA* 2000; **283**:2223–4.
2. Otley CC, Zitelli JA, Review of sentinel lymph node biopsy and systemic interferon for melanoma: promising but investigational modalities. *Dermatol Surg* 2000; **26**:177–80.
3. Editorial, WHO declares lymphatic mapping to be the standard of care for melanoma. *Oncology* 1999; **13**:288.
4. Gershenwald JE, Thompson W, Mansfield PF et al, Multi-institutional melanoma lymphatic mapping experience: the prognostic value of sentinel lymph node status in 612 stage I or II melanoma patients. *J Clin Oncol* 1999; **17**:976–83.
5. Veronesi U, Adamus J, Bandiera DC et al, Delayed regional lymph node dissection in stage I melanoma of the skin of the lower extremities. *Cancer* 1982; **49**:2420–30.
6. Sim FH, Taylor WF, Ivins JC et al, A prospective randomized study of the efficacy of routine elective lymphadenectomy in management of malignant melanoma. *Cancer* 1978; **41**:948–56.
7. Cascinelli N, Morabito A, Santinami M et al, Immediate or delayed dissection of regional nodes in patients with melanoma of the trunk: a randomised trial. WHO Melanoma Programme. *Lancet* 1998; **351**:793–6.
8. Balch CM, Soong S-J, Bartolucci AA et al, Efficacy of an elective regional lymph node dissection of 1 to 4 mm thick melanomas for patients 60 years of age and younger. *Ann Surg* 1996; **224**:255–66.
9. Balch CM, Soong S, Ross MI et al, Long-term results of a multi-institutional randomized trial

comparing prognostic factors and surgical results for intermediate thickness melanomas (1.0 to 4.0 mm). Intergroup Melanoma Surgical Trial. *Ann Surg Oncol* 2000; **7**:87–97.

10. Reintgen DS, Emerging evidence for a survival benefit associated with regional lymph node dissection for melanoma. *Ann Surg Oncol* 2000; **7**:75–6.

11. Reintgen DS, Regional nodal surgery for melanoma impacts recurrence rates and survival. *Ann Surg Oncol* 2000; **7**:80–1.

12. Morton DL, Wen DR, Wong JH et al, Technical details of intraoperative lymphatic mapping for early stage melanoma. *Arch Surg* 1992; **127**:392–9.

13. Essner R, Bostick PJ, Glass EC et al, Standardized probe-directed sentinel node dissection in melanoma. *Surgery* 2000; **127**:26–31.

14. Reintgen D, Cruse CW, Wells K et al, The orderly progression of melanoma nodal metastases. *Ann Surg* 1994; **220**:759–67.

15. Miliotes G, Albertini J, Berman C et al, The tumor biology of melanoma nodal metastases. *Am Surg* 1996; **62**:81–8.

16. Gershenwald JE, Colome MI, Lee JE et al, Patterns of recurrence following a negative sentinel lymph node biopsy in 243 patients with stage I or II melanoma. *J Clin Oncol* 1998; **16**:2253–60.

17. Albertini, JJ, Cruse CW, Rapaport D et al, Intraoperative radiolymphoscintigraphy improves sentinel lymph node identification for patients with melanoma. *Ann Surg* 1996; **223**:217–24.

18. Essner R, Conforti A, Kelley MC et al, Efficacy of lymphatic mapping, sentinel lymphadenectomy, and selective complete lymph node dissection as a therapeutic procedure for early-stage melanoma. *Ann Surg Oncol* 1999; **6**:442–9.

19. Gershenwald JE, Tseng CH, Thompson W et al, Improved sentinel lymph node localization in patients with primary melanoma with the use of radiolabeled colloid. *Surgery* 1998; **124**:203–10.

20. Gennari R, Bartolomei M, Testori A et al, Sentinel node localization in primary melanoma: preoperative dynamic lymphoscintigraphy, intraoperative gamma probe, and vital dye guidance. *Surgery* 2000; **127**:19–25.

21. Morton DL, Thompson JF, Essner R et al, Validation of the accuracy of intraoperative lymphatic mapping and sentinel lymphadenectomy for early-stage melanoma: a multicenter trial. Multicenter Selective Lymphadenectomy Trial Group. *Ann Surg* 1999; **230**:453–63.

22. Brobeil A, Cruse CW, Messina JL et al, Cost analysis of sentinel lymph node biopsy as an alternative to elective lymph node dissection in patients with malignant melanoma. *Surg Oncol Clin N Am* 1999; **8**:435–45.

23. Kirkwood JM, Strawderman MH, Ernstoff MS et al, Interferon alfa-2b adjuvant therapy of high-risk resected cutaneous melanoma: the Eastern Cooperative Oncology Group Trial EST 1684. *J Clin Oncol* 1996; **14**:7–17.

24. Kirkwood JM, Ibrahim J, Sondak V et al, Preliminary analysis of the E1690/S9111/C9190 Intergroup Postoperative Adjuvant Trial of High- and Low-Dose IFNα-2b (HDI and LDI) in High-Risk Primary or Lymph Node Metastatic Melanoma (meeting abstract). *Proc ASCO* 1999; **18**:A2072.

25. Buzaid AC, Ross MI, Balch CM et al, Critical analysis of the current American Joint Committee on Cancer staging system for cutaneous melanoma and proposal of a new staging system. *J Clin Oncol* 1997; **15**:1039–51.

26. Balch CM, Buzaid AC, Atkins MB et al, A new American Joint Committee on Cancer staging system for cutaneous melanoma. *Cancer* 2000; **88**:1484–91.

27. Wang X, Heller R, VanVoorhis N et al, Detection of submicroscopic lymph node metastases with polymerase chain reaction in patients with malignant melanoma. *Ann Surg* 1994; **220**:768–74.

28. Shivers SC, Wang X, Li W, Joseph E et al, Molecular staging of malignant melanoma: correlation with clinical outcome. *JAMA* 1998; **280**:1410–15.

29. Mellado B, Colomer D, Castel T et al, Detection of circulating neoplastic cells by reverse-transcriptase polymerase chain reaction in malignant melanoma: association with clinical stage and prognosis. *J Clin Oncol* 1996; **14**:2091–7.

15

Review of published experience

Mary S Brady and Deena Thayer

The clinical management of patients with cutaneous melanoma has been revolutionized by
the development of sentinel lymph-node mapping. This procedure allows the surgeon to
accurately stage the regional lymph node basin
by excising the first draining, or "sentinel,"
lymph node from a cutaneous melanoma and
submitting it for careful pathologic examination. The status of the sentinel lymph node
(SLN) has been shown to be the most accurate
predictor of prognosis in clinical Stage I and II
melanoma patients.[1] Those with evidence of
metastasis in the SLN (positive SLN) undergo a
staging evaluation and completion lymph-node
dissection, while patients without metastasis
(negative SLN) require no additional operative
therapy. In addition, this highly accurate and
minimally invasive procedure allows the surgeon to identify patients who may benefit from
adjuvant therapy. While it is too early to determine whether the use of SLN mapping will
improve the survival experience of patients
with melanoma, the published experience using
this technique has helped define and reserve its
role in the management of patients with the disease.

THE IMPORTANCE OF REGIONAL LYMPH NODES IN PATIENTS WITH CUTANEOUS MELANOMA

The regional nodal basin is the first site of recurrence in 60–70% of patients with clinically localized melanoma who develop metastases.[2] In
addition, it is well established that the presence
or absence of regional lymph-node metastases is
the most accurate predictor of prognosis in
patients with melanoma.[3,4] Despite the intuitive
appeal of removing the draining lymph nodes in
patients with clinically localized disease, early
prospective, randomized trials failed to demonstrate a survival advantage for this approach.[5,6]
Despite this, many surgeons were reluctant to
abandon elective lymph-node dissection, primarily because retrospective studies suggested a
benefit when compared to wide excision alone in
the management of patients with melanoma.[7–9]
Although a recent prospective, randomized trial
demonstrated no benefit from elective lymph-
node dissection in all of 740 patients with intermediate-thickness melanoma (1–4 mm in depth),
large subgroups of patients had a more favorable outcome following elective lymph-node dis-

section than those treated initially with wide-local excision and therapeutic lymph-node dissection when necessary.[10] It is clear that there is a subset of patients who benefit from removal of regional lymph nodes containing subclinical metastatic melanoma. Until recently, identifying this subset of patients (approximately 20% of patients with melanoma 1–4 mm in depth) has not been possible.

Once regional nodal metastases are palpable, a patient's opportunity for long-term survival is reduced by 20–50% patients those found to have microscopically positive nodes at elective lymph-node dissection.[11] The development of lymphatic mapping with vital blue dye[12] and, more recently, radiolabeled colloid,[13] has provided an appealing compromise between routine elective lymph-node dissection for all patients at risk for metastasis and the delayed therapeutic procedure once regional disease is clinically evident. The use of SLN mapping allows the surgeon to limit the use of complete regional lymph-node dissection to those patients known to have metastatic melanoma in the SLN.

DEVELOPMENT OF LYMPHATIC MAPPING FOR PATIENTS WITH MELANOMA

The development of lymphatic mapping for melanoma began with the use of cutaneous lymphoscintigraphy (LSG) by Donald Morton and colleagues, as described in Chapter 1. Morton went on to demonstrate the value of blue dye in lymphatic mapping.[12] However, SLN mapping using blue dye alone was associated with two disadvantages. The procedure required substantial experience to achieve consistency in finding the SLN. More importantly, additional SLNs deep within the nodal basin were not easily detected if the afferent blue channel was not identified in the skin flaps.

The addition of radiolabeled colloid to facilitate SLN identification represented a significant improvement in the technique of SLN mapping. David Krag and colleagues published the first large multicenter experience with SLN mapping using radiolabeled colloid, and they

demonstrated that SLN mapping using a combination of blue dye and radiolabeled colloid was easily learned by investigators at participating centers.[14] This technical advance led to the rapid application of SLN mapping across the USA, initially at tertiary cancer-referral centers and more recently in many community hospitals.

TECHNICAL SUCCESS

Published reports document a high degree of technical success associated with SLN mapping for melanoma when a radiocolloid and gamma probe are used in addition to blue dye. The largest of these studies, as well as earlier reports using blue dye alone, are summarized in Table 15.1.[1,12,14–19]

Most investigators report success in 95–100% of procedures when a combination of blue dye and radiocolloid is used. Morton and colleagues reported technical success in 99% of patients using both blue dye and radiocolloid compared with 95% when blue dye alone was used.[20] Kapteijn and associates reported technical success in 99% of patients undergoing SLN mapping using blue dye and colloid compared with 84% success when blue dye alone was used.[21] In another large retrospective experience, Gershenwald and colleagues found that the addition of radiocolloid resulted in an increase in the technical success of the procedure from 87% for blue dye alone to 99% when both blue dye and colloid were used.[22]

LESSONS LEARNED FROM LYMPHATIC MAPPING

The widespread use of LSG to facilitate SLN mapping has demonstrated how variant and unpredictable cutaneous lymphatic flow can be, particularly for patients with primary melanoma of the trunk, head, or neck. Norman and colleagues used radiolabeled colloid to visualize lymphatic drainage patterns in 82 patients with nonextremity, intermediate-thickness melanoma.[23] They demonstrated that over

Table 15.1 Clinical experience with lymphatic mapping for cutaneous melanoma

Investigator	Technique	N	Positive SLN (%)	Success (%)
Morton et al (1992)[12]	Blue dye	237[a]	21	82
Thompson et al (1995)[16]	Blue dye	118	21[a]	87
Glass et al (1995)[18]	Blue dye	132	23	99
Krag et al (1995)[14]	Both	121	12	98
Gershenwald et al (1999)[1]	Both	580	15	95
Haddad et al (1999)[17]	Both	693	14	99
Cascinelli et al (2000)[19]	Both[b]	829	18	88
Porter et al (2000)[15]	Both	765[a]	16	99

[a]N, number of lymphatic basins.
[b]Intraoperative gamma probe used in only 17% of patients.

Table 15.2 Clinical experience of patients with drainage to more than one lymphatic basin

Investigator	N	Site/stage	Patients with more than 1 basin on LSG (n)	(%)
Morton et al (1992)[12]	223[a]	All, I & II	14	6
Uren et al (1993)[24]	209	Trunk, >1.5 mm	121	58
Thompson et al (1995)[16]	100	All, I & II	16	16
Mudun et al (1996)[25]	25	All, I & II	8	32
Gershenwald et al (1999)[1]	612	All, I & II	67	11

[a]Only patients with primary melanoma located in ambiguous drainage sites underwent lymphoscintigraphy (LSG).

59% of patients had drainage patterns that differed substantially from classic anatomic teaching.[23]

Drainage to more than one lymphatic basin is also relatively common, as illustrated by a series of 118 patients with melanoma (all sites) undergoing SLN biopsy, in whom 17% had drainage to more than one nodal basin.[14] Several other reports suggest that drainage to multiple basins occurs in 6% to 58% of patients, depending on the location of the primary melanoma (Table 15.2).[1,12,16,24,25] Because lym-phatic drainage is difficult to predict reliably, as well as the fact that drainage to multiple lymphatic basins is relatively common, preoperative LSG is crucial to successful localization of the SLN(s). In addition, a significant number of patients will be found to have in-transit SLNs (nodes found outside of regional basins) which would be more likely to be missed without the assistance of preoperative LSG. Uren and colleagues reported that these nodes have the same risk of harboring micrometastatic melanoma as other SLNs.[26]

TECHNICAL ISSUES

Several different techniques for SLN mapping using radiocolloid have been reported, and all are highly successful in facilitating identification of the SLN. These include the injection of unfiltered technetium-99m-sulfur colloid (Tc-99m-SC) or Tc-99m-human serum albumin (Tc-99m-HSA) injected 24 hours prior to the procedure, and filtered Tc-99m-SC injected on the same day as (4–6 hours prior to) the procedure. A same-day injection of filtered Tc-99m-SC may be somewhat superior to the other two techniques by providing the highest differential counts between the SLN and the remaining basin as well as concordance between the blue-stained and radioactive nodes.[27] Nathanson et al compared Tc-99m-SC and Tc-99m-HSA in a rat model of SLN mapping.[28] They found that Tc-99m-SC was rapidly taken up by the lymphatics and preferentially retained compared with Tc-99m-HSA, which tended to diffuse more rapidly into surrounding tissues.

The publication of the results of SLN mapping at the MD Anderson Cancer Center has allowed further refinement of the technical aspects of the procedure. Porter and colleagues reported the outcome in 633 patients undergoing SLN mapping and biopsy.[15] They found that in the 124 lymphatic basins that contained a positive SLN, 95% of the time the most radioactive node was the positive node. In addition, removal of more than two SLNs did not upstage any patient. They emphasize that pursuing additional radioactive lymph nodes after two SLNs have been removed is unlikely to increase the likelihood of detecting metastatic melanoma, particularly if the remaining nodes have counts that are less than two-thirds that of the SLNs.[15]

ACCURACY OF SLN STAGING

The accuracy of SLN mapping has been demonstrated in two ways. When the procedure was first introduced, it was important to determine that the incidence of false-negative SLN biopsies was low. This was accomplished by following SLN biopsy with a completion lymph-node dissection, regardless of the pathologic status of the SLN. Morton and colleagues reported their experience using the blue-dye technique in 223 patients (237 lymph-node basins).[12] They were able to identify the SLN in 194 of 237 basins (82%). Metastases were present in 47 of 259 (18%) SLNs, or 40 of 194 (21%) lymphatic basins. Nonsentinel lymph nodes were the sole site of metastasis in only 2 of 194 (1%) completion lymph-node dissection specimens. When analyzed by lymph nodes removed, less than 0.1% of non-SLNs removed contained tumor, demonstrating the low false-negative rate of the procedure for staging the lymphatic basin.[20] This low false-negative rate of SLN biopsy has been confirmed by other investigators (Table 15.3).[12,16,29,30]

Table 15.3 Accuracy of SLN mapping for cutaneous melanoma

Investigator	Technique	N	False-negative rate
Morton et al (1992)[12]	Blue dye	237[a]	2/237 (1%)
Morton et al (1993)[29]	Blue dye	72[b]	0
Reintgen et al (1994)[30]	Blue dye	42	0
Thompson et al (1995)[16]	Blue dye	105[a]	2/105 (1.9%)

[a]Lymphatic basins.
[b]Patients with head and neck melanoma; only 34 patients had confirmatory results of lymph-node dissection following SLN identification.

Table 15.4 Sentinel lymph-node basin failure in SLN-negative melanoma patients		
Investigator	Nodal SLN basin failure	Median follow-up (mo)
Gadd et al (1999)[31]	7/89 (8%)	23
Jansen et al (2000)[33]	6/151 (4%)	32
Cascinelli et al (2000)[19]	40/710 (6%)	29
Muller et al (2000)[34]	3/162 (2%)	42
Gershenwald et al (1998)[32]	10/243 (4%)	35

Another indication of the accuracy of SLN mapping is the incidence of nodal-basin failure in patients found to have pathologically negative SLNs. Nodal-basin failure for patients undergoing elective lymph-node dissection who are found to have negative lymph nodes is quite low. McCarthy and colleagues reported recurrence patterns in 3171 node-negative melanoma patients.[2] Of these, 27% ($N = 866$) developed recurrent disease at a mean follow-up of 9.5 years. Regional nodal recurrence was uncommon in patients undergoing elective lymph-node dissection, accounting for less than 10% of initial sites of recurrence in the 866 patients who developed recurrent disease.[2]

Two more recent studies have addressed this issue, although the median follow-up period was relatively short.[31,32] Gadd and colleagues reported regional nodal-basin recurrence in 7 of 89 (8%) patients who underwent SLN mapping and were found to have negative SLNs.[31] Gershenwald found that 10 of 270 (4%) patients with negative SLNs developed nodal-basin recurrence in the previously mapped basin.[32] Both investigators attributed a significant percentage of the false-negative SLNs to errors of pathologic examination. Gadd and colleagues found that when the SLNs from the 7 patients with nodal basin recurrence were pathologically re-examined, evidence of metastatic disease was found in SLNs from 3 of the 7 patients (43%).[31] Gershenwald reported occult evidence of metastatic disease demonstrated on re-review of the SLN in 8 of the 10 patients (80%)

with nodal-basin failure.[32] These and other reports are listed in Table 15.4.[19,31–34] Further follow-up is necessary before an accurate assessment of nodal-basin failure rate in patients undergoing SLN biopsy can be determined with confidence, although these reports suggest that it will be low.

PATIENTS WITH MELANOMA OF THE HEAD AND NECK

Patients undergoing SLN mapping with primary melanoma of the head and neck warrant special consideration. Lymphatic drainage patterns are even less predictable than in patients with melanoma arising on the trunk or extremities. Multiple drainage basins are common, and intraparotid SLNs provide technical challenges. Several investigators have published their experiences in this subgroup of melanoma patients. In general, technical success rates are high, and morbidity is uncommon. These data are summarized in Table 15.5.[35–38]

The parotid gland is a common site of drainage in patients with cutaneous melanoma of the head and neck. Intraparotid lymph nodes tend to be small, and parotid background uptake of radioactivity can make identification of these SLNs challenging. Ollila et al reported the experience of the John Wayne Cancer Center with SLN mapping in 39 patients with melanoma of the scalp, ear, or face.[39] Thirty-seven of 39 patients (95%) showed mapping to

Table 15.5 Sentinel lymph-node biopsy in patients with melanoma of the head and neck				
Investigator	N	Technical success (%)	Positive SLN	Positive non-SLN
Carlson et al (2000)[35]	58	96	10/58 (17%)	3/10 (30%)
Wells et al (1997)[36]	58	95	6/58 (10%)	0
Jansen et al (2000)[37]	30	90	8/27 (30%)	0
Wagner et al (2000)[38]	70	99	12/70 (17%)	5/12 (42%)

a lymph node in the parotid region. In only two patients could the SLN not be located in the parotid region, and these patients required a superficial parotidectomy. The procedure-related morbidity was low, with only one case of temporary facial-nerve paresis. Ollila et al concluded that SLN mapping is safe and efficacious for patients with primary melanoma of the ear, face or scalp that drains to the parotid region.[39] A similar conclusion was reached by Carlson and colleagues, who reported intra-parotid SLNs in 24% of 58 patients with melanoma of the head and neck.[35] They were unsuccessful in localizing the SLN in the parotid region in only 17% of cases. They reported no cases of facial-nerve damage. Wagner and colleagues reported their experience with SLN mapping in patients with melanoma of the head and neck.[38] They found that compared with other patients with melanoma, patients with primary melanoma of the head and neck mapped to significantly more nodal basins, and were found to have significantly more SLNs (mean 3.5) compared with those who did not have head and neck primaries (mean 2.3). The incidence of positive SLNs in patients with melanoma of the head and neck is no different from that found in patients with melanoma of the extremities or trunk.[35,38] Other reports suggest, however, that additional positive non-SLNs are more common in patients with head and neck melanoma than in those with melanoma arising elsewhere.[35,38]

MORBIDITY OF SLN MAPPING

The morbidity of SLN mapping using blue dye and radiocolloid is small. The most common complication of the procedure is seroma formation following SLN removal. An uncommon complication of SLN biopsy using blue dye is anaphylaxis;[40] this is reported much more commonly in patients undergoing SLN mapping for breast cancer, and is probably related to the volume of dye injected. Lymphedema can also occur following SLN biopsy. Wrone and colleagues reported an incidence of 1.7% in their experience with 235 procedures.[41]

FACTORS ASSOCIATED WITH SLN POSITIVITY

Only two factors have been reported to be predictive of SLN positivity. By far the most important of these is the Breslow depth of the primary tumor. Indeed, there is a linear relationship between increasing tumor depth and risk of lymph-node metastasis. These data are summarized in Table 15.6,[1,17,42,43] which shows that patients with primary melanoma less than 1.5 mm in Breslow depth have a low risk ($<$10%) of metastatic melanoma in the SLN node. In contrast, patients with deep primary melanoma ($>$4 mm Breslow depth) have a 30–35% chance of having a positive SLN. When all patients with melanoma between 1 mm and 4 mm in depth are considered, the risk of SLN positivity ranges from 15% to 20%.

Table 15.6 Percentage of patients with positive SLN based on depth of primary lesion

Breslow depth (mm)	Patients with positive SLNs (%)	No. of patients	Investigator
<0.76	0	0/14	Joseph et al (1998)[42]
	0	0/20	Haddad et al (1999)[17]
	0	0/70	Landi et al (2000)[43]
0.76–1.0	6	5/83	Joseph et al (1998)[42]
	5.3	4/94	Haddad et al (1999)[17]
1.1–1.5	7	12/169	Joseph et al (1998)[42]
	8	15/188	Haddad et al (1999)[17]
<1.5	4.8	230	Gershenwald et al (1999)[1]
	6	19/302	Haddad et al (1999)[17]
1.5–4	19.2	271	Gershenwald et al (1999)[1]
	18	48/267	Joseph et al (1998)[42]
	19	59/315	Haddad et al (1999)[17]
>4	34.4	64	Gershenwald et al (1999)[1]
	30	19/62	Joseph et al (1998)[42]
	29	22/76	Haddad et al (1999)[17]
Total	15	565	Gershenwald et al (1999)[1]
	14.4	693	Haddad et al (1999)[17]

There is some controversy as to whether patients with thin melanoma (<1 mm in depth) should undergo SLN mapping. Most investigators agree that it is reasonable to perform the procedure in patients with melanoma less than 1 mm in Breslow depth if it is a Clark's Level IV lesion, has undergone regression, or is ulcerated. Bedrosian and colleagues have recently reported that the presence of vertical growth-phase (VGP) melanoma may serve to identify patients with thin melanoma at higher risk of nodal metastases.[44] Indeed, they observed a 5.6% incidence of positive SLNs in patients with melanoma of Breslow depth less than or equal to 1 mm when VGP tumor was present. Indeed, in the Sydney Melanoma Unit experience, the incidence of positive SLNs in patients with melanomas less than 1.5 mm thick was 4.6%.[45] Pathologic consistency in quantitating VGP is not strong, however, and other more commonly used features are of more practical

use in identifying thin lesions at higher risk for metastasis. These include ulceration, Clark's level, mitotic count, and regression.

The largest series to report the risk of SLN metastasis in patients with thin melanoma is that of Haddad and colleagues at the H Lee Moffitt Cancer Center.[17] In their experience, no patient with melanoma less than 0.76 mm in depth had SLN metastasis. Patients with melanoma between 0.76 mm and 1 mm in Breslow depth had a 5.6% chance of having a positive SLN. Corsetti and colleagues examined the risk of recurrence in a small group of patients with thin melanoma (≤1 mm), Clark's Level III or IV, and found that lesions recurred in 3 out of 25 patients with Clark's Level III melanoma.[46] They argue that this justifies SLN mapping in this group of patients. It is interesting to note, however, that only two of the three patients developed "regional" recurrence (presumably nodal), and one developed distant recurrence. It is unclear whether SLN mapping would have altered the natural history of the disease in these patients.

The only other factor reported to affect the risk of SLN positivity is the number of drainage basins identified on LSG. Patients with drainage to multiple nodal basins may be at increased risk of having a positive SLN. Porter and colleagues from the MD Anderson Cancer Center observed that patients with truncal melanoma that drained to multiple lymphatic basins had a higher risk of SLN metastases compared with patients who had primaries that drained to a single lymphatic basin.[47] They reported that in 281 patients who underwent SLN mapping, drainage to multiple nodal basins was present in 31% of patients. The relative risk of a positive SLN was 1.9 in these patients ($p < 0.03$) compared with those with truncal melanoma that drained to one basin.

PATHOLOGIC EVALUATION OF THE SLN

Pathologic analysis of the SLN in melanoma patients ranges from a routine hematoxylin-and-eosin (H&E) examination of the bivalved SLN to analysis using polymerase chain reaction (PCR) analysis on nucleic acid extracted from the SLN. Routine histologic examination involves taking one or two sections from the central cross-section of the node and staining with H&E, an examination that involves less than 1% of the volume of the node. This is the extent of examination historically used for determining whether lymph nodes contain tumor. There is little doubt that the use of routine H&E only will underestimate SLN positivity. In addition, reported series demonstrate that the use of serial sectioning and immunohistochemical (IHC) staining will increase the number of positive nodes identified.[32,39] Cochran and colleagues have demonstrated that 14 of 100 melanoma patients found to have pathologically "negative" lymph nodes by routine H&E were upstaged when IHC was performed using S-100 and a confirmatory monoclonal antibody NK1/C3.[48] Baisden and colleagues evaluated the use of HMB-45 for

identifying additional positive SLNs among specimens that were negative for metastatic disease by serial sectioning.[49] Of 54 patients with histologically negative SLNs, 4 were found to have HMB-45-positive cells consistent with metastatic melanoma (7%). The authors found no HMB-45-positive nodes in 244 lymph nodes sampled from patients without melanoma.[49] Considerable controversy surrounds the question of which methodology is appropriate for clinical decision-making. Currently, most centers perform serial sectioning and IHC staining for at least two melanoma-associated antigens (commonly S-100 and HMB-45) when evaluating the SLN in melanoma patients.

There is tremendous interest in using PCR techniques to evaluate the otherwise negative SLN in patients with melanoma. Wang and colleagues demonstrated that 8 of 18 patients with pathologically "negative" lymph nodes were positive by PCR using reverse transcriptase-PCR (RT-PCR) with tyrosinase-specific primers.[50] Importantly, none of the negative controls (lymph nodes from patients with tumors other than melanoma) was positive for tyrosinase by PCR. Bostick and colleagues found that 36% of patients ($N = 55$) with histopathologically negative SLNs had PCR evidence of metastatic melanoma in their SLNs.[51] They also demonstrated that these patients were at higher risk of relapse than patients whose SLNs were negative by PCR analysis. Shivers and colleagues reported a significant difference in recurrence rates in patients with histologically negative lymph nodes based on whether the lymph nodes were PCR-positive or negative.[52] Polymerase chain reaction will undoubtedly play an increasingly important role in the evaluation of the SLN, particularly when more effective adjuvant therapies become available. These studies are highlighted in Table 15.7.[12,48–50,52]

THERAPEUTIC VALUE OF SLN MAPPING AND BIOPSY FOR PATIENTS WITH MELANOMA

Despite its technical ease, minimal morbidity, and intuitive appeal, the technique of SLN

Table 15.7 Methods used to increase the sensitivity of pathologic detection of micrometastases in lymph nodes

Investigator	Technique	No. of patients	Patients upstaged	
			(*n*)	(%)
Cochran et al (1988)[48]	IHC	100	14	14
Morton et al (1992)[12]	IHC	194[a]	NA	9[a]
Wang et al (1994)[50]	PCR	29	8	28
Shivers et al (1998)[52]	PCR	114	47	41
Baisden et al (2000)[49]	IHC	66	4	6

[a]Lymphatic basins.
IHC, immunohistochemistry; NA, not applicable; PCR, polymerase chain reaction.

mapping and SLN-directed regional lymph-node dissection offers no proven survival advantage in the management of patients with cutaneous melanoma over wide-local excision and nodal observation. Morton and colleagues are conducting an ongoing trial, the Multicenter Selective Lymphadenectomy Trial (MSLT), to determine whether the use of SLN mapping in patients with cutaneous melanoma results in improved survival.[20] Eligible patients for the MSLT are those with primary cutaneous melanoma 1 mm or greater in Breslow depth or Clark's Level IV lesions. Patients are randomized to receive either wide-local excision or wide-local excision and regional lymph-node dissection if the SLN is positive. The major goal of the trial is to determine whether SLN mapping will provide a survival advantage over wide-local excision and nodal observation.

While it remains to be seen whether SLN mapping will improve the survival of patients with melanoma, it certainly does not reduce it. Patients undergoing SLN mapping and selective regional lymph-node dissection have a similar survival experience as historical control groups undergoing elective lymph-node dissection when stratified for depth, stage, anatomic site of the primary lesion, sex, and age.[53]

CONTROVERSIES

Is SLN mapping accurate in patients with a prior wide-local excision?

The procedure of lymphatic mapping with SLN biopsy is highly accurate in patients who have undergone an excisional or incisional biopsy only, as demonstrated in Morton's initial study using the blue-dye technique.[12] Karakousis and Grigoropoulos reported on a small series of patients in whom SLN mapping did not appear to be compromised by a prior wide excision as long as no rotation flap had been created.[54] Ideally, however, the option of SLN mapping should be discussed with patients prior to resection of their primary lesion. Wide excision of the primary lesion should only be undertaken if the patient chooses not to undergo the procedure.

Is SLN mapping appropriate in patients with primary melanoma greater than 4 mm in Breslow depth?

Patients with deep primary melanoma are at significant risk for occult systemic metastasis. Some argue that because the risk of occult systemic disease is so high in this group of patients, SLN mapping is unlikely to provide a significant therapeutic benefit.

Gershenwald and colleagues reported their results in 131 patients with primary melanoma 4 mm or greater in depth.[55] They found that 39% of the patients had a positive SLN, and that SLN status was the most important predictor of outcome. The 3-year disease-free survival rate of patients with negative SLNs was 82% compared with 58% for patients found to have positive SLNs. The patient's SLN status was the most important predictor of overall survival in this group, suggesting that it may identify a relatively favorable subgroup of patients with deep primary melanoma.

Is completion lymph-node dissection necessary in all patients with positive SLNs?

There is considerable interest in identifying patients with minimal risk of harboring additional positive lymph nodes following excision of the SLN(s). The hope is that these patients may be spared the morbidity of complete lymph-node dissection.

Three factors are reportedly associated with the risk of disease in non-SLNs at completion lymph-node dissection. These include the depth of the primary melanoma, the number of lym-

phatic basins draining the primary, and the number of SLNs with metastatic melanoma. Joseph et al reported that all patients with positive SLNs who were found to have additional positive lymph nodes at completion lymph-node dissection had primary tumors greater than 3 mm in depth.[42] In contrast, Wagner and colleagues reported no association between primary-tumor depth and risk of additional disease in non-SLNs in 275 patients undergoing SLN biopsy.[56] They found that more than one positive SLN was the only factor that increased the likelihood that additional disease would be found in the lymphatic basin at completion lymph-node dissection.[24,39]

In a series of 121 patients undergoing SLN biopsy, 10 of 15 patients with positive SLNs (67%) had no additional positive nodes at subsequent lymph-node dissection.[12] Other investigators have reported that between 7% and 42% of patients will be found to have additional positive nodes at completion lymph-node dissection (Table 15.8).[14,17,38,42,56]

Until effective adjuvant therapies capable of eradicating residual microscopic disease with less morbidity become available, identification of a positive SLN should almost always be followed by a complete regional lymph-node dissection. It must be remembered that with the pathologic assessment of nodal disease subject to the particular techniques applied, removal of

Table 15.8 Incidence of additional positive nodes in SLN-positive patients at completion lymph node dissection

Investigator	No. of patients with additional positive non-SLNs/ patients with positive SLNs
Haddad et al (1999)[17]	6/81 (7%)
Krag et al (1995)[14]	5/15 (33%)
Wagner et al (2000)[56]	15/53 (28%)
Wagner et al (2000)[38 a]	5/12 (42%)[a]
Joseph et al (1998)[42]	5/64 (8%)

[a]SLNs in the head and neck.

remaining "pathologically negative" nodes which may harbor disease detectable only by specialized techniques is certainly justified. Exceptions to this may be patients with positive SLNs in three or more lymphatic basins. Treatment must be individualized in these patients based on the likelihood of surgical cure. Radiologic surveillance, particularly using positron-emission tomography, may be a reasonable alternative in these patients.

SUMMARY

Sentinel lymph-node mapping for patients with melanoma should be considered the standard of care for patients with intermediate-thickness cutaneous melanoma. Patients with thin melanoma should be offered SLN mapping if their primary melanoma is a Clark's Level IV lesion, and SLN mapping should be considered in patients with Clark's Level III lesions less than 1 mm in depth when there is evidence of regression or ulceration. The risk of SLN metastasis is directly related to the depth of the lesion, and for all patients with intermediate-thickness melanoma it is approximately 20%. Patients found to have positive SLNs should undergo a completion lymph-node dissection, because 10–50% of these patients will be found to have additional positive lymph nodes in the draining basin.

CONCLUSION

Surgical oncologists are entering a new era in the management of patients with cutaneous melanoma. The technique of SLN mapping provides the surgeon with the ability to stage patients accurately, as well as to reserve early regional lymph-node dissection for only those patients with microscopic evidence of nodal involvement. It is premature to speculate whether the identification and removal of SLNs and selective lymph-node dissection in patients in whom the SLN is positive will provide patients with a survival benefit over those undergoing wide excision only. Despite this, the technique can be used for accurate staging of patients with minimal morbidity. In addition, the reassurance provided to those found to have negative SLNs is clearly of significant value.

REFERENCES

1. Gershenwald JE, Thompson W, Mansfield PF et al, Multi-institutional melanoma lymphatic mapping experience: the prognostic value of sentinel lymph node status in 612 stage I or II melanoma patients. *J Clin Oncol* 1999; **17**:976–83.
2. McCarthy WH, Shaw HM, Thompson JF, Milton GW, Time and frequency of recurrence of cutaneous stage I malignant melanoma with guidelines for follow-up study. *Surg Gynecol Obstet* 1988; **166**:497–502.
3. Veronesi V, *Prognostic Factors in Malignant Melanoma.* Academic Press: Orlando, 1987.
4. Balch CM, Soong S-J, Shaw HW et al, *An Analysis of Prognostic Factors in 4000 Patients with Cutaneous Melanoma.* Lippincott: Philadelphia, 1985.
5. Sim FH, Taylor WF, Ivins JC et al, A prospective randomized study of the efficacy of routine elective lymphadenectomy in management of malignant melanoma. Preliminary results. *Cancer* 1978; **41**:948–56.
6. Veronesi U, Adamus J, Bandiera DC et al, Delayed regional lymph node dissection in stage I melanoma of the skin of the lower extremities. *Cancer* 1982; **49**:2420–30.
7. Balch CM, Soong SJ, Milton GW et al, A comparison of prognostic factors and surgical results in 1786 patients with localized (stage I) melanoma treated in Alabama, USA, and New South Wales, Australia. *Ann Surg* 1982; **196**:677–84.
8. Balch CM, Murad TM, Soong SJ et al, Tumor thickness as a guide to surgical management of clinical stage I melanoma patients. *Cancer* 1979; **43**:883–8.
9. Milton GW, Shaw HM, McCarthy WH et al, Prophylactic lymph node dissection in clinical stage I cutaneous malignant melanoma: results of surgical treatment in 1319 patients. *Br J Surg* 1982; **69**:108–11.
10. Balch CM, Soong SJ, Bartolucci AA et al, Efficacy of an elective regional lymph node dissection of 1 to 4 mm thick melanomas for patients 60 years of age and younger. *Ann Surg* 1996; **224**:255–66; discussion 263–6.

11. Ross MI, The case for elective lymphadenectomy. *Surg Clin N Am* 1992; **1**:205–22.

12. Morton DL, Wen DR, Wong JH et al, Technical details of intraoperative lymphatic mapping for early stage melanoma. *Arch Surg* 1992; **127**:392–9.

13. Alex JC, Weaver DL, Fairbank JT et al, Gamma-probe-guided lymph node localization in malignant melanoma. *Surg Oncol* 1993; **2**:303–8.

14. Krag DN, Meijer SJ, Weaver DL et al, Minimal-access surgery for staging of malignant melanoma. *Arch Surg* 1995; **130**:654–8; discussion 659–60.

15. Porter GA, Ross MI, Berman RS et al, How many lymph nodes are enough during sentinel lymphadenectomy for primary melanoma? *Surgery* 2000; **128**:306–11.

16. Thompson JF, McCarthy WH, Bosch CM et al, Sentinel lymph node status as an indicator of the presence of metastatic melanoma in regional lymph nodes. *Melanoma Res* 1995; **5**:255–60.

17. Haddad FF, Stall A, Messina J et al, The progression of melanoma nodal metastasis is dependent on tumor thickness of the primary lesion. *Ann Surg Oncol* 1999; **6**:144–9.

18. Glass LF, Fenske NA, Messina JL et al, The role of selective lymphadenectomy in the management of patients with malignant melanoma. *Dermatol Surg* 1995; **21**:979–83.

19. Cascinelli N, Belli F, Santinami M et al, Sentinel lymph node biopsy in cutaneous melanoma: the WHO Melanoma Program experience. *Ann Surg Oncol* 2000; **7**:469–74.

20. Morton DL, Thompson JF, Essner R et al, Validation of the accuracy of intraoperative lymphatic mapping and sentinel lymphadenectomy for early-stage melanoma: a multicenter trial. Multicenter Selective Lymphadenectomy Trial Group. *Ann Surg* 1999; **230**:453–63; discussion 463–5.

21. Kapteijn BA, Nieweg OE, Liem I et al, Localizing the sentinel node in cutaneous melanoma: gamma probe detection versus blue dye. *Ann Surg Oncol* 1997; **4**:156–60.

22. Gershenwald JE, Tseng CH, Thompson W et al, Improved sentinel lymph node localization in patients with primary melanoma with the use of radiolabeled colloid. *Surgery* 1998; **124**:203–10.

23. Norman J, Cruse CW, Espinosa C et al, Redefinition of cutaneous lymphatic drainage with the use of lymphoscintigraphy for malignant melanoma. *Am J Surg* 1991; **162**:432–7.

24. Uren RF, Howman-Giles RB, Shaw HM et al, Lymphoscintigraphy in high-risk melanoma of the trunk: predicting draining node groups, defining lymphatic channels and locating the sentinel node. *J Nucl Med* 1993; **34**:1435–40.

25. Mudun A, Murray DR, Herda SC et al, Early stage melanoma: lymphoscintigraphy, reproducibility of sentinel node detection, and effectiveness of the intraoperative gamma probe. *Radiology* 1996; **199**:171–5.

26. Uren RF, Howman-Giles R, Thompson JF et al, Interval nodes: the forgotten sentinel nodes in patients with melanoma. *Arch Surg* 2000; **135**:1168–72.

27. Essner R, Bostick PJ, Glass EC et al, Standardized probe-directed sentinel node dissection in melanoma. *Surgery* 2000; **127**:26–31.

28. Nathanson SD, Anaya P, Karvelis KC et al, Sentinel lymph node uptake of two different technetium-labeled radiocolloids. *Ann Surg Oncol* 1997; **4**:104–10.

29. Morton DL, Wen DR, Foshag LJ et al, Intraoperative lymphatic mapping and selective cervical lymphadenectomy for early-stage melanomas of the head and neck. *J Clin Oncol* 1993; **11**:1751–6.

30. Reintgen D, Cruse CW, Wells K et al, The orderly progression of melanoma nodal metastases. *Ann Surg* 1994; **220**:759–67.

31. Gadd MA, Cosimi AB, Yu J et al, Outcome of patients with melanoma and histologically negative sentinel lymph nodes. *Arch Surg* 1999; **134**:381–7.

32. Gershenwald JE, Colome MI, Lee JE et al, Patterns of recurrence following a negative sentinel lymph node biopsy in 243 patients with stage I or II melanoma. *J Clin Oncol* 1998; **16**:2253–60.

33. Jansen L, Nieweg OE, Peterse JL et al, Reliability of sentinel lymph node biopsy for staging melanoma. *Br J Surg* 2000; **87**:484–9.

34. Muller MG, Borgstein PJ, Pijpers R et al, Reliability of the sentinel node procedure in melanoma patients: analysis of failures after long-term follow-up. *Ann Surg Oncol* 2000; **7**:461–8.

35. Carlson GW, Murray DR, Greenlee R et al, Management of malignant melanoma of the head and neck using dynamic lymphoscintigraphy and gamma probe-guided sentinel lymph node biopsy. *Arch Otolaryngol Head Neck Surg* 2000; **26**:433–7.

36. Wells KE, Rapaport DP, Cruse CW et al, Sentinel lymph node biopsy in melanoma of the head and neck. *Plast Reconstr Surg* 1997; **100**:591–4.

37. Jansen L, Koops HS, Nieweg OE et al, Sentinel node biopsy for melanoma in the head and neck region. *Head Neck* 2000; **22**:27.

38. Wagner JD, Park HM, Coleman JJ et al, Cervical sentinel lymph node biopsy for melanomas of the head and neck and upper thorax. *Arch Otolaryngol Head Neck Surg* 2000; **126**:313–21.

39. Ollila DW, Foshag LJ, Essner R et al, Parotid region lymphatic mapping and sentinel lymphadenectomy for cutaneous melanoma. *Ann Surg Oncol* 1999; **6**:150–4.

40. Woltsche-Kahr I, Komericki P, Kranke B et al, Anaphylactic shock following peritumoral injection of patent blue in sentinel lymph node biopsy procedure. *Eur J Surg Oncol* 2000; **26**: 313–14.

41. Wrone DA, Tanabe KK, Cosimi AB et al, Lymphedema after sentinel lymph node biopsy for cutaneous melanoma: a report of 5 cases. *Arch Dermatol* 2000; **136**:511–14.

42. Joseph E, Brobeil A, Glass F et al, Results of complete lymph node dissection in 83 melanoma patients with positive sentinel nodes. *Ann Surg Oncol* 1998; **5**:119–25.

43. Landi G, Polverelli M, Moscatelli G, Sentinel lymph node biopsy in patients with primary cutaneous melanoma: study of 455 cases. *J Eur Acad Dermatol Venereol* 2000; **14**:35–45.

44. Bedrosian I, Faries MB, Guerry D et al, Incidence of sentinel node metastasis in patients with thin primary melanoma (< or = 1 mm) with vertical growth phase. *Ann Surg Oncol* 2000; **7**:262–7.

45. Thompson JF, Shaw HM, Sentinel node metastasis from thin melanomas with vertical growth phase (editorial; comment). *Ann Surg Oncol* 2000; **7**:251–2.

46. Corsetti RL, Allen HM, Wanebo HJ, Thin < or = 1 mm level III and IV melanomas are higher risk lesions for regional failure and warrant sentinel lymph node biopsy. *Ann Surg Oncol* 2000; **7**:456–60.

47. Porter GA, Ross MI, Berman RS et al, Significance of multiple nodal basin drainage in truncal melanoma patients undergoing sentinel lymph node biopsy. *Ann Surg Oncol* 2000; **7**:256–61.

48. Cochran AJ, Wen DR, Morton DL, Occult tumor cells in the lymph nodes of patients with pathological stage I malignant melanoma. An immunohistological study. *Am J Surg Pathol* 1988; **12**:612–18.

49. Baisden BL, Askin FB, Lange JR, Westra WH, HMB-45 immunohistochemical staining of sentinel lymph nodes: a specific method for enhancing detection of micrometastases in patients with melanoma. *Am J Surg Pathol* 2000; **24**:1140–6.

50. Wang X, Heller R, VanVoorhis N et al, Detection of submicroscopic lymph node metastases with polymerase chain reaction in patients with malignant melanoma. *Ann Surg* 1994; **220**: 768–74.

51. Bostick PJ, Morton DL, Turner RR et al, Prognostic significance of occult metastases detected by sentinel lymphadenectomy and reverse transcriptase-polymerase chain reaction in early-stage melanoma patients. *J Clin Oncol* 1999; **17**:3238–44.

52. Shivers SC, Wang X, Li W et al, Molecular staging of malignant melanoma: correlation with clinical outcome. *JAMA* 1998; **280**:1410–15.

53. Essner R, Conforti A, Kelley MC et al, Efficacy of lymphatic mapping, sentinel lymphadenectomy, and selective complete lymph node dissection as a therapeutic procedure for early-stage melanoma. *Ann Surg Oncol* 1999; **6**:442–9.

54. Karakousis CP, Grigoropoulos P, Sentinel node biopsy before and after wide excision of the primary melanoma. *Ann Surg Oncol* 1999; **6**: 785–9.

55. Gershenwald JE, Mansfield PF, Lee JE, Ross MI, Role for lymphatic mapping and sentinel lymph node biopsy in patients with thick (> or = 4 mm) primary melanoma. *Ann Surg Oncol* 2000; **7**:160–5.

56. Wagner JD, Gordon MS, Chuang TY et al, Predicting sentinel and residual lymph node basin disease after sentinel lymph node biopsy for melanoma. *Cancer* 2000; **89**:453–62.

Part III
Sentinel Lymph-Node Biopsy for Breast Cancer

16

Surgical aspects

Hiram S Cody III

The surgical treatment of breast cancer over the last fifty years has become increasingly conservative, and a series of landmark clinical trials support this conservatism.[1-4] As a result, radical mastectomy is no longer the "gold standard," internal mammary node dissection has been abandoned, and breast-conservation therapy has proved to be feasible and safe for an increasing proportion of patients. Throughout this period, axillary lymph-node dissection (ALND) has remained the standard of care.

The historic role of axillary clearance has rested upon three observations: first, the well-documented imprecision of clinical assessment, with as many as 40% of clinically node-negative patients proving to be node-positive;[5] second, a substantial rate of axillary relapse in patients treated without ALND;[3] and third, a significant rate of nodal metastasis for patients with even the smallest invasive cancers: for T1a (0–0.5 cm) breast cancers, 20% from the era of clinical detection[6] and 10% in the current era of mammographic screening.[7]

Breast cancer has a long natural history and a wide spectrum of clinical behavior, and is responsive to both local and systemic treatment. In this setting, the rationale for ALND is three-fold: prognosis, local control, and the possibility of a survival benefit. First and most important, virtually all studies identify axillary node status as by far the strongest prognostic indicator in breast cancer,[8] and as an indispensable guide to the choice of both regional and systemic adjuvant therapies. Second, local recurrence necessitating reoperation develops in as many as 20% of invasive breast cancer patients treated without ALND,[3] and this rate of reoperation should be as unacceptable in patients with cancer as in those having surgery for any other reason. Finally, after an era in which it was axiomatic that local control and survival were unrelated,[9] recent prospective randomized trials persuasively link the two, finding significantly better survival rates in the groups with the least local recurrence.[10,11] While this last point remains a matter of debate,[12] few would disagree that patients with negative axillary nodes cannot possibly benefit from their removal.

BACKGROUND

The phrase "sentinel lymph node" (SLN) first appears in a 1960 paper by Gould et al,[13]

Table 16.1 Statistical measures of SLN biopsy	
Measure	**Definition**
Success rate	successful mappings/total cases
Specificity	true-negative/(true-negative + false-positive)
Negative predictive value	true-negative/(true-negative + false-negative)
Positive predictive value	true-positive/(true-positive + false-positive)
Sensitivity	true-positive/(true-positive + false-negative)
False-negative rate	false-negative/(true-positive + false-negative)
Accuracy	(true-positive + true-negative)/total cases

suggesting its benefit, if negative, in preventing radical neck dissection for cancer of the parotid. Apparently unaware of this report, Cabanas used the term "sentinel lymph node" in 1977 in a report on penile cancer,[14] as did Morton in a 1992 report on melanoma.[15] Morton's classic study used blue dye to identify the SLN, incorporated a full regional node dissection as validation for the technique, demonstrated an accuracy of 95%, and has served as the template for all of the subsequent studies applying SLN biopsy to breast cancer (see Chapter 7). The first of these was David Krag's landmark 1993 paper from the University of Vermont, using a technique of radioisotope mapping,[16] and the second was Armando Giuliano's 1994 report from the John Wayne Cancer Institute,[17] using Morton's blue-dye method (see Chapter 18). Albertini et al from the H. Lee Moffitt Cancer Center first reported in 1996 a technique combining isotope and blue dye (see Chapter 20).[18] To date, more than forty published series, all validated by backup ALND and representing the authors' initial experience in more than 4000 breast-cancer patients, confirm that the SLN can be found in more than 90% of procedures and that it correctly stages the axilla in 93% of node-positive cases and in 97% of all cases (see Chapter 27).[19]

STATISTICAL ISSUES

The intent of SLN biopsy is to accurately stage the axilla in a given patient. For clarity, the proper denominator is *number of patients* and not (as is sometimes reported) *number of SLNs*. Like any diagnostic test, SLN biopsy is subject to the standard measures of sensitivity, specificity, negative predictive value, and positive predictive value. To these one might add success rate, accuracy, and false-negative rate (Table 16.1). Because false-positive results are rare, the most relevant of these for patient and physician alike are those that use as the denominator either *node-positive cases* or *total number of cases*.

Success rate

The success rate is simply the proportion of all cases in which an SLN could be identified (number of successful mappings/total number of cases), and it answers the question: How likely is the procedure to find an SLN? Each failed mapping represents an ALND that might not have been necessary, and for this reason, the surgeon's primary objective should be to pursue a technique that maximizes the likelihood of success. The collective literature, reflecting the early experience of most authors, reports a success rate of 90%.

Specificity

Specificity is the proportion of all node-negative cases in which the SLN is also negative. Because false-positive results are exceedingly rare (in one of our first 1000 procedures, a benign nevus rest was mistaken for metastasis at frozen-section analysis), virtually all authors report a specificity of 100%.

Negative predictive value

The negative predictive value (the proportion of SLN-negative cases in which the axilla proved to be truly negative) answers the question: if the SLN biopsy is negative, how likely is the axilla to be truly negative?

Positive predictive value

The positive predictive value (the proportion of SLN-positive cases in which the axilla is truly positive) answers the question: if the SLN biopsy is positive, how likely is the axilla to be truly positive? Because false-positives are exceedingly rare (and limited largely to intraoperative frozen-section analysis, where we have observed only one false-positive result in our first 1000 SLN procedures), positive predictive value is of limited usefulness.

Sensitivity

Sensitivity (the proportion of node-positive cases correctly identified by the SLN) answers the question: if the axillary nodes are positive, how likely is the SLN to determine this? By using node-positives as the denominator, sensitivity is a rigorous measure of the procedure, and in the collective literature is 93% overall.

False-negative rate

The false-negative rate (1.0 − sensitivity) is the proportion of node-positive cases in which the SLN was negative: false-negative/(true-positive + false-negative). Using the same denominator as sensitivity, this is an equally rigorous measure. The collective literature reports a false-negative rate of 7%.

Accuracy

Accuracy is the proportion of all cases correctly staged by using the SLN biopsy: (true-positive + true-negative)/total cases. Accuracy as the sole measure of SLN biopsy can be misleading. The value of the procedure is in its ability to detect nodal metastases; to the degree that it is performed selectively in very early stage node-negative cases, little will be learned despite an impression of great accuracy. The collective literature reports an accuracy of 97%.

STRUCTURING AN SLN BIOPSY PROGRAM

Sentinel lymph-node biopsy poses a series of unique challenges for the institution or surgeon wishing to set up such a program. The procedure is highly multidisciplinary, requiring close collaboration between specialists in nuclear medicine, surgery, and pathology. It poses a new set of technical issues for each specialty, none of which has been completely resolved. Finally, as a new operation, SLN biopsy carries a medicolegal risk. The long-term morbidity of the procedure (and particularly the axillary relapse rate), while universally assumed to be small, is unknown.

The early experience of each surgeon (and institution) with SLN biopsy should be conducted under a formalized protocol with Institutional Review Board approval. A clear definition of patient eligibility is essential, as is informed consent. The nuclear medicine, surgical, and pathologic protocols should be described in detail and followed in all cases. Each surgeon's early experience requires backup ALND to audit success and false-negative rates. Finally, long-term follow-up is essential to monitor patterns of surgical morbidity and local relapse; while both are assumed to be minimal, neither is known with certainty.

THE LEARNING CURVE

The SLN biopsy procedure has a distinct learning curve, as measured by two indices: successful localization of the SLN and a low false-negative rate. By the first of these measures, Cox et al demonstrated that surgeons at their own institution (using dye plus isotope) required on average 23 procedures to achieve a 90% success rate, and 53 to reach 95% success.[20] In a multicenter validation trial, Krag et al reported the results of 443 SLN biopsy procedures done by 11 surgeons at 11 different institutions using isotope alone.[21] Sentinel lymph nodes were found in 93% of cases (range 82–98%), and surgeons using the procedure frequently found the SLN more often. Our own success in finding the SLN increased from 90% in our first 100 cases to 96% in our fifth 100.[22]

Using the second and more definitive criterion, Cox et al reported only a single false-negative procedure among 186 patients having planned backup ALND, for a false-negative rate of 2% (1 of 54 node-positive cases).[20] On a more cautionary note, Krag's multicenter study had a false-negative rate of 11.4%,[21] and one of the three surgeons performing the procedure most often had the highest false-negative rate, 28%. Our own false-negative rate of 10.6% fell to 5.2% if each surgeon's *first six cases* were excluded.[22] Half of these "false-negative" cases had clinically obvious nodal disease found at surgery. Most authorities recommend that each surgeon's first 25–30 SLN biopsy procedures be followed by a backup ALND to confirm high success and low false-negative rates.[23,24] The difficulty is that far more procedures are required to establish with statistical confidence a high sensitivity/low false-negative rate (denominator equals node-positives) than a high success rate (denominator equals all cases). As Table 16.2 illustrates, if one performs 30 SLN biopsies, the lower limit of the 95% confidence interval for the success rate is 74%, and for sensitivity, it is 52%! Even after 100 procedures, the lower limit of success is 82%, while for sensitivity it is 78%.

The above studies reflect not only the learning curves of the individual surgeons, but also the evolution of the SLN biopsy technique itself. Once the SLN is found successfully under a well-defined protocol *using a mature methodology*, the accuracy of the result may be relatively independent of the surgeon's experience. McMasters et al, in a multi-institutional trial comprising 806 SLN biopsy procedures by 99 surgeons, demonstrated identical success (88% and 90%) and false-negative rates (7.6% and 9.3%) whether the participating surgeon had performed fewer than ten, or ten or more procedures prior to entering the trial (see Chapter 26).[25]

MORBIDITY OF A FAILED PROCEDURE

The most significant consequence of a failed SLN mapping is the performance of a conventional ALND that might not have been needed. This is disappointing for both surgeon and patient. For the surgeon, it represents a failure of technique requiring default to a larger operation, and for the patient a fear of greater surgical morbidity. This fear has been greatly exaggerated in the SLN era, with a disproportionate emphasis on the risk of lymphedema and infection following conventional ALND.

First, patients should be informed that while the morbidity of SLN biopsy is certainly less than that of ALND, it remains a real operation, with the possibility of hematoma, seroma, wound infection, pain, shoulder stiffness, sensory loss, and even lymphedema in a very small fraction of patients. Blue-dye allergy may cause a striking blue urticaria in about 1% of patients and hypotension in fewer than 1%.[26,27] While no true tattooing occurs, a faint blue stain may persist in the breast for a year or longer.

Second, the morbidity of a conventional ALND is quite reasonable, as Roses et al demonstrated in a detailed study (one of very few in the literature) of 200 patients following Levels I and II ALND.[28] With a median follow-up of 3 years, significant lymphedema (>2 cm difference in arm circumference) developed in 6% to 13.5% of patients, and infection developed in 5.5%. Prolonged pain occurred in only 3% of patients, and postoperative sensory

Table 16.2 Confidence intervals for success and sensitivity of SLN biopsy by number of procedures done

(A) *Assuming 90% success in locating the SLN*

No. of procedures	95% confidence intervals for success rate
10	0.555–0.997
20	0.68–0.99
30	0.74–0.98
50	0.78–0.97
100	0.82–0.95
200	0.85–0.94
500	0.87–0.92

(B) *Assuming that the SLN identifies a positive axilla with 93% sensitivity and that 30% of patients are node-positive*

No. of procedures	No. of node-positive cases	95% confidence interval for sensitivity
10	3	0.3–10.0
20	6	0.54–10.0
30	9	0.52–0.997
50	15	0.68–0.998
100	30	0.78–0.99
200	60	0.84–0.98
500	150	0.88–0.97

phenomena improved or resolved completely in 82% of cases. In a multivariate analysis, only arm infection and heavy/obese body habitus predicted lymphedema.

MORBIDITY OF A FALSE-NEGATIVE PROCEDURE

There are two consequences of a false-negative SLN biopsy: the possibility of an axillary relapse requiring reoperation, and the possibility of systemic undertreatment of a patient incorrectly thought to be node-negative.

Neither has proved to be as significant as initially thought.

Relapse in the regional node basin after a negative SLN biopsy for melanoma has been reported by Gershenwald et al to occur in 4% of 243 patients.[29] Reanalysis of the "negative" SLNs by enhanced pathological techniques found that they contained tumor in eight of the ten patients who experienced local recurrence. In breast cancer, the "worst-case scenario" is represented by series in which no ALND was done at all. In the historic National Surgical Adjuvant Breast and Bowel Project (NSABP) B-04 trial (1971–4),[3] axillary recurrence developed in 17.8% of patients randomized to receive total mastectomy without ALND (about half of the expected proportion with positive nodes). Based on this experience, later NSABP protocols all included ALND. A more recent report from Milan of 401 breast cancer patients treated without ALND is more reassuring.[30] Axillary relapse at 5 years was 6.7% overall and highly correlated with tumor size, ranging from 2% for patients with T1a (≤0.5 cm) to 20% for T2 (2.1–5.0 cm) cancers. With only a single published report of 67 cases,[31] *no axillary recurrences have yet been reported after a negative SLN biopsy for breast cancer.* Such recurrences will almost certainly occur, but the frequency will most probably be comparable to that after a conventional ALND, 1% or less.[8]

In a disease with effective systemic adjuvant therapy, systemic undertreatment is of greater concern than local recurrence, particularly if 7% of node-positive cases will not be identified by SLN biopsy. Fortunately, current breast-cancer treatment guidelines dictate systemic adjuvant treatment for all patients with invasive cancers 1 cm or larger and for patients with even smaller tumors having unfavorable histopathology, regardless of nodal status.[32] *To date, there are no reports of a false-negative SLN biopsy for a breast cancer smaller than 1 cm.* In the SLN era, conventional pathologic techniques, which miss prognostically significant micrometastases in 10–20% of cases,[33] will be the source of more false-negative results than SLN biopsy itself (see Chapter 6).

PATIENT ELIGIBILITY FOR SLN BIOPSY

Sentinel lymph-node biopsy works well for the overwhelming majority of breast-cancer patients, those who have T1–2 tumors and clinically negative axillae. The success and accuracy of the procedure is in general unrelated to method of biopsy, excision size, tumor size, location, or histopathologic features.[34,35] Routine exclusions in most SLN protocols are pregnancy, ductal carcinoma in situ (DCIS), multicentric disease, or clinically positive axillary nodes. None of these is an absolute contraindication.

Pregnancy

The risk of SLN biopsy in pregnancy is indeed unknown but would seem to be very small, basically that of exposure to a very small dose of radioisotope (1 mCi or less) or the possibility of an urticarial (1%) or hypotensive (<1%) allergic reaction to blue dye. Certain pregnant patients, fully informed, may choose to proceed in this context.

Ductal carcinoma in situ

The risk of axillary metastasis in DCIS (as assessed by conventional pathologic techniques) is 1% or less,[36–38] despite which a small fraction of DCIS patients (1.5% in the NSABP B-17 protocol[39]) will die of distant metastatic disease. Sentinel lymph-node biopsy with enhanced pathologic analysis demonstrates occult nodal metastases in 6% of consecutive unselected DCIS patients[40] and in 12% of "high-risk" DCIS cases[41] (those with extensive lesions in whom the presence of occult invasion cannot be excluded). It seems reasonable that the few DCIS patients who develop metastasis may actually have had occult invasive cancers, and that the finding of SLN micrometastasis in "DCIS" identifies this higher-risk subset of patients at risk for distant relapse.

Multifocality

Veronesi's influential report of 163 SLN biopsy procedures, in which two of four patients with false-negative SLNs had "multifocal" tumors,[42] raised the possibility of separate tumor foci draining to different SLNs and has led most centers to exclude patients with multiple foci of disease. Increasing evidence (elegantly summarized by Borgstein[43] and consistent with work at the author's institution[44] and Montgomery LL (unpublished work)) supports the concept that most of the breast drains to *the same sentinel node or (nodes)*, and that the procedure may be as suitable for multifocal as for unifocal disease.

Clinically positive axilla

Clinical assessment of the axilla entails false-positive as well as false-negative results, particularly in previously biopsied patients with reactive nodes. Fisher et al reported clinically positive axillae in 27% of pathologically node-negative cases.[5] Sentinel lymph-node biopsy may have a role in the clinically node-positive patient, as long as the surgeon maintains a low threshold for default to ALND on the grounds of intraoperative suspicion. Nodes grossly involved by tumor may not take up dye and isotope normally,[22,35] and suspicious non-SLNs should always be biopsied.

There are a very few situations that preclude SLN biopsy, but these include patients with very large tumors and/or extensive lymphatic damage from earlier surgery.

T3–4 Cancers

While suitable for patients with T1 and T2 cancers,[35,45,46] the procedure is less accurate for those with T3 (>5.0 cm) tumors, a group in whom we have observed a disproportionate number of false-negative results,[47] or for patients with T4 (or inflammatory) breast cancer, where the overwhelming majority will be node-positive. Even in locally advanced cases, Kuerer et al suggest a role for SLN biopsy following neoadjuvant chemotherapy as a means of identifying patients who have had complete chemotherapeutic eradication of their nodal disease and thus might not require ALND.[48]

Lymphatic disruption

Sentinel lymph-node biopsy is critically dependent upon intact lymphatic pathways between the tumor site and the axilla. Extensive lymphatic disruption by prior surgery (a large upper outer quadrant biopsy cavity, a mastectomy done for DCIS or a prophylactic mastectomy in which invasive cancer is found unexpectedly) precludes accurate lymphatic mapping. As for most clinically apparent cancers, patients with upper outer quadrant lesions are best diagnosed by either fine-needle aspiration or core needle biopsy, with SLN biopsy done immediately prior to tumor excision (while the lymphatic channels are still intact). Similarly, mastectomy for prophylaxis[49] or for extensive DCIS[40,41] should be immediately preceded by SLN biopsy.

DYE, ISOTOPE, OR BOTH?

A crucial goal for the surgeon performing SLN biopsy is to define the technical elements of the procedure. Isotope, blue dye, or a combination of the two all work well, as detailed in subsequent chapters.

Isotope mapping, as first described by Krag,[16] allows the performance of a preoperative lymphoscintigram to identify unexpected patterns of lymphatic drainage and has the advantages of a high early-success rate and easier intraoperative localization of the SLN, especially in patients with a difficult axilla. Isotope has disadvantages that are both logistical and technical. Isotope localization requires a separate procedure for the patient and may delay the start of surgery. Many variables relating to both isotope preparation and technique of injection will affect results; patient factors and other variables (as yet undefined) almost certainly have a role as well.

Blue dye, as first described by Giuliano,[17] has the outstanding advantage of simplicity, requiring only an injection given immediately prior to surgery and no special instrumentation. The method has the disadvantages of a lower initial success rate and a longer learning curve than isotope mapping. Even with experience, identification of a blue SLN (or *all* of the blue nodes) in a large, fatty axilla can be very challenging.

The combination of isotope and dye, as first described by Albertini et al,[18] anticipates complementarity of the two methods, with each making up for the deficiencies of the other. The experience of our own first 60,[50] 500,[35] and 1000 procedures[26,51] supports this hypothesis (see the MSKCC approach described in Chapter 23).

DEFINING THE SUCCESSFUL PROCEDURE

Exactly what constitutes a "successful" lymphatic mapping procedure? During the rapid parallel evolution of SLN biopsy at many centers, no widely accepted "standard" definition of success has emerged, nor is it clear that any one definition is superior to another.

For isotope mapping, all authors define the SLN as one containing isotope counts higher than the axillary background. Some define this liberally, requiring a node/background ratio of 4–5 : 1,[35,50] others more stringently at 10 : 1,[21] and many do not specify a threshold at all. A ratio that is too low will be more inclusive but runs a theoretical risk of including additional lymph nodes which are not "true" SLNs; conversely, a ratio that is too high may exclude "true" SLNs from consideration. While no study has sought to define optimal node-to-background ratios, the above studies, using either a liberal[35] or a more stringent definition[21] of isotope success, report comparable frequency of successful mapping, false-negative results, and number of SLNs obtained. A precise definition of isotope success may be less important for the surgeon than simply removing all relatively "hot" nodes.

For blue dye, all authors have followed Giuliano's lead[17,52] in defining successful mapping as the identification of a blue lymph node, a blue lymphatic leading to a blue node, or a blue lymphatic leading directly to a node that has not yet turned blue. While dye results are usually unambiguous, the coloration of SLNs may on occasion be so subtle as to be indistinguishable from normal coloring. In this setting, a consensus judgement by the operating team may resolve any uncertainty.

TECHNICAL NUANCES

As with defining a successful procedure, the definition of procedural technique for isotope, dye, and the combined method is subject to considerable variation. Technetium-99m has emerged universally as the isotope of choice, but isotope dose, carrier particle, and particle size vary widely, as do the timing, route, site, volume, and distribution of isotope injection. Blue dye is subject to the same variation. Subsequent chapters present in detail the techniques used by major institutions worldwide that have the largest experience in SLN biopsy in breast cancer.

In general, the published techniques of SLN biopsy for breast cancer are based more on anecdote and personal preference than on comparative data. While comparative studies are much needed, the similarity of results observed with such a wide variety of techniques strongly affirms, first, that the SLN hypothesis is valid, and second, that the methodology is robust.

PATHOLOGIC ISSUES

Sentinel lymph-node biopsy requires the participation of an expert surgical pathologist, both for intraoperative frozen-section analysis and for enhanced pathologic analysis of the SLNs (including serial sections and immunohistochemical stains).

Once a surgeon has passed the validation phase, in which all SLN patients undergo a backup ALND, intraoperative frozen-section analysis (if positive) allows an immediate ALND and saves the patient a return to the operating room. The sensitivity of frozen-section analysis in detecting SLN metastases is dependent on tumor size and ranges from 40% for T1a cancers to 76% for T2 lesions. Most false-negative frozen sections represent a failure to detect micrometastatic disease.[53]

Many retrospective studies using lymph-node serial sectioning and/or immunohistochemical (IHC) staining for cytokeratins demonstrate that conventional pathologic analysis of axillary lymph nodes with a single section stained with hematoxylin and eosin (H&E) misses micrometastases in 10–20% of patients.[33] Given adequate size and length of follow-up, the same studies find a significantly worse survival rate in "node-negative" patients found to have micrometastases after the fact. Sentinel lymph-node biopsy for the first time allows enhanced pathologic studies of the lymph nodes to be done on a routine basis, and large prospective studies are currently under way to determine whether micrometastases detected in this setting are also prognostically significant (see Chapter 25).

RECORD-KEEPING AND DATA MANAGEMENT

Like any other medical procedure, an SLN biopsy requires careful documentation appropriate to the technique employed. For isotope localization, the nuclear medicine physician's report should detail the dose, preparation, volume, time, and site or sites of injection, as well as the technique and results of all lymphoscintigraphic studies. Operative records should indicate time of procedure, the volume and type of blue dye injected, whether any allergic phenomena were observed, and what treatment, if any, was given. The surgeon's operative note should indicate in detail the number and location of the SLNs, and whether they contained blue dye, isotope, or both. The ex vivo isotope counts of each SLN and the postexcision axillary bed counts should be noted. The surgeon should note whether intraoperative palpation revealed any suspicious sentinel or nonsentinel nodes. The pathologic report should detail the results of intraoperative frozen-section analysis, as well as the results of both H&E and IHC staining of the SLNs. If possible, the volume of nodal metastasis should be categorized as a macrometastasis (>2 mm), a micrometastasis (≤2 mm), or individual tumor cell(s).

Our own practice has been to maintain a prospective database of all SLN biopsy procedures. Simple data sheets are filled out immediately during the nuclear medicine and surgical procedures (Figures 16.1 and 16.2). A paper chart for each case incorporates lymphoscintigrams, data sheets, operating-room records, operative notes, and the pathologic report. Each patient's complete data are then entered into a dedicated secure SLN database. For consistency and to avoid duplication of work, individual queries are routed through a data manager.

PATIENT FOLLOW-UP

All breast-cancer patients, including those who have had SLN biopsy, require lifelong follow-up, with physical examination at least every 6 months and annual mammography. Particular attention must be paid to the axilla in patients who have had a negative SLN biopsy and no ALND. While no axillary recurrences have yet been observed in this group, the only published follow-up study included just 67 patients.[31] Pending the results of larger trials, the rate of axillary recurrence after SLN biopsy remains unknown.

Sentinel lymph-node biopsy is presumed to have less long-term morbidity than a conventional ALND, and the subjective impression of most observers confirms this. Many patients develop transient lymphedema of the breast, and in a minority this persists. Postoperative pain, loss of sensation, wound infection, seroma, shoulder stiffness, and even lymphedema of the arm can all occur after SLN biopsy. How often? Existing prospective studies promise definitive answers over the years to come.

DATE: _____   **NAME:** _____

MRN: _____

Injection: no. given   _____

             intramammary   _____

             intradermal   _____

Protocol: one day: [ ]   two day: [ ]

Dose: Colloid: _____ mCi   Volume: _____ ml

Filtered: [ ]   Unfiltered: [ ]   Initials: [ ]

	Time	Person making entry
Time of injection		
Time of end of last image		
Time of knife to skin		
Time of blue dye		

Time post prior procedure: [   ]

Nature of prior procedure: [   ]

Complications of prior procedure:

[   ]

Figure 16.1 Nuclear medicine data sheet, Memorial Sloan-Kettering Cancer Center.

SLN DATA SHEET/BREAST SERVICE

Measure arm circumference 10 cm above and 5 cm below olecranon process while patient is supine with arms alongside her body. **Take each measurement twice.**

Right Lower Arm: _____ cm _____ cm   Left Lower Arm: _____ cm _____ cm
Right Upper Arm: _____ cm _____ cm   Left Upper Arm: _____ cm _____ cm

STUDY: 1. *(Planned ALND or ALND done despite negative SLN)*
             2. *(SLN Positive ⇨ ALND)*

FROZEN-SECTION ANALYSIS: 0. No   1. Yes, planned FS 2. Yes, intraoperative finding (unplanned)
PRE-OP CHEMO: 0. No   1. Yes
ISOTOPE: 1. One-day study 2. Two-day study
SIDE: 1. Right   2. Left   3. Bilateral
PALP MASS: 0. No   1. Yes
PREV. BX. OUTSIDE: 0. No   1. Yes
Dx BY: 1. FNA   2. Core   3. Surg bx/prior 4. Surg bx (concurrent)
TUMOR LOCATION: 1. UOQ   2. LOQ   3. UIQ   4. LIQ   5. CENTRAL

CLINICAL SIZE: _____.____ cm (UNK = 99.9)

PATH SIZE: _____.____ cm (UNK = 99.9)

DATE OF PROCEDURE: _____/_____/_____

LYMPHOSCINTIGRAM: 0. Negative   1. Positive

LSG SITES POSITIVE: 0. Neg 1. Aux only 2. Ax+IM 3. Ax+IM+SC 4. IM only 5. N/A

COUNTS*:   INJECTION SITE   _____
(*if >1 reading taken, use highest no. of counts)

	SLN SITE 1	SLN SITE 2*	SLN SITE 3*	SLN SITE 4*	SLN SITE 5*
Location (level) of nodes					
Blue dye? 0. No 1. Yes					
Counts over skin					
Specimen counts ex vivo					
Bed counts postexcision					

*use for 2nd – 5th hot spot anatomically separate from 1st site.

Figure 16.2 Surgical data sheet.

REFERENCES

1. Veronesi U, Valagussa P, Inefficacy of internal mammary nodes dissection in breast cancer surgery. *Cancer* 1981; **47**:170–5.
2. Veronesi U, Banfi A, Del Vecchio M, Comparison of Halsted mastectomy with quadrantectomy, axillary dissection, and radiotherapy in early breast cancer: long-term results. *Eur J Cancer Clin Oncol* 1986; **22**:1085–19.
3. Fisher B, Redmond C, Fisher E, Ten-year results of a randomized clinical trial comparing radical mastectomy and total mastectomy with or without radiation. *N Engl J Med* 1985; **312**:674–81.
4. Fisher B, Redmond C, Poisson R, Eight-year results of a randomized clinical trial comparing total mastectomy and lumpectomy with or without irradiation in the treatment of breast cancer. *N Engl J Med* 1989; **320**:822–8.
5. Fisher B, Wolmark N, Banes M, The accuracy of clinical nodal staging and of limited axillary dissection as a determinant of histologic nodal status in carcinoma of the breast. *Gynecol Obstet* 1981; **152**:765–72.
6. Carter CL, Allen C, Henson DE, Relation of tumor size, lymph node status, and survival in 24 740 breast cancer cases. *Cancer* 1989; **63**:181–7.
7. Rush-Port E, Tan LK, Borgen PI, Van Zee KJ, Incidence of axillary lymph node metastases in T1a and T1b breast carcinoma. *Ann Surg Oncol* 1998; **5**:23–7.
8. Petrek JA, Blackwood MM, Axillary dissection: current practice and technique. *Curr Probl Surg* 1995; **32**:259–323.
9. Fisher B, Laboratory and clinical research in breast cancer: a personal adventure: The David A. Karnofsky memorial lecture. *Cancer Res* 1980; **40**:3863–74.
10. Ragaz J, Jackson SM, Le N et al, Adjuvant radiotherapy and chemotherapy in node-positive premenopausal women with breast cancer. *N Engl J Med* 1997; **337**:956–62.
11. Overgaard M, Hansen PS, Overgaard J et al, Postoperative radiotherapy in high-risk premenopausal women with breast cancer who receive adjuvant chemotherapy. *N Engl J Med* 1997; **337**:949–55.
12. Cady B, A contemporary view of axillary dissection. *Ann Surg* 2000; **232**:8–9.
13. Gould EA, Winship T, Philbin PH, Kerr H, Observations on a "sentinel node" in cancer of the parotid. *Cancer* 1960; **13**:77–8.
14. Cabanas R, An approach for the treatment of penile carcinoma. *Cancer* 1977; **39**:456–66.
15. Morton DL, Wen DR, Wong JH et al, Technical details of intraoperative lymphatic mapping for early stage melanoma. *Arch Surg* 1992; **127**:392–9.
16. Krag DN, Weaver DL, Alex JC et al, Surgical resection and radiolocalization of the sentinel lymph node in breast cancer using a gamma probe. *Surg Oncol* 1993; **2**:335–40.
17. Giuliano AE, Kirgan DM, Guenther JM, Morton DL, Lymphatic mapping and sentinel lymphadenectomy for breast cancer. *Ann Surg* 1994; **220**:391–401.
18. Albertini JJ, Lyman GH, Cox C et al, Lymphatic mapping and sentinel node biopsy in the patient with breast cancer. *JAMA* 1996; **276**:1818–22.
19. Cody HS, Clinical aspects of sentinel node biopsy. *Breast Cancer Res* 2001; **3**:104–8.
20. Cox CE, Bass SS, Boulware D et al, Implementation of new surgical technology: outcome measures for lymphatic mapping of breast carcinoma. *Ann Surg Oncol* 1999; **6**:553–61.
21. Krag D, Weaver D, Ashikaga T et al, The sentinel node in breast cancer—a multicenter validation study. *N Engl J Med* 1998; **339**:941–6.
22. Cody HS, Hill ADK, Tran KN et al, Credentialing for breast lymphatic mapping—how many cases are enough? *Ann Surg* 1999; **229**:723–8.
23. Giuliano AE, See one, do twenty-five, teach one: the implementation of sentinel node dissection in breast cancer. *Ann Surg Oncol* 1999; **6**:520–1.
24. Hill ADK, Mann GB, Borgen PI, Cody HS, Sentinel lymphatic mapping in breast cancer. *J Am Coll Surg* 1999; **188**:545–9.
25. McMasters KM, Tuttle TM, Carlson DJ et al, Sentinel lymph node biopsy for breast cancer: a suitable alternative to routine axillary dissection in multi-institutional practice when optimal technique is used. *J Clin Oncol* 2000; **18**:2560–6.
26. Cody HS, Borgen PI, State-of-the-art approaches to sentinel node biopsy for breast cancer: study design, patient selection, technique, and quality control at Memorial Sloan-Kettering Cancer Center. *Surg Oncol* 1999; **8**:85–91.
27. Leong SPL, Donegan E, Heffernon W et al, Adverse reactions to isosulfan blue during selective sentinel lymph node dissection in melanoma. *Ann Surg Oncol* 2000; **7**:361–6.
28. Roses DF, Brooks AD, Harris MN et al, Complications of level I and II axillary dissection in the treatment of carcinoma of the breast. *Ann Surg* 1999; **230**:194–201.

29. Gershenwald JE, Colome MI, Lee JE et al, Patterns of recurrence following a negative sentinel lymph node biopsy in 243 patients with stage I or II melanoma. *J Clin Oncol* 1998; **16:** 2253–60.

30. Greco M, Agresti R, Cascinelli N et al, Breast cancer patients treated without axillary surgery: clinical implications and biologic analysis. *Ann Surg* 2000; **232:**1–7.

31. Giuliano AE, Haigh PI, Brennan M et al, Prospective observational study of sentinel lymphadenectomy without further axillary dissection in patients with sentinel node-negative breast cancer. *J Clin Oncol* 2000; **18:**2553–9.

32. Carlson RW, Anderson BO, Bensinger W et al, Update: NCCN practice guidelines for the treatment of breast cancer. *Oncology* 1999; **13:**187–212.

33. Dowlatshahi K, Fan M, Snider HC, Habib FA, Lymph node micrometastases from breast carcinoma: reviewing the dilemma. *Cancer* 1997; **80:** 1188–97.

34. Haigh PI, Hansen NM, Qi K, Giuliano AE, Biopsy method and excision volume do not effect success rate of subsequent sentinel lymph node dissection in breast cancer. *Ann Surg Oncol* 2000; **7:**21–7.

35. Hill ADK, Tran KN, Akhurst T et al, Lessons learned from 500 cases of lymphatic mapping for breast cancer. *Ann Surg* 1999; **229:**528–35.

36. Silverstein MJ, Gierson ED, Waisman JR et al, Axillary lymph node dissection for T1a breast carcinoma: is it indicated? *Cancer* 1994; **73:**664–7.

37. Yiangou C, Shousha S, Sinnett HD, Primary tumor characteristics and axillary lymph node status in breast cancer. *Br J Cancer* 1999; **80:** 1974–8.

38. Solin LJ, Kurtz J, Fourquet A et al, Fifteen-year results of breast-conserving surgery and definitive breast irradiation for the treatment of ductal carcinoma in situ of the breast. *J Clin Oncol* 1996; **14:**754–63.

39. Fisher B, Dignam J, Wolmark N et al, Lumpectomy and radiation therapy for the treatment of intraductal breast cancer: findings from the National Surgical Adjuvant Breast and Bowel Project B-17. *J Clin Oncol* 1998; **16:**441–52.

40. Pendas S, Dauway E, Giuliano AE et al, Sentinel node biopsy in duct carcinoma in situ patients. *Ann Surg Oncol* 2000; **7:**15–20.

41. Klauber-DeMore N, Tan LK, Liberman L et al, Sentinel lymph node biopsy: is it indicated in patients with high-risk ductal carcinoma-in-situ and ductal carcinoma-in-situ with microinvasion? *Ann Surg Oncol* 2000; **7:**636–42.

42. Veronesi U, Paganelli G, Galimberti V et al, Sentinel-node biopsy to avoid axillary dissection in breast cancer with clinically negative lymphnodes. *Lancet* 1997; **349:**1864–7.

43. Borgstein P, Meijer S, Historical perspective of lymphatic tumour spread and the emergence of the sentinel node concept. *Eur J Surg Oncol* 1998; **24:**85–9.

44. Linehan DC, Hill ADK, Akhurst T et al, Intradermal radiocolloid and intraparenchymal blue dye injection optimize sentinel node identification in breast cancer patients. *Ann Surg Oncol* 1999; **6:**450–4.

45. Olson J, Fey J, Winawer J et al, Sentinel lymphadenectomy accurately predicts nodal status in T2 breast cancer. *J Am Coll Surg* 2000; **191:**592–9.

46. Bedrosian I, Reynolds C, Mick R et al, Accuracy of sentinel lymph node biopsy in patients with large primary breast tumors. *Cancer* 2000; **88:** 2540–5.

47. Boolbol SK, Fey J, Borgen PI et al, Intradermal isotope injection: a highly accurate method of lymphatic mapping in breast carcinoma. *SSO Ann Surg Oncol* 2001; **8:**20–4.

48. Kuerer HM, Sahin AA, Hunt KK et al, Incidence and impact of documented eradication of breast cancer axillary lymph node metastases before surgery in patients treated with neoadjuvant chemotherapy. *Ann Surg* 1999; **230:**72–8.

49. Dupont EL, McCann C, Shons AR et al, The role of sentinel lymph node biopsy in women undergoing prophylactic mastectomy. *Eur J Nucl Med* 1999; **26**(suppl):S72.

50. O'Hea BJ, Hill ADK, El-Shirbiny A et al, Sentinel lymph node biopsy in breast cancer: initial experience at Memorial Sloan-Kettering Cancer Center. *J Am Coll Surg* 1998; **186:**423–7.

51. Cody HS, Fey J, Akhurst T et al, Complementarity of blue dye and isotope in sentinel node localization for breast cancer: univariate and multivariate analysis of 966 procedures. *Ann Surg Oncol* 2001; **8:**13–19.

52. Giuliano AE, Jones RC, Brennan M, Statman R, Sentinel lymphadenectomy in breast cancer. *J Clin Oncol* 1997; **15:**2345–50.

53. Weiser MR, Montgomery LL, Susnik B et al, Is routine intraoperative frozen-section examination of sentinel lymph nodes in breast cancer worthwhile? *Ann Surg Oncol* 2000; **7:**651–5.

17

Pathologic aspects

Roderick R Turner

Sentinel lymph-node (SLN) biopsy represents an important and timely advance in accurate pathologic staging of breast cancer. Effective screening programs, most notably mammography, have led to the early detection of breast cancer and smaller average tumor sizes at diagnosis.[1] Patients with small, invasive carcinomas who undergo complete axillary lymph-node dissection (ALND) with standard pathologic examination are likely to have negative lymph nodes. Sentinel lymph-node biopsy reliably determines the tumor status of the axilla, spares many patients the potential morbidity of ALND, and is well suited to detect early nodal metastases.

The accuracy of the SLN concept is supported by the observation that if only one axillary lymph node is positive, it is most likely to be the SLN.[2] Since many centers examine the SLNs more intensively than they do the non-SLNs, the validity of that comparison is limited. The most convincing pathologic validation studies have applied the same sensitive cytokeratin immunohistochemistry (IHC) techniques to both SLNs and non-SLNs.[3–5] Turner et al described a single-institution study of 103 patients who underwent SLN biopsy by an experienced surgeon.[3] He focused on 70 consecutive cases that were SLN-negative by hematoxylin-and-eosin (H&E) examination. Among the 60 patients who remained SLN-negative after cytokeratin-IHC examination, only one patient had a non-SLN metastasis, for an overall accuracy of 99% and a false-negative rate of 2% (1/44). Weaver et al[4] described a multi-institutional trial with variable surgeon and pathologist experience and reported overall accuracy of 91% for SLN staging, with a false-negative rate of 12% (14/118); metastasis in a non-SLN was 13.4 times more likely for SLN-positive than SLN-negative patients.[4]

The pathologist depends on the surgeon's expertise to correctly identify the SLN, since current techniques do not permit the pathologist to determine independently if the submitted lymph node is the true SLN. There is an important role on the team, however, for dedicated pathologists intent on detecting early metastatic carcinoma, since that finding decreases false-negative results,[6] and may affect recommendations for adjuvant therapies. Several good reviews of pathologic techniques applied to SLN examination have been published.[7–12]

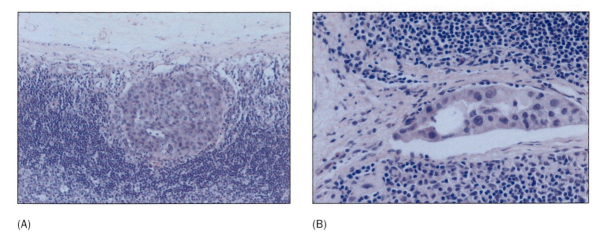

(A)   (B)

Figure 17.1 A 0.3-mm micrometastasis (A) displaces SLN parenchyma, (B) expands the SLN sinus.

DIAGNOSTIC EVALUATION

General

Careful pathologic examination increases the sensitivity and accuracy of SLN staging. Larger SLNs are more likely to contain metastasis than smaller SLNs, but exceptions are common. Gross tissue sections should be approximately 2 mm thick, and all grossly negative SLN tissue should be embedded. Loss of diagnostic tissue for molecular biology studies may cause a falsely negative histopathology result.[13] The SLN is usually sectioned longitudinally because this reduces the number of tissue slices for the histotechnologist to embed flat and allows for more accurate measurement of metastasis size. Some pathologists prefer transverse sections, however, because it may not be possible to cut longitudinal sections from the outer cortex through the hilum to assess afferent and efferent lymphatic vessels.[10]

Routine H&E examination of the SLN detects more micrometastases (≤2.0 mm) than does standard evaluation of nodes removed during complete ALND. The historical incidence of micrometastasis in routinely examined ALND specimens is approximately 8–15% of node-positive patients;[14,15] in contrast, H&E-detected micrometastasis represents 20–25% of SLN-positive patients,[16] and, with the addition of cytokeratin-IHC, approximately 50% of SLN-positive patients.[17,18]

Hematoxylin-and-eosin examination

Detection of H&E micrometastasis is easily accomplished in most cases with the visualization of cohesive clusters of carcinoma cells that displace SLN parenchyma or expand an SLN sinus (Figure 17.1). With small micrometastases, capable and expert pathologists may overlook the finding (Figure 17.2), or incorrectly interpret benign cells as malignant owing to the histologic similarity of small aggregates or single carcinoma cells and nodal mesenchymal cells, such as reactive histiocytes, lymphocytes, endothelial cells, or nodal nevus cells (Figure 17.3).

A multi-institutional study with central pathology review of H&E slides in 431 cases revealed that the diagnosis at the original institution was falsely negative in 2.6% (8/309) cases, for a false-negative rate of 6% (8/128). Original results were falsely positive in 1.6% (2/122) of patients.[4]

Benign epithelial inclusions,[19] commonly found in pelvic and cervical lymph nodes, are

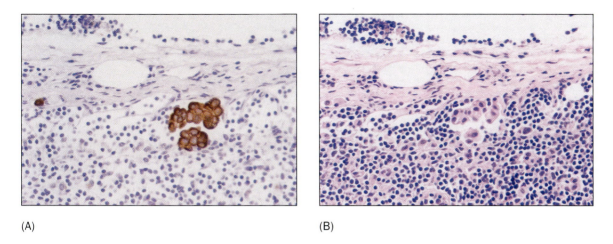

(A)   (B)

Figure 17.2 Occult metastasis, less than 0.1 mm, detected initially (A) on cytokeratin-IHC stained and retrospectively (B) on H&E-stained section.

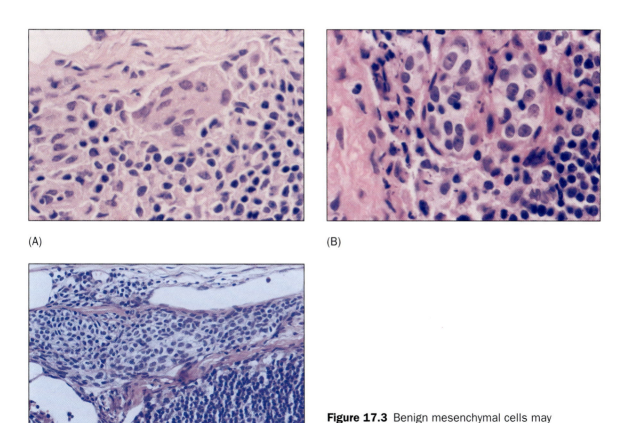

(A)   (B)

(C)

Figure 17.3 Benign mesenchymal cells may occasionally mimic small metastases; these include (A) a multinucleated histiocyte, (B) reactive endothelial cells, and (C) capsular nevus cells (H&E stains).

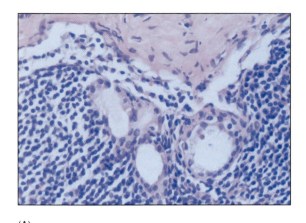

(A)

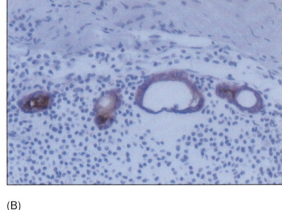

(B)

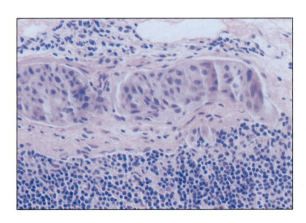

(C)

Figure 17.4 Micrometastasis, 0.2 mm, mimics a benign glandular rest. (A) Bland epithelial cells are (B) cytokeratin-positive and (C) similar to the patient's low-grade infiltrating ductal carcinoma with tubular features. The epithelial cells in the SLN lacked a myoepithelial layer on actin IHC and were present in the nodal sinus on deeper sections.

described in less than 0.5% of ALNDs.[20] These cytokeratin-positive cells may be macroscopic or microscopic and are typically seen on H&E-stained sections as cytologically bland squamous or apocrine rests, commonly cystic, or as a benign breast lobule within the lymph-node capsule. Although these can generally be identified confidently, micrometastases of low-grade ductal carcinoma with good tubule formation may mimic benign epithelial inclusions (Figure 17.4). If the epithelium is in the SLN and is morphologically similar to the patient's primary tumor, it is best regarded as a micrometastasis. Occasionally, a micrometastasis may appear to be in the SLN capsule or extracapsular soft tissue, owing to plugging of the afferent lymphatic vessel, and may be difficult to distinguish from benign epithelial cells (Figure 17.5). The absence

Figure 17.5 A 0.4-mm micrometastasis limited to afferent lymphatic vessel within SLN capsule (H&E stain).

of an actin-positive myoepithelial cell layer provides evidence against a benign epithelial cell rest.

Step-section levels

Serial or step sections and IHC methods, which have not been routine for ALND specimens, are commonly used in SLN evaluation with little added effort or expense. The combination of step sections and IHC methods applied to standard ALND has converted approximately 20% of node-negative patients to node-positive status,[21] and similar results have been reported for SLN biopsies. Sentinel lymph-node micrometastases undetected on first-level H&E have been found in approximately 10% of patients with step-section H&E, 8–15% with one-level cytokeratin-IHC, and approximately 15–20% with step-section cytokeratin-IHC.[3,4,8,12,22–25] Current practice is highly variable and ranges from a single H&E-stained section to multiple step-section levels with cytokeratin-IHC examination. The number and depth of step-section levels and IHC stains affect the incidence of micrometastasis.

It is not well understood where in the subcapsular sinus region opposite the hilum small metastases are likely to be found. It has been suggested, but not yet confirmed, that blue dye, if present focally on gross visual examination, may target the region likely to contain micrometastasis.[26] Alternatively, the use of a carbon dye may provide a histologic marker to assist tumor-cell detection and confirm a true SLN.[27]

It is appealing to apply mathematical models to determine statistically the depth and number of levels needed to reach a satisfactory degree of confidence; however, mathematical models that base calculations on the detection of a single metastatic deposit provide misleading statistical probabilities,[25,28] because most SLNs with micrometastasis have multiple small aggregates or single tumor cells that can be visualized with cytokeratin-IHC at multiple levels of the SLN.[29] It appears that most SLNs that contain micrometastasis can be detected

using two to four IHC levels separated by 100–250 μm;[22,25,29] this degree of sectioning is not currently necessary. A standard SLN protocol that specifies the number and depth of H&E and cytokeratin-IHC levels to be examined will not be developed until there is consensus on the prognostic and therapeutic implications of micrometastases of various sizes.

CYTOKERATIN IMMUNOHISTOCHEMISTRY

Whether to obtain cytokeratin-IHC stains is the most controversial issue in pathologic diagnosis of SLNs. Although the method is commonly used, some have advised against it outside research trials.[4,10,30] Reasons include the conflicting data from standard ALND studies on the significance of IHC-detected micrometastases. The size of micrometastases does appear to be prognostically important, and IHC-detected micrometastases are usually very small; IHC-detected tumor-cell clusters are on average one-tenth the size of H&E-detected micrometastases (0.1 mm vs 1.0 mm).[4,17] Second, adjuvant therapy protocols are based on relapse and survival data from standard H&E examination of axillary lymph nodes; IHC detection of micrometastases not found in routine histologic examination causes a stage shift and unnecessary chemotherapy. Additionally, technical and interpretive concerns with cytokeratin-IHC make it difficult to exclude the possibility of a false-positive result.

The case in favor of IHC argues that most recent studies with adequate numbers of patients and long-term follow-up demonstrate that the presence of micrometastasis conveys a small but significant adverse effect on disease-free and, to a lesser degree, overall survival. As tumors and related metastases become smaller at diagnosis, micrometastasis may become more significant in the future. Second, this sensitive approach may help to reduce the surgical false-negative rate and improve the accuracy of SLN staging. Nonsentinel lymph nodes are more likely to be positive in patients with H&E-negative SLNs that contain cytokeratin-IHC micrometastases.[3–5] Third, pathologists understand that micrometastases are easier to find on good-quality IHC stains, which in turn may enhance the accuracy and reproducibility of pathologic diagnoses. Atypical-appearing mesenchymal cells, such as histiocytes, endothelial cells, and nodal nevocytes, can be confidently excluded with a negative cytokeratin-IHC stain.

Technical factors

The enzyme pretreatment of tissue sections and monoclonal antibody titers routinely employed in surgical pathology laboratories for tumor diagnosis may not be optimal for lymph-node staining. Meticulous attention to these factors enhances the specificity of SLN examination. Cytokeratin monoclonal antibody cocktails are highly specific for epithelial cells in lymph nodes, but may also weakly stain fibroblastic reticular cells (FRC), the mesenchymal cells that support the nodal framework and contain cytokeratin 8 and 18 filaments.[31,32] Staining of FRC is observed commonly with CAM 5.2[33] and mixtures of multiple antibody cocktails, but it is generally not observed with carefully titred AE-1/AE-3 (Table 17.1).[31-34] Pathologists using cytokeratin-IHC should be aware of FRC stain-

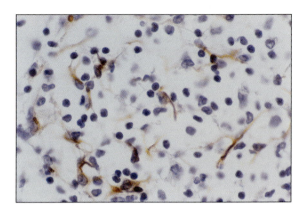

Figure 17.6 Fibroblastic reticular cells may stain weakly with cytokeratin antibodies but are easily distinguished from micrometastases.

ing and recognize it by the meshwork pattern, the bland cytologic features, and the weak staining relative to epithelial cells (Figure 17.6). With poor IHC-staining techniques, other cell types may also stain positively. Automated instruments, now widely available, improve consistency of IHC stains. It is helpful to have H&E and IHC stains on adjacent tissue sections to facilitate morphologic assessment of cells that are immunoreactive.

Table 17.1 Commonly used cytokeratin antibodies	
	Moll number[a]
Commonly used cytokeratin antibodies	
CAM 5.2	8, 18, 19
AE-1	10, 14–16, 19
AE-3	1–8
MAK-6	1, 14–16, 18, 19
Cytokeratin-positive cells in SLN immunostains	
Breast carcinoma[34]	7, 8, 18, 19
Fibroblastic reticular cells[31-33]	8,18

[a]Moll cytokeratin numbers 1 through 8 are basic, high molecular weight; numbers 9 through 19 are acidic, low molecular weight.

Interpretation

Cytokeratin-detected carcinoma cells should be strongly immunoreactive and morphologically similar to the patient's primary tumor cells. They are commonly found as small aggregates of cells in SLN sinuses and less commonly in nodal parenchyma. Up to 30% of patients with IHC-detected micrometastasis have only single (individual) scattered tumor cells;[17] lobular carcinoma metastases are well known to demonstrate this pattern with a "buckshot" appearance in SLN parenchyma and sinuses (Figure 17.7), while single-cell in-transit metastases of aggressive ductal carcinomas are more likely to be seen only in nodal sinuses (Figure 17.8).

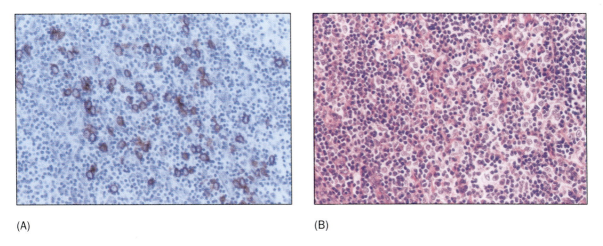

(A) (B)

Figure 17.7 Lobular carcinoma cells in SLN are highlighted on (A) cytokeratin-IHC stain but difficult to visualize on (B) H&E stain.

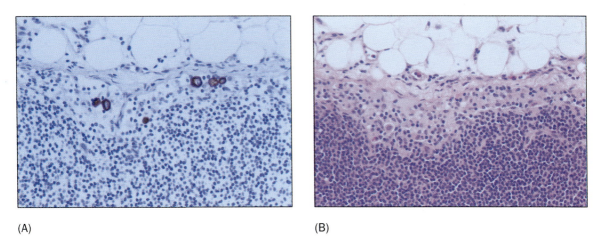

(A) (B)

Figure 17.8 Ductal carcinoma single-cell metastases. (A) Cytokeratin-IHC stain highlights carcinoma cells; (B) histiocytic inflammation obscures the SLN finding on H&E stains. This patient had similar cells in ten SLNs and non-SLNs.

Needle biopsy of the breast may displace fragments of epithelium into breast stroma.[35] Concern has been expressed that these malignant or benign epithelial cells could drain through lymphatic vessels and result in a positive SLN without a documented invasive lesion of the breast.[36,37] The paradox of ductal carcinoma in situ (DCIS) with SLN micrometastasis may also be explained by the difficulty in pathologic detection of early stromal invasion in some DCIS cases. Because displaced epithelial cells are commonly seen in the breast, surrounded by granulation tissue at the biopsy site, lymphatic clearance of these displaced cell clusters appears to be infrequent. One of the advantages of cytokeratin-IHC over molecular diagnostic approaches is the ability to evaluate morphologic features of a positive signal; if the stained cells do not appear compatible with the patient's primary tumor, the finding can be discounted. Most pathologists regard cells in the SLNs that demonstrate strong cytokeratin-IHC staining and morphologic features compatible with carcinoma cells as evidence of early metastasis, recognizing that their clinical significance is not clearly understood.

MOLECULAR BIOLOGY TECHNIQUES

Reverse transcriptase–polymerase chain reaction (RT-PCR) provides highly sensitive detection of breast carcinoma through amplification of a nucleic acid signal.[38,39] However, RT-PCR and other molecular diagnostic approaches are currently limited in breast cancer by the lack of a specific marker, which raises the likelihood of false-positive results.[40,41] A positive signal cannot be confirmed morphologically and may represent benign mesenchymal cells or nonviable tumor-cell debris. Additionally, RT-PCR techniques currently require fresh or frozen tissue. If a gross slice or bisected SLN is provided for molecular studies, histopathologic diagnosis may be falsely negative.[13]

Molecular techniques for SLN biopsy are still experimental and should be used only in research protocols. Cytokeratin-IHC already provides highly sensitive and more specific SLN evaluation. In future clinical practice, molecular techniques may find a role in the serial testing of bone marrow or blood samples.

INTRAOPERATIVE ASSESSMENT

Intraoperative assessment of the SLN has been recognized as a problem since an early SLN study reported that frozen-section results were falsely negative in 24% of cases.[42] Intraoperative assessment will remain problematic as long as surgical protocols direct patients with SLN micrometastasis to further lymphadenectomy. Intraoperative cytology or frozen-section techniques reliably identify SLN macrometastasis but often fail to detect micrometastasis, whereas more intensive and accurate intraoperative techniques with rapid cytokeratin-IHC increase the detection of micrometastasis but delay the surgical procedure. Standard intraoperative-cytology and frozen-section techniques are currently subject to detrimental inaccuracy, discussed further in the following section. If therapeutic ALND is recommended more selectively in the future, however, primarily for patients with macrometastases (thereby sparing some patients with SLN micrometastasis undetected at surgery an ALND), the clinical accuracy of standard intraoperative-cytology and frozen-section techniques, the methods by which macrometastases are usually detected, will improve.

Intraoperative cytology

Combined with a careful examination of thinly cut gross sections, cytologic assessment is the preferred approach because of its speed and ease of preparation, and because it avoids consumption of tissue and frozen-section artifacts on subsequent paraffin sections. Initial studies used imprint cytology ("touch preps"),[43–45] as has been applied to low axillary samples, whereas more recent reports have favored scrape smears,[46,47] which more closely resemble fine-needle aspiration cytology. If a suspicious focus is visualized grossly, the scrape-smear technique enhances cellular yield of the focus.

The widely varying sensitivity of cytologic

techniques[43–45,47–50] reflects not only the differences in paraffin-section protocols but also the difficulties in interpreting these cytology slides. An aggressive approach may achieve an intraoperative-cytology sensitivity of 80–90% compared with H&E paraffin-section findings, which is equivalent to frozen-section results, but which will eventually yield a false-positive. In contrast, a conservative approach will probably avoid false-positives but will yield only a 40–70% sensitivity and cause more indeterminate (suspicious) results. Experience may help a pathologist to reduce, but not eliminate, these problems. The frequency of indeterminate intraoperative-cytology results has not yet been reported in clinical practice. Clusters of benign cells in lymph nodes, such as germinal center cells and reactive endothelial cells, may be difficult to distinguish from a small cluster of carcinoma cells (Figure 17.9), and single carcinoma

cells cannot be definitively detected among reactive histiocytes and lymphocytes. These problems are also encountered with frozen-section techniques. Rapid cytokeratin-IHC of cytology slides has been used to detect some small metastases and improve the sensitivity of intraoperative-cytology evaluation,[51] but requires additional time, cost, and personnel, and presents different technical challenges.

Frozen-section analysis

Most pathologists, even including experienced cytopathologists, are more confident making a diagnosis of SLN metastasis on a tissue section than a cytology slide. Therefore, frozen-section analysis may have an important role with SLNs that are grossly negative but positive or suspicious on intraoperative cytology (Table 17.2).

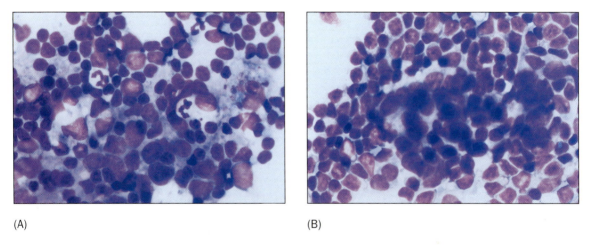

(A) (B)

Figure 17.9 Intraoperative imprint cytology. A germinal center (A) may be difficult to distinguish from a carcinoma-cell aggregate (B).

Table 17.2 Intraoperative techniques versus paraffin-section H&E results		
Technique	Negative predictive value (%)	Estimated sensitivity (%)
Cytology[43–45,47,48]	81–99	60–70 (range, 29–96)
Frozen-section analysis[42,49,50,52,53]	91–94	80 (range, 74–91)

Some institutions have routinely used frozen-section analysis, alone or in combination with intraoperative cytology, for intraoperative examination of SLNs because it provides an added degree of assurance and interpretive consistency. Reported sensitivity is approximately 80–90% compared with H&E-stained paraffin sections, or 50% to 80% compared with final cytokeratin-IHC stains.[49,50,52,53] Frozen-section analysis of only half of the SLNs is less accurate but consumes less tissue. Rapid cytokeratin-IHC may be used to improve the sensitivity of the intraoperative frozen-section evaluation but delays the surgical procedure.[54–56] False-positive results, not yet reported with frozen-section analysis, are unlikely if suspicious or indeterminate results are regarded by the surgeon as negative until confirmed positive (Figure 17.10). Indeterminate or suspicious results have been reported in 2% of cases.[50] Because loss of diagnostic tissue and subsequent frozen-tissue artifacts on paraffin sections are major concerns, institutions that cannot carefully control personnel factors and the cryostat instrument used in frozen-section preparation should avoid this technique, particularly for small SLNs.

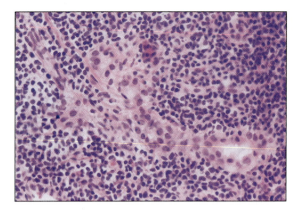

Figure 17.10 Frozen-section analysis. Small tubular structures led to an indeterminate (suspicious) frozen-section result but this proved to be endothelial cells on paraffin IHC stains (cytokeratin-negative, CD31-positive).

Surgeons intent on having a final diagnosis at surgery, to avoid a second operation, may be willing to wait while more intensive examination is undertaken. Viale et al have developed a protocol with complete step-sections at 50 μm through the SLN, if initial sections are negative, and stained with rapid cytokeratin-IHC as needed for any suspicious cells.[56] This technique requires about 40–50 minutes and has an intraoperative positivity rate of 50%; however, the absence of paraffin tissue sections makes it difficult to assess accuracy. While this technique works well at a large referral institution, its time, cost, and personnel requirements make it unlikely to be adopted for widespread use.

Patient selection

Most melanoma centers have discontinued intraoperative examination of SLNs, in part because results are positive in less than 10% of patients with intermediate-risk primary melanomas. Breast cancer, in contrast, has a higher frequency of SLN metastasis, with positive frozen-section results in approximately 15–20% of cases, which accounts in part for the continued use of intraoperative examination. Since patients with small breast tumors are unlikely to have a positive SLN by standard intraoperative-cytology or frozen-section techniques, it would be reasonable to forgo intraoperative frozen-section examination in these cases. Intraoperative examination may also be avoided in patients who will not undergo further axillary surgery even if there is SLN metastasis.

RADIATION SAFETY

In the United States, radiopharmaceutical use requires compliance with Nuclear Regulatory Commission and state laws that include licensure and approved handling procedures; the aim is to keep radiation exposures to individuals and releases into the environment as low as is reasonably achievable.

Standard doses of technetium-99m-sulfur

colloid (Tc-99m-SC), approximately 1 mCi (37 MBq) per case, impart only minimal radiation exposure to pathology department personnel who handle the lumpectomy and SLN specimens.[57–59] The level of radiation emitted from breast specimens is 10 to 100 times greater than that from SLN specimens, which are usually near background levels. While exposure is greater to the pathologist's hands than to the torso, doses to the torso are very low. It has been estimated that a pathologist could perform 14 705 hours of procedural work per year without reaching maximum allowable radiation exposure.[57] Since gross handling of breast lumpectomy and SLN specimens is usually accomplished in approximately 20 minutes, and expected annual procedural time is well below the allowable level, no delay in tissue processing is necessary. Monitoring of specific areas of the laboratory has demonstrated that the cryostat instrument, SLN-tissue cassettes, paraffin blocks, and slides do not exceed background levels and no special precaution or maintenance is required.

After gross examination, breast-tissue cassettes and unprocessed tissue in formalin should be placed behind a lead shield or removed from the work area to reduce continued exposure. Since Tc-99m has a half-life of approximately 6 hours, conservative estimates indicate that radioactivity will decay to background levels within 3 days.[60] A written procedure, prepared in conjunction with the Radiation Safety Committee, for the handling and disposal of these specimens is recommended.

PROGNOSIS AND THERAPEUTIC DECISIONS

Accuracy

Treatment recommendations for patients with breast cancer must be based on highly accurate staging information. Although axillary status has historically been regarded as the single best predictor of survival, 20–30% of patients whose axillary nodes are negative by standard histologic evaluation will develop recurrence; for this reason, medical oncologists recommend chemotherapy for many node-negative patients. There is good evidence that SLN biopsy with cytokeratin-IHC provides more accurate staging than standard axillary node examination.[61] With surgical expertise and careful pathologic evaluation, overall staging accuracy with SLN biopsy approaches 98%, with a false-negative rate of less than 5% and a negative predictive value of approximately 96–98%. Many centers now believe that a negative SLN represents adequate surgical staging and therapy of axillary regional nodes. Although this has not been tested with extended clinical follow-up, preliminary data suggest a very low rate of axillary recurrence after negative SLN biopsy;[62] long-term distant recurrence rates for SLN-negative patients are unknown.

Therapeutic axillary dissection

Pathologic characteristics of the SLN metastasis and primary tumor may permit identification of patients who are at greatest risk of additional non-SLN macrometastases or micrometastases.[17,18,63] Size of the SLN metastasis is an important predictor of further metastases in non-SLNs; the risk of non-SLN involvement is significantly higher when the SLN metastasis is macrometastatic rather than micrometastatic, and approximately half of cases with SLN macrometastasis have non-SLN macrometastasis. The number of positive SLNs is another measure of SLN tumor volume; multiple positive SLNs correlate with non-SLN metastasis, but may be less significant when controlled for maximal size of SLN metastasis. Extranodal soft-tissue invasion is observed as SLN hilar-tissue invasion or efferent vascular invasion in approximately half of cases with SLN macrometastases, and is usually associated with non-SLN macrometastases (Figure 17.11).[17] Among primary tumor characteristics, larger tumor size and peritumoral lymphatic vascular invasion (LVI) are associated with additional metastases in non-SLNs. Clinical follow-up studies after standard ALND demonstrated that primary tumor size, peritumoral LVI,

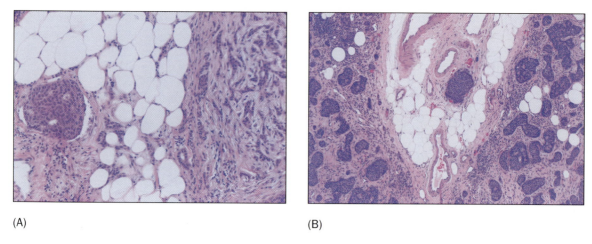

(A)   (B)

Figure 17.11 Extranodal soft-tissue invasion by the SLN metastasis may be seen as (A) extranodal hilar-tissue invasion or (B) efferent vascular invasion. This finding is strongly associated with non-SLN metastases.

number of positive nodes, size of nodal metastases, and extranodal soft-tissue invasion are associated with greater risk of relapse and death from disease.

Further ALND is indicated when the SLN contains established metastases, because tumor cells have already demonstrated adhesion and proliferation properties for growth in the lymph-node environment. If tumor cells are found only in SLN sinuses, however, and appear to be in transit (isolated tumor cells), it is less clear that ALND would be of benefit.

Along with surgical expertise, careful pathologic examination of the primary tumor and SLN metastasis may permit selection of SLN-positive patients who are at low risk of additional axillary metastasis and may be safely spared ALND. Patients with a T1 primary tumor (≤2.0 cm) and SLN micrometastasis (N1a) are unlikely to have non-SLN macrometastasis (0–4%).[5,17,18,63] In the author's experience, non-SLN macrometastasis is also infrequent (2%) in patients with a T1 or T2 tumor that is associated with no peritumoral LVI and only micrometastatic involvement of the SLN.[17] Clinical studies are needed to determine whether these patients can be safely treated with axillary radiation or no further axillary-directed therapy.

Prognostic information

The most important prognostic information that might be obtained from SLN examination is the risk of distant metastasis and death. Highly sensitive techniques for detecting nodal micrometastases could alter the staging process upon which adjuvant protocols are based. The use of cytokeratin-IHC to detect axillary micrometastasis may provide useful prognostic information but fails to identify some patients who subsequently relapse.[64] Primary tumor size and grade, and the tumor status of bone marrow, represent other important prognostic factors. Identification of metastasis in the bone marrow is strongly associated with an adverse outcome, and the combination of bone marrow and nodal assessments may greatly enhance the precision of staging and the selection of patients for adjuvant therapies.[65–68] Clinical studies are evaluating the significance of occult metastases detected in bone marrow and SLNs,[69] and their results will help determine whether these techniques are sufficiently accurate to direct systemic therapies.

Techniques for detection of occult tumor cells may be more sensitive than is clinically necessary. This is most apparent with in situ and small invasive carcinomas, in which SLN stag-

Table 17.3 SLN cytokeratin-positive metastases in small breast carcinomas

Tumor stage by AJCC/UICC criteria[74]	References	Reported SLN-positive average (range) (%)	Estimated distant-relapse rate (%)
Tis	70, 71	6	1–3
T1mic	71, 72	21 (9–33)	3–5
T1a	5, 22, 24, 50, 71, 73	17 (6–83)	5–15
T1b	5, 22, 24, 50, 71, 73	18 (16–42)	10–20
T1c	5, 22, 24, 50, 71, 73	32 (26–40)	20–30

ing with IHC identifies more patients with metastasis than would be expected to relapse (Table 17.3).[5,22,24,50,70–73] The finding of a few cytokeratin-positive cells in the SLN, the fates of which are unknown, is best regarded as a potential risk factor, not an indicator, of future relapse, and should be viewed in the context of the primary tumor findings.

Advances in microstaging will determine if these SLN and marrow techniques have a future role in management of breast cancer patients, or may be replaced by molecular techniques on blood samples. Continued advances in prognostic studies of primary tumors, with improved IHC markers and development of molecular techniques, such as microarray analysis, will help assign patients to low- or high-risk groups who may be spared SLN or bone-marrow staging studies.

REPORTING SLN RESULTS

The American Joint Committee on Cancer (AJCC)/International Union Against Cancer (Union Internationale Contre le Cancer, UICC) staging system is well designed for macrometastases and provides a useful framework for nodal staging (Table 17.4),[74] but it has only one group for patients with micrometastasis (N1a), defined as any number of metastases less than or equal to 2 mm in size. Since the size

and number of micrometastases and the method of detection employed may be clinically important, there should be a separate staging classification for metastases detected with IHC or molecular techniques. Descriptive terms for minimal tumor involvement have included occult, circulating or in-transit metastases, and isolated tumor cells. Variable methods have also been applied to measure small metastases in SLNs, with an ocular micrometer measurement preferred to a count of the malignant cells. Reynolds et al summed the diameters of multiple deposits, and if greater than 2.0 mm, considered it a macrometastasis;[18] while Turner et al measured the maximal dimension of the largest cohesive cluster of carcinoma cells, without adjustment for the number of clusters.[17]

The UICC has proposed criteria for distinguishing isolated tumor cells (defined as single cells or small clusters) from micrometastases.[75] These criteria are based primarily on the presence of cells within lymphatic vessels or nodal sinuses. The recommended nodal staging for isolated tumor cells would be pN0, with an additional symbol to represent the results of morphologic (IHC) or molecular (RT-PCR) examination. The College of American Pathologists has also recommended that cytokeratin-positive cells should not be considered a micrometastasis in the absence of a histologically identified tumor-cell cluster.[76,77]

The problem with a distinction based on

Table 17.4 Regional lymph nodes AJCC/UICC pathologic staging	
Stage	**Definition**
pN0	No regional lymph node metastasis
pN1	Metastasis to movable ipsilateral axillary lymph node(s)
pN1a	Only micrometastasis (none larger than 0.2 cm)
pN1b	Metastasis to lymph node(s), any larger than 0.2 cm
pN1bi	Metastasis in 1 to 3 lymph nodes, any more than 0.2 cm and all less than 2 cm in greatest dimension
pN1bii	Metastasis to 4 or more lymph nodes, any more than 0.2 cm and all less than 2 cm in greatest dimension
pN1biii	Extension of tumor beyond the capsule of a lymph node metastasis less than 2 cm in greatest dimension
pN1biv	Metastasis to a lymph node 2 cm or more in greatest dimension
pN2	Metastasis to ipsilateral axillary lymph nodes that are fixed to one another or to other structures
pN3	Metastasis to ipsilateral internal mammary lymph node(s)

From reference 74.

detection method (H&E vs IHC) is that careful search of the H&E-stained adjacent tissue sections usually reveals comparable cells, which leads to interpretive variation. The proposed UICC criteria[75] seem too complex for reliable interpretation. A more consistent and reproducible system would be based on the maximal size of the largest cell cluster. Page et al have suggested this approach, with a cutoff of 0.2 mm; metastases no greater than 0.2 mm would be stage N0, whereas those measuring 0.21 mm to 2.0 mm would be N1a.[78] This arbitrary cutoff is easily adapted to current AJCC/UICC nodal staging, excludes the majority of metastases detected primarily by cytokeratin-IHC, and represents a good compromise until a consensus is reached on the clinical significance of tiny nodal metastases.

FUTURE DIRECTIONS

Pathology protocols
Current practice patterns employ diverse gross- and microscopic-section techniques, with variable use of step-sections and cytokeratin-IHC. As physicians begin to understand which metastases are clinically important, pathology protocols can be devised accordingly.

Micrometastasis staging
Definitions and patterns of micrometastases are being developed for the AJCC/UICC nodal staging system.

Intraoperative consultation
Surgeons will continue to put pressure on pathologists to find SLN metastases at intraoperative examination as long as ALND is used for SLN-positive cases. If ALND is used selectively in the future, mainly for patients with SLN macrometastasis, the accuracy of intraoperative evaluation by standard cytologic or frozen-section techniques will improve, since

macrometastases are usually detected with these methods.

Immunohistochemical ultrastaging

Micrometastasis detection in SLNs and bone marrow may be sufficiently accurate, along with primary tumor prognostic factors, to identify high-risk patients for adjuvant therapies.

New staging approaches

As advances in imaging studies or molecular techniques applied to primary tumors and blood or bone marrow are proposed to replace surgical staging of axillary lymph nodes, lessons learned from SLN staging will provide a valuable basis for comparison.

CONCLUSIONS

1. Sentinel lymph-node biopsy represents an important advance in the management of breast cancer patients, because it provides more accurate axillary staging than standard ALND, and for many patients it avoids the potential morbidity of ALND.
2. It marks the beginning of an era in which micrometastasis detection, combined with advances in primary tumor prognostic factors, will permit a more targeted approach to axillary and systemic therapies.
3. Pathologic methods for SLN evaluation vary greatly and affect the incidence of micrometastasis, which in turn affects treatment recommendations and study results. Accurate descriptions of pathology techniques are needed to better determine their roles.
4. The high sensitivity of SLN and bone-marrow staging with IHC will provide new insights into the biologic behavior of various breast cancers; the proposed definition of nodal micrometastases as those 0.21 mm to 2.0 mm in size may help to avoid therapeutic dilemmas with minimal metastases.

REFERENCES

1. Cady B, Stone MD, Schuler JG et al, The new era in breast cancer. Invasion, size, and nodal involvement dramatically decreasing as a result of mammographic screening. *Arch Surg* 1996; **131**:301–8.
2. Roumen RMH, Valkenburg JGM, Geuskens LM, Lymphoscintigraphy and feasibility of sentinel node biopsy in 83 patients with primary breast cancer. *Eur J Surg Oncol* 1997; **23**:495–502.
3. Turner RR, Ollila DW, Krasne DL, Giuliano AE, Histopathologic validation of the sentinel lymph node hypothesis for breast carcinoma. *Ann Surg* 1997; **226**:271–8.
4. Weaver DL, Krag DN, Ashikaga T et al, Pathologic analysis of sentinel and nonsentinel lymph nodes in breast carcinoma. *Cancer* 2000; **88**:1099–107.
5. Czerniecki BJ, Scheff AM, Callans LS et al, Immunohistochemistry with pancytokeratins improves the sensitivity of sentinel lymph node biopsy in patients with breast cancer. *Cancer* 1999; **85**:1098–103.
6. Liberman L, Pathologic analysis of sentinel lymph nodes in breast carcinoma. *Cancer* 1999; **88**:971–7.
7. Pfeifer JD, Sentinel lymph node biopsy. *Am J Clin Pathol* 1999; **112**:599–602.
8. Van Diest PJ, Peterse HL, Borgstein PJ et al, Pathological investigation of sentinel lymph nodes. *Eur J Nucl Med* 1999; **26**(suppl):S43–9.
9. Noguchi M, Tsugawa K, Bando E et al, Sentinel lymphadenectomy in breast cancer: identification of sentinel lymph node and detection of metastases. *Breast Cancer Res Treat* 1999; **53**:97–104.
10. Lee AHS, Ellis IO, Pinder SE et al, Pathological assessment of sentinel lymph node biopsies in patients with breast cancer. *Virchows Arch* 2000; **436**:97–101.
11. Turner RR, Giuliano AE, Hoon DSB et al, Pathologic examination of the sentinel lymph node for breast carcinoma. *World J Surg* 2000; **25**:798–805.
12. Ku NNK, Pathologic examination of sentinel lymph nodes in breast cancer. *Surg Oncol Clin N Am* 1999; **8**:469–79.
13. Smith PAF, Harlow SP, Krag DN, Weaver DL, Submission of lymph node tissue for ancillary studies decreases the accuracy of conventional breast cancer axillary node staging. *Mod Pathol* 1999; **12**:781–5.

14. Fisher ER, Palekar A, Rockette H et al, Pathologic findings from the national surgical adjuvant breast project (protocol no. 4). V. Significance of axillary nodal micro- and macrometastases. *Cancer* 1978; **42**:2032–8.

15. Clayton F, Hopkins CL, Pathologic correlates of prognosis in lymph node-positive breast carcinomas. *Cancer* 1993; **71**:1780–90.

16. Giuliano AE, Dale PS, Turner RR et al, Improved axillary staging of breast cancer with sentinel lymphadenectomy. *Ann Surg* 1995; **222**:394–401.

17. Turner RR, Chu KU, Qi K et al, Pathologic features associated with nonsentinel lymph node metastases in patients with metastatic breast cancer in a sentinel lymph node. *Cancer* 2000; **89**:574–81.

18. Reynolds C, Mick R, Donohue JH et al, Sentinel lymph node biopsy with metastasis: can axillary dissection be avoided in some patients with breast cancer? *J Clin Oncol* 1999; **17**:1720–6.

19. Rosen PP, Pathology of axillary and intramammary lymph nodes. In: *Rosen's Breast Pathology,* pp. 801–15. Lippincott-Raven: Philadelphia, 1997.

20. McGuckin MA, Cummings MC, Walsh MD et al, Occult axillary metastases in breast cancer: their detection and prognostic significance. *Br J Cancer* 1996; **73**:88–95.

21. Dowlatshahi K, Fan M, Snider HC, Habib FA, Lymph node micrometastases from breast carcinoma: reviewing the dilemma. *Cancer* 1997; **80:** 1188–97.

22. Cserni G, Metastases in axillary sentinel lymph nodes in breast cancer as detected by intensive histopathological work-up. *J Clin Pathol* 1999; **52**:922–4.

23. Schreiber RH, Pendas S, Ku NN et al, Microstaging of breast cancer patients using cytokeratin staining of the sentinel lymph node. *Ann Surg Oncol* 1999; **6**:95–101.

24. Dowlatshahi K, Fan M, Bloom KJ, Occult metastases in the sentinel lymph nodes of patients with early stage breast carcinoma. A preliminary study. *Cancer* 1999; **86**:990–6.

25. Van Diest PJ, Histopathological workup of sentinel lymph nodes: how much is enough? *J Clin Pathol* 1999; **52**:871–3.

26. Cserni G, Mapping metastases in sentinel lymph nodes of breast cancer. *Am J Clin Pathol* 2000; **113**:351–4.

27. Lucci A, Turner RR, Morton DL, Carbon dye as an adjunct to isosulfan blue dye for sentinel lymph node dissection. *Surgery* 1999; **126**:48–53.

28. Meyer JS, Sentinel lymph node biopsy: strategies for pathologic examination of the specimen. *J Surg Oncol* 1998; **69**:212–8.

29. Turner RR, Ollila DW, Stern S, Giuliano AE, Optimal histopathologic examination of the sentinel lymph node for breast carcinoma staging. *Am J Surg Pathol* 1999; **23**:263–7.

30. Allred DC, Elledge RM, Caution concerning micrometastatic breast carcinoma in sentinel lymph nodes. *Cancer* 1999; **86**:905–7.

31. Doglioni C, Dell'Orto P, Zanetti G et al, Cytokeratin-immunoreactive cells of human lymph nodes and spleen in normal and pathological conditions. An immunohistochemical study. *Virchows Arch A Pathol Anat Histopathol* 1990; **416**:479–90.

32. Gould VE, Bloom KJ, Franke WW et al, Increased numbers of cytokeratin-positive interstitial reticulum cells (CIRC) in reactive, inflammatory, and neoplastic lymphadenopathies: hyperplasia or induced expression? *Virchows Arch* 1995; **425**:617–29.

33. Luzzolino P, Bontempini L, Doglioni C, Zanetti G, Keratin immunoreactivity in extrafollicular reticular cells of the lymph node. *Am J Clin Pathol* 1989; **91**:239–40.

34. Nagle RB, Intermediate filaments. Efficacy in surgical pathology diagnosis. *Am J Clin Pathol* 1989; **91**(suppl 1):S14–8.

35. Youngson BJ, Liberman L, Rosen PP, Displacement of carcinomatous epithelium in surgical breast specimens following stereotaxic core biopsy. *Am J Clin Pathol* 1995; **103**:598–602.

36. Carter BA, Jensen RA, Simpson JF, Page DL, Benign transport of breast epithelium into axillary lymph nodes after biopsy. *Am J Clin Pathol* 2000; **113**:259–65.

37. Rogers LW, Ries SG, Another variable in lymph node biopsy. *Am J Clin Pathol* 2000; **114**:293–5.

38. Min CJ, Tafra L, Verbanac KM, Identification of superior markers for polymerase chain reaction detection of breast cancer metastases in sentinel lymph nodes. *Cancer Res* 1998; **58**:4581–4.

39. Bostick PJ, Huynh K, Sarantou T et al, Detection of metastases in sentinel lymph nodes of breast cancer patients by multiple-marker RT-PCR. *Int J Cancer (Pred Oncol)* 1998; **79**:645–51.

40. Zippelius A, Kufer P, Honold G et al, Limitations of reverse-transcriptase polymerase chain reaction analyses for detection of micrometastatic epithelial cancer cells in bone marrow. *J Clin Oncol* 1997; **15**:2701–8.

41. Bostick PJ, Chatterjee S, Chi DD et al, Limitations of specific reverse-transcriptase polymerase

chain reaction markers in the detection of metastases in the lymph nodes and blood of breast cancer patients. *J Clin Oncol* 1998; **16**:2632–40.

42. Veronesi U, Paganelli G, Galimberti V et al, Sentinel node biopsy to avoid axillary dissection in breast cancer with clinically negative lymph nodes. *Lancet* 1997; **349**:1864–7.

43. Ku NN, Ahmad N, Smith PV et al, Intraoperative imprint cytology of sentinel lymph nodes in breast cancer. *Acta Cytol* 1997; **41**:1606–7.

44. Rubio IT, Korourian S, Cowan C et al, Use of touch preps for intraoperative diagnosis of sentinel lymph node metastases in breast cancer. *Ann Surg Oncol* 1998; **5**:689–94.

45. Ratanawichitrasin A, Biscotti CV, Levy L, Crowe JP, Touch imprint cytological analysis of sentinel lymph nodes for detecting axillary metastases in patients with breast cancer. *Br J Surg* 1999; **86**: 1346–9.

46. Silverberg SG, Intraoperative assessment of sentinel nodes in breast cancer. *Histopathol* 2000; **36**: 185–6.

47. Moes GS, Guibord RS, Weaver DL et al, Intraoperative cytologic evaluation of sentinel lymph nodes in breast cancer patients. *Mod Pathol* 2000; **13**:28 (Abstract).

48. Litz C, Miller R, Ewing G et al, Intraoperative sentinel lymph node touch imprints are not sensitive in detecting metastatic carcinoma. *Mod Pathol* 2000; **13**:26 (Abstract).

49. Van Diest PJ, Torrenga H, Borgstein PJ et al, Reliability of intraoperative frozen section and imprint cytological investigation of sentinel lymph nodes in breast cancer. *Histopathol* 1999; **35**:14–8.

50. Turner RR, Hansen NM, Stern SL, Giuliano AE, Intraoperative examination of the sentinel lymph node for breast carcinoma staging. *Am J Clin Pathol* 1999; **112**:627–34.

51. Ahmad N, Ku NNK, Nicosia SV et al, Evaluation of sentinel lymph node imprints in breast cancer: role of intraoperative cytokeratin immunostaining in breast cancer staging. *Acta Cytol* 1998; **42**:1218 (Abstract).

52. Flett MM, Going JJ, Stanton PD et al, Sentinel node localization in patients with breast cancer. *Br J Surg* 1998; **85**:991–3.

53. Chiu A, DeLellis R, Swistel A et al, Frozen section examination of axillary sentinel nodes: is it predictive of status of other axillary nodes? *Mod Pathol* 2000; **13**:19 (Abstract).

54. Richter T, Nahrig J, Komminoth P et al, Protocol for ultrarapid immunostaining of frozen sections. *J Clin Pathol* 1999; **52**:461–3.

55. Hyjek E, Chiu A, Chadburn A et al, Rapid intraoperative immunostaining for cytokeratin of sentinel lymph nodes in breast cancer. *Mod Pathol* 2000; **13**:223 (Abstract).

56. Viale G, Bosari S, Mazzarol G et al, Intraoperative examination of axillary sentinel lymph nodes in breast cancer patients. *Cancer* 1999; **85**:2433–8.

57. Stratmann SL, McCarty TM, Kuhn JA, Radiation safety with breast sentinel node biopsy. *Am J Surg* 1999; **178**:454–7.

58. Glass EC, Basinski JE, Krasne DL, Giuliano AE, Radiation safety considerations for sentinel node techniques. *Ann Surg Oncol* 1999; **6**:10–1.

59. Fitzgibbons PL, LiVolsi VA, Recommendations for handling radioactive specimens obtained by sentinel lymphadenectomy. Surgical Pathology Committee of the College of American Pathologists, and the Association of Directors of Anatomic and Surgical Pathology. *Am J Surg Pathol* 2000; **24**:1549–51.

60. Miner TJ, Shriver CD, Flicek PR et al, Guidelines for the safe use of radioactive materials during localization and resection of the sentinel lymph node. *Ann Surg Oncol* 1999; **6**:75–82.

61. Giuliano AE, Dale PS, Turner RR et al, Improved axillary staging of breast cancer with sentinel lymphadenectomy. *Ann Surg* 1995; **222**:394–9.

62. Giuliano AE, Haigh PI, Brennan MB et al, Prospective observational study of sentinel lymphadenectomy without further axillary dissection in patients with sentinel node-negative breast cancer. *J Clin Oncol* 2000; **18**: 2553–9.

63. Chu KU, Turner RR, Hansen NM et al, Do all patients with sentinel node metastasis from breast carcinoma need complete axillary node dissection? *Ann Surg* 1999; **229**:536–41.

64. Cote RJ, Peterson HF, Chaiwun B et al, Role of immunohistochemical detection of lymph-node metastases in management of breast cancer. *Lancet* 1999; **354**:896–900.

65. Braun S, Pantel K, Muller P et al, Cytokeratin-positive cells in the bone marrow and survival of patients with stage I, II, or III breast cancer. *N Engl J Med* 2000; **342**:525–33.

66. Pantel K, Cote RJ, Fodstad O, Detection and clinical importance of micrometastatic disease. *J Natl Cancer Inst* 1999; **91**:1113–24.

67. Diel IJ, Cote RJ, Bone marrow and lymph node assessment for minimal residual disease in

patients with breast cancer. *Cancer Treat Rev* 2000; **26**:53–65.

68. Liu D, Shi SR, Taylor CR et al, The prognostic significance of lymph node and bone marrow micrometastases (LNM, BMM) in node-negative breast cancer. *Proc Amer Assoc Cancer Res* 1998; **39**:268–9 (Abstract).

69. Reintgen DS, Cox CE, National protocols for lymphatic mapping. *Surg Oncol Clin N Am* 1999; **8**:511–4.

70. Pendas S, Dauway E, Giuliano R et al, Sentinel node biopsy in ductal carcinoma *in situ*. *Ann Surg Oncol* 2000; **7**:15–20.

71. Pendas S, Dauway E, Cox CE et al, Sentinel node biopsy and cytokeratin staining for the accurate staging of 478 breast cancer patients. *Am Surg* 1999; **65**:500–6.

72. Zavotsky J, Hansen N, Brennan MB et al, Lymph node metastasis from ductal carcinoma *in situ* with microinvasion. *Cancer* 1999; **85**:2439–43.

73. Hill ADK, Tran KN, Akhurst T et al, Lessons learned from 500 cases of lymphatic mapping for breast cancer. *Ann Surg* 1999; **229**:528–35.

74. Fleming ID, Cooper JS, Henson DE et al, Breast. In: American Joint Committee on Cancer, eds, *Cancer Staging Manual*, 5th edn, 171–80. Lippincott-Raven: Philadelphia, 1997.

75. Hermanek P, Hutter RVP, Sobin LH, Wittekind C, Classification of isolated tumor cells and micrometastasis. *Cancer* 1999; **86**:2668–73.

76. Fitzgibbons PL, Page DL, Weaver D et al, Prognostic factors in breast cancer. College of American Pathologists Consensus Statement 1999. *Arch Pathol Lab Med* 2000; **124**:966–78.

77. Hammond MEH, Fitzgibbons PL, Compton C et al, College of American Pathologists Conference XXXV: Solid tumor prognostic factors: which, how, and so what? *Arch Pathol Lab Med* 2000; **124**:958–65.

78. Page DL, Anderson TJ, Carter BA, Minimal solid tumor involvement of regional and distant sites: when is a metastasis not a metastasis? *Cancer* 1999; **86**:2589–92 (Editorial).

18

The blue-dye technique

Armando E Giuliano

The John Wayne Cancer Institute technique for SLN Biopsy in breast cancer			
Technique	Dye (combination technique used only in medial tumors)	**Isotope**	See Technical Details section, page 211
Dye	*Type*: Isosulfan blue dye (1%) *Volume*: 5 ml (cc)		
Injection site	*Dye*: Adjacent and lateral to breast mass		

The status of the axillary lymph nodes remains the single best prognostic indicator in patients with early-stage breast cancer. Dissection of axillary nodes in Levels I and II is traditionally used to determine the presence or absence of nodal metastasis. This operation can cause numbness, lymphedema, and limitation of arm motion, however, as well as other potentially significant problems. A less-invasive surgical staging technique is sentinel lymph-node (SLN) biopsy, originally introduced by Morton et al for the identification of regional metastasis in patients with primary cutaneous melanoma.[1] The SLN in melanoma, breast cancer, and any other tumor that drains via the lymphatics, is defined as the first lymph node in the regional drainage basin to harbor tumor cells metastasizing from the primary lesion.

Since our group at the John Wayne Cancer Institute (JWCI) first described dye-directed SLN biopsy for the staging of primary breast cancer,[2] several different dye-directed and/or probe-directed studies have reported successful identification of axillary SLNs.[3–7] As a result, SLN biopsy is rapidly becoming standard practice—despite the absence of a standard technique. Moreover, most of the reports in the literature are based on cumulative experience with techniques in evolution. This chapter therefore begins with the caveat that no surgeon should undertake SLN biopsy without routine completion axillary lymph-node dissection (ALND) until that individual has documented a consistently high rate of SLN identification using the same mapping agent and mapping technique.

DEVELOPMENT OF DYE-DIRECTED MAPPING FOR BREAST CANCER

Our group adapted the dye-directed SLN biopsy technique in melanoma (a cutaneous tumor system) for use in primary breast cancer (a parenchymal tumor system), and in October 1991 we initiated a feasibility study of lymphatic mapping with isosulfan blue dye in patients with primary breast cancer. Because there was no prior study of dye-directed SLN biopsy in breast cancer, the initial portion of the study was a developmental period during which technical aspects of the procedure were defined. Among the factors affecting the success of SLN biopsy were patient selection, injection technique, dissection technique, and histopathologic evaluation of the SLN.

In 1994, we reported the results of this feasibility study.[2] The study included 172 participants, several of whom had advanced tumors and grossly involved nodes—characteristics that we have since identified as exclusion criteria. Two of the 172 patients had synchronous bilateral breast cancer. All patients underwent completion ALND (Levels I and II) immediately after SLN biopsy. Mapping with a 1% solution of isosulfan blue identified SLNs in 114 (66%) procedures. These SLNs accurately predicted the status of the entire axillary basin in 109 (96%) of the 114 cases. Since then we have improved the technique and systematically studied its application. Dye-directed mapping is the only SLN biopsy technique that has been studied in this stepwise fashion, and therefore it is not surprising that the highest accuracy rates are reported with vital dye.

The five false-negative results in our feasibility study occurred in the first 87 procedures, and two occurred in the first 10 procedures. In three cases, dye-stained axillary fat was misidentified as an SLN. This prompted the routine use of frozen-section analysis to confirm lymph-node recovery. In another case, micrometastasis was identified when the SLN was re-examined using immunohistochemical staining (IHC) with anti-cytokeratin antibodies. Only one of the five apparently false-negative SLNs was a true false-negative. Thus, there was only a single case of non-SLN metastasis in the absence of SLN metastasis.

Critics of dye-directed mapping continue to refer to the "low" SLN detection rate and "high" false-negative rate reported in our feasibility trial. Remember, however, that this trial was undertaken to develop the procedure and establish guidelines that previously were nonexistent. During the study, we were constantly identifying and redefining different aspects of the technique until we developed a reliable, accurate protocol—a protocol that in retrospect would have excluded many of the reported cases (e.g., patients with locally advanced tumors or clinically involved nodes).

Our next report was a comparison of SLN biopsy with enhanced histopathology (using IHC) versus ALND followed by routine processing of nodal tissue.[8] The SLN group contained 162 patients undergoing successful SLN biopsy followed by completion ALND; the ALND group included 134 patients undergoing ALND alone. All SLNs were evaluated by serial sections using hematoxylin-and-eosin (H&E) staining and anti-cytokeratin IHC; non-SLNs were evaluated by H&E alone. Both groups had comparable clinical characteristics and underwent excision of similar numbers of axillary nodes. The rate of axillary metastasis was 42% in the SLN group versus 28% in the ALND group. This significant difference ($p < 0.05$) was primarily due to the incremental detection of SLN micrometastases (<2 mm) by IHC. Sixteen per cent of SLN patients had micrometastases, compared with 3% of ALND patients. Detection of micrometastases by both H&E (9% versus 3%) and IHC (7% vs 0%) increased with examination of the SLN. These findings indicate that when compared with ALND, SLN biopsy can increase the accuracy of axillary staging. Sentinel lymph-node biopsy allows the highly focused examination of a few nodes, an examination that would be too costly and time-consuming for an entire ALND specimen.

After completing the developmental stage of SLN biopsy, we undertook a study of our mature technique in a series of 107 patients.[9] The rate of SLN identification was 94%. With no false-negative or false-positive results, the sensitivity and specificity were 100%. We then conducted an exhaustive histopathologic analysis of non-SLNs to confirm that the SLN was truly the first node to harbor metastases and not an artifact of greater histopathologic scrutiny.[10] We found that when the SLN was tumor-free by both routine H&E and IHC and the non-SLNs were subjected to the same intensive analysis, only 1 of 1087 non-SLNs contained tumor. This finding validates the SLN hypothesis in breast cancer and shows that the risk of non-SLN involvement is extremely low when the SLN is tumor-free.

Based on these findings, we began a study of SLN biopsy without routine completion ALND. Between October 1995 and July 1997, a total of 133 women who had primary invasive breast tumors clinically 4 cm or less in diameter and no axillary lymphadenopathy (consecutive cases) were prospectively entered into a trial of SLN biopsy using isosulfan blue dye.[11] Sentinel lymph nodes were examined by standard microscopy or IHC. Sentinel lymph-node biopsy was the only axillary surgery if the SLNs were tumor-free; completion ALND was performed if the SLNs contained metastases or if no SLN was identified. Excluded from subsequent analysis were patients with unsuspected multifocal carcinoma and those who refused completion ALND. Sentinel lymph-node biopsy succeeded in 132 of 133 patients (99%). Eight patients were excluded from further analysis. Of the 125 evaluable patients, 57 had tumor-positive SLNs and one had an unsuccessful SLN mapping procedure. These patients underwent completion ALND. In the remaining 67 (54%) patients, SLN biopsy was the only axillary surgery. The rate of complications was significantly higher when SLN biopsy was followed by ALND (35% vs 3% for SLN biopsy alone; $p = 0.001$), and most importantly, there were no local or axillary recurrences in the SLN-only patients at a median follow-up of 32 months. This prospective observational study was the first to demonstrate the safety of SLN biopsy as the sole axillary staging procedure. These results support SLN biopsy as an accurate staging alternative for breast cancer and suggest that routine ALND can be safely eliminated for patients with histopathologically negative SLNs.

TECHNICAL DETAILS OF DYE-DIRECTED SLN BIOPSY

At the John Wayne Cancer Institute (JWCI), we use a dye-directed mapping technique for SLN biopsy in patients with breast cancer; a combination of dye and radioisotope is used only in patients with medial tumors. Candidates for SLN biopsy are patients whose primary breast tumors do not exceed 4 cm in diameter by physical examination or mammography. Sentinel lymph-node biopsy should not be attempted in patients with multifocal tumors, locally advanced disease, or disease diagnosed by large excisional biopsies or quadrant resections. Patients with medial-hemisphere lesions should undergo preoperative breast lymphoscintigraphy (LSG) to document lymphatic drainage to the axilla and to rule out internal mammary drainage. In rare cases, tumors in the medial half of the breast will drain only to internal mammary nodes, decreasing the likelihood of finding an axillary SLN. No study has yet demonstrated the effectiveness of SLN biopsy for internal mammary nodes. At JWCI, we attempt to identify an axillary SLN, and if one is not found, we perform a standard ALND. If the LSG has documented internal mammary drainage we recommend that the internal mammary nodes be included in the radiation port.

Our technique of dye-directed SLN biopsy can be performed under local anesthesia with sedation, or under general anesthesia. A 1% solution of isosulfan blue dye is injected adjacent and just lateral to the breast mass, and just below the subcutaneous fat to avoid tattooing the overlying skin. If the primary tumor is not palpable, dye is injected through a needle inserted under mammographic guidance for tumor localization. If an excisional biopsy has been performed previously, dye is injected into the wall of the biopsy cavity at its periphery.

Immediately after injection of the dye, the breast is gently compressed for 5–7 minutes to enhance lymph flow. The duration of compression depends on the distance of the primary tumor from the axilla. A transverse incision is then made just below the hair-bearing area in the axilla. Dissection proceeds to the interface of subcutaneous adipose tissue with the axillary lymphatic tissue. In this plane of dissection, but anterior, the tail of the breast is encountered as it enters the axilla. Dye-stained lymphatic vessels are identified at the tail of the breast and followed to all blue-stained SLNs (Figure 18.1). Even if a dye-stained node is immediately obvious, the afferent lymphatic vessels should be traced back to the tail of the breast to assure that this node is the most proximal node and that there is no bifurcation that could lead to other SLNs. If more than one dye-filled lymphatic tract is identified, each is followed. These tracts usually drain to the same node or to additional neighboring SLNs. After confirmation of the SLN, the procedure is completed and the SLN specimen is sent separately for pathologic evaluation. Segmental or total mastectomy is then performed as needed.

Completion ALND is performed at the time of SLN biopsy if no SLN is identified or if a frozen section of the SLN contains tumor cells. Axillary lymph-node dissection is performed as a secondary procedure if permanent sections of the SLN are positive by either H&E and/or IHC staining. We have shown that dye-directed SLN biopsy is highly accurate,[2,8–10] and we do not perform ALND in patients whose SLNs are considered tumor-free. Conventional closed-suction drainage of the axilla is used for all patients undergoing ALND, but is not required after SLN biopsy alone.

We recommend a 1% solution of isosulfan blue dye, largely because of previous studies showing no local toxicity for 1% solutions of triphenylmethane dyes but widespread tissue necrosis for solutions with concentrations exceeding 3%. Mild hypersensitivity reactions

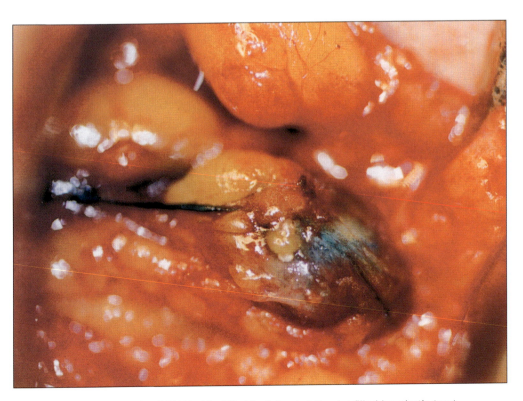

Figure 18.1 The blue-stained SLN is identified by following the dye-filled lymphatic tract.

to isosulfan blue have been reported but tend to be self-limited, and may be uncommon with SLN biopsy because most of the injected dye is removed during segmental resection. A recent report describes three cases of anaphylaxis after intradermal injection of isosulfan blue in 406 patients who underwent SLN biopsy for melanoma,[12] an incidence of 1%. Residual systemic dye is excreted primarily by the biliary system and the kidneys. Patients should be informed that the dye produces a transient blue discoloration of both the skin and the urine; these phenomena are minimized when the volume of injection is limited and extraneous dye is promptly removed. Residual deep-tissue staining is rare if dye injection is limited to those tissues intended for resection.

In some cases, the SLN cannot be found. The reasons for this may be multifactorial. Egress of dye from the primary site may be impeded by edema, infection, or tumor. Injection into a previous biopsy cavity or injection into large tumors may retard flow of dye. Drainage to high Level II or III axillary nodes may follow routes undetectable by present methods. Patients may have nonaxillary lymphatic drainage; preoperative LSG can demonstrate uptake in the internal mammary, supraclavicular, or other anomalous sites. Another possibility is that lymphatic vessels may be transected prematurely, preventing dye from reaching the SLN. Proximity of primary tumors to lymph-node regions at risk and inappropriate injection of tissues other than the breast may impair lymphatic mapping. The possibility of nonlocalization of the SLN (and hence an appropriate contingency plan) should always be discussed with the patient preoperatively. Failed SLN mappings should not exceed 15% in experienced hands.

Because the SLN specimen contains only one or two lymph nodes on average, it can be routinely examined in multiple sections with IHC using anti-cytokeratin antibodies. Each SLN is bisected and examined during surgery by frozen-section analysis: if the node contains tumor, completion ALND is performed immediately. The SLN is then processed routinely for permanent section with H&E. Each node is blocked individually, with preparation of two permanent-section levels per paraffin block. If H&E staining is negative for tumor cells, the SLN is examined with IHC using an antibody cocktail (MAK-6) directed against cytokeratin of low and intermediate molecular weight. Approximately six to eight histologic sections (including the frozen section) of each SLN are examined. The ALND specimen is examined using standard pathologic technique; lymph nodes are identified visually or with manual palpation, and no node-clearing solution is employed. Non-SLNs greater than 3–4 mm are grossly sectioned and all nodal tissue is embedded in paraffin. One or two H&E-stained histologic sections are prepared, as IHC stains are not routinely used to examine these non-SLNs.

PUBLISHED STUDIES AND ONGOING TRIALS OF DYE-DIRECTED SLN BIOPSY

Results of dye-directed SLN biopsy validated by ALND have been reported by other investigators (Table 18.1). Among 145 patients who underwent SLN biopsy followed by ALND, Guenther et al successfully identified an SLN in 71% (103 of 145).[13] This study should be interpreted as a feasibility trial, since it included tumors ranging from T0 to T4, and the technique of SLN biopsy was not standardized in the initial phase of the study. Nonetheless, the SLN accurately reflected the axillary status in 100 of 103 patients (97%), and the three false-negatives occurred in the early phase of this study. Dale and Williams reported their initial SLN biopsy experience in 20 patients who underwent dye-directed SLN biopsy (one of these bilateral) followed by ALND.[14] Sentinel lymph nodes were identified in 14 of 21 basins (66%) and were 100% predictive of axillary nodal status. Koller et al reported their experience using either methylene blue 1% or patent blue-V dye to map lymphatic drainage from a primary breast cancer.[15] Sentinel lymph nodes were found in 96 of 98 cases (98%), accurately predicting the node status in 93 (97%).

Albertini et al combined blue dye with a radiopharmaceutical, filtered technetium-99m-

Table 18.1 Studies using blue dye with or without radiopharmaceutical for mapping the SLN in breast cancer

Study	N	Mapping technique	SLN staining technique	Rate of SLN identification	Accuracy of SLN as indicator of axillary tumor status
Giuliano[2]	174	Dye	H&E	114/174 (66%)	109/114 (96%)
Albertini[4]	62	Dye + probe	H&E	57/62 (92%)	57/57 (100%)
Giuliano[9]	107	Dye	H&E + IHC	100/107 (94%)	100/100 (100%)
Guenther[13]	145	Dye	H&E	103/145 (71%)	100/103 (97%)
Dale[14]	21	Dye	H&E	14/21 (66%)	14/14 (100%)
Barnwell[6]	42	Dye + probe	H&E	38/42 (90%)	38/38 (100%)
O'Hea[7]	59	Dye + probe	H&E	55/59 (93%)	52/55 (95%)
Cox[16]	466	Dye + probe	H&E + IHC	440/466 (94%)	—
Koller[15]	98	Dye	—	96/98 (98%)	93/96 (97%)
Hill[17]	492	Dye + probe	H&E + IHC	458/492 (93%)	99/104(95%)[a]
Giuliano[11]	125	Dye	H&E/IHC	124/125 (99%)	—[a]

[a]Not all patients underwent axillary lymph-node dissection.
H&E, hematoxylin-and-eosin staining; IHC, immunohistochemical staining.

sulfur colloid (Tc-99m-SC), in 62 patients undergoing SLN biopsy for primary breast cancer.[4] The SLN was blue-stained in 73% of the patients and radioactive in an additional 19%, increasing the total SLN detection rate to 92%. Sensitivity was 100%, and there were no false-negative SLNs. Barnwell et al reported their experience with this combination approach in 42 patients; SLNs were detected in 90% and accurately predicted axillary status in 100%.[6] O'Hea et al identified SLNs in 55 of 59 (93%) patients, with 95% accuracy in predicting axillary metastasis.[7] Finally, Cox et al compiled results for 466 patients enrolled in three breast SLN biopsy protocols, with SLNs identified in 94% (440 of 466).[16]

The results of these studies using dual-agent mapping have led many to conclude that the combination of dye and pharmaceutical is superior to either agent alone, especially for sur-geons just starting the procedure.[17] Adding a radiocolloid does not necessarily increase map-ping accuracy, however, and may introduce additional technical problems such as "shine-through" when the tumor is near the axillary nodal basin. In this case, SLNs cannot be detected by the probe without special tech-niques such as removing the primary site or shielding the probe with a collimator. Moreover, many authors who comment on the difficulty of performing SLN biopsy with blue dye alone have never actually seen the tech-nique performed correctly. While it is true that identification of SLNs may be increased by adding isotope to blue dye, the surgeon should consider the possibility that in combining the two mapping techniques, neither is optimal because the results of each method may to some extent influence the other. Only by achieving a consistently high rate of SLN identification using the *same* mapping agent and mapping technique can a surgeon obtain optimal results. Standardization and consistency are of paramount importance.

The controversy over mapping agent and technique does not invalidate the SLN hypothesis. Breast cancer does metastasize preferentially to a single node, and this SLN is the first node to harbor axillary metastases in patients with clinically localized breast cancer. The SLN concept is not Halstedian because no implication is made about the systemic spread of breast cancer, nor is it suggested that breast cancer does not spread directly via the bloodstream. Rather, if breast cancer spreads to the lymph nodes, it can be tracked to an SLN. This SLN is usually in Level I, but may be in Level II of the axilla.[2] Level III SLNs are unlikely to be easily detected with any of the above technologies. The concept of "skip" metastases is not valid because the SLN is defined as the first node to contain metastases and therefore cannot be skipped; that is, "skip" metastases are in actuality SLNs. Failure to identify the SLN is far more likely to be on the basis of surgical or pathologic issues than on the basis of anomalous anatomy.

Although a tumor-free SLN indicates node-negative breast cancer in at least 95% of cases performed by an experienced SLN team, the procedure should not be accepted as an alternative to routine ALND until each surgeon has performed a sufficient number of cases with concurrent ALND to document staging accuracy. How many cases of SLN biopsy plus completion ALND must the surgeon perform before switching to SLN biopsy alone? Morton recommended approximately 60–80 cases to develop an "acceptable level of technical skill (90% accuracy in identifying sentinel node)."[18] He noted that the experience required for this level of proficiency does not match the number of breast-cancer patients in most community practice situations or the number of breast operations performed by surgeons not working in major cancer centers. The author's estimate of the number of cases would be closer to 25 or 30, however.[19] Both estimates are of course completely arbitrary. Surgical fellows training at

JWCI generally learn dye-directed SLN biopsy after about 10–15 cases, and visiting surgeons who observe our technique usually find it easy to master when they return to their practice. Most surgeons just starting SLN biopsy will probably use both blue dye and radiocolloid, feeling more secure with a "backup" mapping agent that allows a "second chance" to identify the SLN. Quick-learning surgeons who have performed many axillary operations will master SLN biopsy after fewer cases, whereas others may never develop the skills necessary to identify the SLN accurately. Once surgeons prove their accuracy, and have assembled a team committed to the procedure, SLN biopsy may become the axillary staging procedure of choice and benefit many patients by allowing accurate staging with minimal morbidity.

The most important question resulting from the emergence of SLN technology is whether SLN biopsy should replace routine ALND. Published data support SLN biopsy as the sole axillary staging procedure when the breast tumor is small, the axillary nodes are clinically normal, and the SLNs are free of tumor by both H&E and IHC. The case for SLN biopsy without ALND is less clear when IHC identifies micrometastases in the SLN. In our experience these patients have a higher risk of non-SLN metastasis (primarily micrometastases) than do patients whose SLNs are tumor-free by IHC.[20] The clinical significance of these axillary micrometastases is currently under dispute.[21] Since all breast-cancer staging has been based on H&E results, however, routine IHC of SLNs is not appropriate at present. Indeed, routine IHC of SLNs can increase the risk of false-positive results,[22] since approximately 5–10% of patients with pure ductal carcinoma in situ are found to have "metastases." Alternatively, this phenomenon may indicate not a false-positive SLN, but rather a "false-negative" diagnosis of in situ cancer in a patient with occult invasive disease.

Although our previous studies using IHC demonstrated the absence of tumor in non-SLNs, these patients still could have non-SLN micrometastases that might eventually become clinically significant. Two large multicenter trials in North America are actively accruing patients to study the clinical impact of micrometastatic nodal disease. The National Surgical Adjuvant Breast and Bowel Project (NSABP) B-32 trial randomizes patients with invasive breast cancer and negative SLNs to ALND or no ALND. The American College of Surgeons Oncology Group (ACSOG) Z0010 trial is a prospective evaluation of the significance of bone-marrow and SLN micrometastases in breast cancer patients whose SLNs are negative when processed by H&E; while these patients have SLN biopsy only, the SLNs and bone marrow are examined at a central laboratory with IHC and reverse transcriptase–polymerase chain reaction (RT-PCR), with patient and clinician masked to the result. The ASCOG Z0011 trial randomizes patients whose SLNs are positive by H&E to receive either ALND or no ALND. The hope is that these trials will definitively determine whether SLN biopsy can replace ALND in the management of many patients with breast cancer.

Even if the SLN is positive on H&E staining, a reasonable case can be made for not performing ALND. In 40–60% of cases the SLN is the only involved lymph node. In addition, if one views ALND as a staging procedure only, then SLN biopsy alone will provide accurate staging. Finally, breast radiation therapy using opposing tangential fields may treat the lower axillary lymph nodes in a substantial fraction of patients, destroying any tumor cells in low-axillary non-SLNs. Thus it may be possible to "treat" patients with SLN biopsy, postoperative chemotherapy, and radiation therapy—without ALND. Complete ALND might be reserved only for patients with clinically positive axillae, either at the time of diagnosis, or in a delayed fashion after SLN biopsy alone.

Until multicenter trials determine the relative roles of SLN biopsy and of ALND and establish the clinical significance of micrometastases in early breast cancer, centers with experienced SLN biopsy teams may *consider* abandoning routine ALND in selected patients whose SLNs are tumor-free. However, ALND must remain routine until each member of the SLN team using a standardized technique is able to achieve acceptably high success rates and an acceptably low incidence of false-negative results.

REFERENCES

1. Morton DL, Wen D-R, Wong JH et al, Technical details of intraoperative lymphatic mapping for early stage melanoma. *Arch Surg* 1992; **127:**392–9.

2. Giuliano AE, Kirgan DM, Guenther JM, Morton DL, Lymphatic mapping and sentinel lymphadenectomy for breast cancer. *Ann Surg* 1994; **220:**391–401.

3. Krag DN, Weaver DL, Alex JC, Fairbank JT, Surgical resection and radiolocalization of the sentinel node in breast cancer using gamma probe. *Surg Oncol* 1993; **2:**335–40.

4. Albertini JJ, Lyman GH, Cox C et al, Lymphatic mapping and sentinel node biopsy in the patient with breast cancer. *JAMA* 1996; **276:**1818–22.

5. Veronesi U, Paganelli G, Galimberti V et al, Sentinel-node biopsy to avoid axillary dissection in breast cancer with clinically negative lymphnodes. *Lancet* 1997; **349:**1864–7.

6. Barnwell JM, Arredondo MA, Kollmorgen D et al, Sentinel node biopsy in breast cancer. *Ann Surg Oncol* 1998; **5:**126–30.

7. O'Hea BJ, Hill ADK, El-Shirbiny AM et al, Sentinel lymph node biopsy in breast cancer: initial experience at Memorial Sloan-Kettering Cancer Center. *J Am Coll Surg* 1998; **186:**423–7.

8. Giuliano AE, Dale PS, Turner RR et al, Improved axillary staging of breast cancer with sentinel lymphadenectomy. *Ann Surg* 1995; **222:**394–401.

9. Giuliano AE, Jones RC, Brennan M, Statman R, Sentinel lymphadenectomy in breast cancer. *J Clin Oncol* 1997; **15:**2345–50.

10. Turner RR, Ollila DW, Krasne DL, Giuliano AE, Histopathologic validation of the sentinel lymph node hypothesis for breast carcinoma. *Ann Surg* 1997; **226:**271–8.

11. Giuliano AE, Haigh PI, Brennan MB et al, Prospective observational study of sentinel lymphadenectomy without further axillary dissection in patients with sentinel node-negative breast cancer. *J Clin Oncol* 2000; **18:**2553–9.

12. Leong SP, Donegan E, Heffernon W et al, Adverse reactions to isosulfan blue during selective sentinel lymph node dissection in melanoma. *Ann Surg Oncol* 2000; **7:**361–6.

13. Guenther JM, Krishnamoorthy M, Tan LR, Sentinel lymphadenectomy for breast cancer in a

community managed care setting. *Cancer J Sci Am* 1997; **3**:336–40.

14. Dale PS, Williams JT, Axillary staging utilizing selective sentinel lymphadenectomy for patients with invasive breast carcinoma. *Am Surg* 1998; **64**:28–32.

15. Koller M, Barsuk D, Zippel D et al, Sentinel lymph node involvement—a predictor for axillary node status with breast cancer—has the time come? *Eur J Surg Oncol* 1998; **24**:166–8.

16. Cox CE, Pendas S, Cox JM et al, Guidelines for sentinel node biopsy and lymphatic mapping of patients with breast cancer. *Ann Surg* 1998; **227**:645–53.

17. Hill AD, Tran KN, Akhurst T et al, Lessons learned from 500 cases of lymphatic mapping for breast cancer. *Ann Surg* 1999; **229**:528–35.

18. Morton DL, Intraoperative lymphatic mapping and sentinel lymphadenectomy: community standard care or clinical investigation? *Cancer J Sci Am* 1997; **3**:328–30.

19. Giuliano AE, Mapping a pathway for axillary staging: a personal perspective on the current status of sentinel lymph node dissection for breast cancer. *Arch Surg* 1999; **134**:195–9.

20. Chu KU, Turner RR, Hansen NM et al, Sentinel node metastasis in patients with breast carcinoma accurately predicts immunohistochemically detectable nonsentinel node metastasis. *Ann Surg Oncol* 1999; **6**:756–61.

21. Rose DM, Giuliano AE, Micrometastatic nodal disease in breast cancer – the dilemma continues. *J Surg Oncol* 2000; **74**:87–9.

22. Pendas S, Dauway E, Giuliano R et al, Sentinel node biopsy in ductal carcinoma in situ patients. *Ann Surg Oncol* 2000; **7**:15–20.

19

The isotope technique

Virgilio Sacchini, Wolfgang Gatzemeier, Viviana Galimberti, Giovanni Paganelli and Umberto Veronesi

---

The European Institute of Oncology technique for SLN Biopsy in breast cancer

Technique	Isotope	**Isotope**	*Type*: Tc-99m-CA (human albumin particles)
Injection site	*Isotope*: Intradermal		*Filtered*: Yes (200–1000 nm)
			Dose: 0.135–0.27 mCi (5–10 MBq)
			Volume: 0.2–0.4 ml (cc)

Classic anatomic studies demonstrate that the lymphatic flow of the breast follows preferred lymphatic pathways,[1] and that the predominance of this flow—97% in the classic studies of Turner-Warwick and others[2,3]—is to the axilla. More recent work by Borgstein confirms that the breast functions as a single biologic unit with lymphatic drainage to the axilla.[4] The idea that one or a few regional nodes receive this drainage first has been suggested for a variety of solid tumors,[5–10] and out of this background the sentinel lymph node (SLN) hypothesis has emerged.

Krag,[11] using radioisotope localization, Giuliano,[12] using blue dye, and Albertini,[13] using a combination of the two methods, have pioneered the application of SLN biopsy to breast cancer. Sandrucci et al reviewed the published results of 4790 SLN biopsy procedures done between 1993 and 1999 using a variety of techniques and reported a wide variation in results.[14] Using dye, isotope, and the combina-tion method, SLNs were found in 65–95%, 67–99%, and 81–95% of patients, respectively, with negative predictive values of 89% to 100%. The results of selected larger series using isotope (with or without blue dye) report greater success (Table 19.1).[11,13,15–22]

At the European Institute of Oncology in Milan, we began to perform SLN biopsy for breast cancer in March 1996, adopting the radioisotope technique. Here we report the rationale, technique, and results of this methodology as it has evolved over the last 4 years at our center.

ISOTOPE VS BLUE DYE: PROS AND CONS

SLN targeting

As suggested by Borgstein et al,[4,16] there is a fundamental difference between the targeting

Table 19.1 Selected clinical studies of SLN biopsy using isotope localization, with or without blue dye guidance

Author	Year of publication	Detection rate (%)	False-negative rate (%)	Method
Krag[11]	1993	82	0	PG
Albertini[13]	1996	92	0	PG, VDG
Veronesi[15]	1997	98	5	PG, LSG
Borgstein[16]	1998	94	2	PG, LSG
O'Hea[17]	1998	93	15	PG, LSG, VDG
Bass[18]	1999	95	1	PG, VDG
Cody[19]	1999	93	11	PG, VDG
Pendas[20]	1999	95	0	PG, VDG
Winchester[21]	1999	90	9	PG, LSG
Veronesi[22]	1999	99	7	PG, LSG

PG, probe-guided; LSG, lymphoscintigraphy; VDG, vital-dye-guided.

mechanisms of isotope and blue dye. Radiocolloids have to be actively phagocytosed, retained, and accumulated in the lymph node, and therefore require the node to have at least some degree of normal functional capacity.[4,16] This mechanism is disrupted by the presence of extensive nodal metastasis. In contrast, the lymphatic uptake of the very small dye particles is predominantly passive. For this reason, dye may be more effective than isotope in identifying grossly positive SLNs; however, massively involved nodes may block lymphatic flow to such an extent that neither method can identify the SLN.

Choice of agent

Technetium-99m is universally the isotope of choice for SLN mapping, but a wide variety of carrier particles have been used, as reviewed by Wilhelm.[23] Sentinel lymph nodes can be identified by Tc-99m-sulfur colloid (Tc-99m-SC), Tc-99m-antimony trisulfide colloid (Tc-99m-ATC),

and Tc-99m-nanocolloidal human albumin (Tc-99m-CA). Technetium-99m-sulfur colloid and Tc-99m-CA are both available in Europe, whereas Tc-99m-SC is the only registered radio-pharmaceutical for lymphoscintigraphy in the United States. Although Tc-99m-SC and Tc-99m-CA identify the SLN equally often, Tc-99m-CA may provide faster and better visualization.[24]

Timing of injection

Blue dye passes quickly from the lymphatic vessels to the SLN and is thus injected several minutes before carrying out the operation. Radiopharmaceuticals take longer, and the literature reports injection-to-surgery times ranging from 30 minutes to 24 hours. Winchester et al reported that SLNs were found more often after overnight migration of the tracer than following injection on the day of surgery (96% vs 85%),[21] while Cody et al found the SLN equally often with day-before and same-day injection.[25]

Site of injection

Krag et al described injecting 37 MBq (1 mCi) of unfiltered Tc-99m-SC in 4 ml (cc) of isotonic saline at four sites around the tumor or biopsy cavity.[11,26] Intralesional, subdermal, intradermal, or subareolar injection of isotope have been reported by others.[4,27–30] While intradermal injection may have greater success in the identification of axillary SLNs, nonaxillary lymphatic drainage (especially to the internal mammary nodes) is better identified by peri- or intratumoral injection.[30,31] By identifying sites of nonaxillary drainage, especially the internal mammary nodes, isotope mapping may increase the accuracy of staging.

Surgery

There is a clear learning curve for SLN biopsy. This is especially true for the blue-dye method, which leaves the surgeon entirely dependent on identifying the SLN intraoperatively. Morton et al have suggested that the dye technique for melanoma requires the performance of 30–50 SLN procedures (with a backup axillary lymph-node dissection) to reach full competence.[10] Isotope speeds the learning process by allowing preoperative identification of the SLN site in most patients, guiding the placement of the skin incision, and facilitating the intraoperative exploration as well.

CASE SELECTION FOR SLN BIOPSY

We have performed SLN biopsy in patients with T1–3 invasive breast cancers and clinically negative axillary nodes. Biopsy technique (fine-needle aspiration, core, or excisional) has not compromised the success of the procedure except in a few patients, in whom a very large excision in the upper outer quadrant of the breast had been done previously.[25,32,33] While Pendas et al[34] report a role for SLN biopsy in patients with ductal carcinoma in situ (DCIS), we have found only a single case of SLN involvement (by a micrometastasis) in 81 consecutive SLN biopsies done for DCIS. We do perform SLN biopsy for DCIS patients with microinvasion and for patients in whom microinvasion cannot be ruled out. We have excluded patients with multifocal or multicentric lesions because of uncertainty about which node is the "true" SLN. In fact, a disproportionate number of patients with false-negative SLNs in our early experience had multicentric tumors.[15] Mertz et al have recently reported SLN biopsy in multifocal cancers using a subareolar injection technique.[35]

NUCLEAR MEDICINE TECHNIQUE

We initially chose to use Tc-99m-labelled colloidal albumin given in a dose of 5–10 MBq (0.135–0.27 mCi) and a volume of 0.2–0.4 ml, injected into the breast parenchyma adjacent to the tumor. The injection was subdermal for superficial tumors and peritumoral if the lesion was deep. We injected the isotope between 2 hours and 24 hours preoperatively, usually the day before surgery.

In our first published series of 163 patients, we used colloidal albumin with a particle-size range of 50 nm to 200 nm, and a total volume of 0.2 ml.[15] Subsequent experience proved that the detection of SLNs was easier with particles of a larger size, 200 nm to 1000 nm, and a volume of 0.4 ml.[36,37]

We obtained lymphoscintigrams routinely, taking 20-minute and 3-hour images in both anterior and oblique projections, and marking the lymphatic pathway and SLN site on the skin. We identified internal mammary nodes as a site of lymphatic drainage exclusively in 2% of cases.[36,37]

SURGICAL TECHNIQUE

Intraoperatively, we have used three different types of probes. In all models, the intensity and frequency of the auditory signal are directly proportional to the level of radioactivity detected. When the tumor site is close to the axilla or in case of mastectomy, SLN biopsy and tumor excision are performed through the same incision. Otherwise, the incisions for the SLN biopsy and tumorectomy are separate.

We carefully preserve the intercostobrachial and other nerves to avoid the postoperative sensory sequelae of axillary lymph-node dissection (ALND). In our series, no axillary-flap necrosis or scar retraction was reported. The SLN must be dissected carefully, avoiding damage to the capsule and keeping an intact specimen for a meticulous histopathologic workup. We have closed the axillary incision without drainage in 98% of patients following exclusive SLN biopsy. In accordance with the findings of other investigators,[38] we have found substantially lower morbidity after SLN biopsy than after conventional ALND.

RADIOGUIDED BIOPSY OF NONPALPABLE LESIONS

The small, nonpalpable breast cancer, in which the risk of axillary involvement is low, represents an ideal application of SLN biopsy. Most nonpalpable breast cancers are localized prior to surgery by the placement of a guidewire, and SLN biopsy works well in this setting.[39] At the European Institute of Oncology, we have developed a method for radiolocalization of both the nonpalpable lesion and the SLN *at the same time*. Under stereotactic or ultrasound guidance, one day before surgery we inject tracers with two different molecular weights: 0.05 mg of serum-albumin macroaggregates (up to 1000 nm in diameter) plus microaggregates (less than 80 nm), labeled with 3.7 MBq (0.1 mCi) of Tc-99m at a specific activity of 74 MBq/mg. Ninety-five per cent of the radioactivity binds to the macroaggregate. The Tc-isotope mixture (in 0.2 ml of saline) is injected into the center of the suspicious lesion using mammographic (stereotactic) guidance when only microcalcifications are present, or ultrasonographic guidance for masses. The large particles of the macroaggregate remain at the site of injection, allowing localization of the tumor by the gamma probe, while the smaller particles of the microaggregate migrate to the SLN in the normal fashion.

Excisional biopsy is performed the following day using the gamma probe for guidance rather than a localizing wire. With the probe, the surgeon identifies the ideal site of skin incision, and the location of the suspicious focus within the breast. The edges of the excision are defined as the locus of points surrounding the "hot spot" where radioactivity falls off sharply. Following excision of the specimen, residual hot spots allow the removal of wider margins where appropriate. Having removed the nonpalpable tumor, the surgeon then proceeds to perform the SLN biopsy as outlined above. We have found that this radioguided approach allows the surgeon to achieve better concentricity of the cancer within the surgical specimen.[40,41]

RADIATION SAFETY ISSUES

Radioguided SLN biopsy is a safe procedure from the standpoint of radiation safety. We have found that SLN biopsy performed according to our protocols involves minimal radiation exposure,[22,42] and that only routine precautions are necessary in this setting. A surgical team performing 50 SLN biopsies per year can be classified using the criteria of the International Commission on Radiological Protection and EURATOM as nonexposed workers (Table 19.2).

RESULTS OF SLN BIOPSY

In our first study at the European Institute of Oncology,[15] 163 patients with T1–3 breast cancers and clinically negative axillae had SLN biopsy followed immediately by complete ALND. Sentinel lymph nodes were found in 98% of cases (160/163) and correctly predicted axillary node status in 97.5% (156/160) of cases. In 5% of node-positive patients (4/85), the SLN was falsely negative. There were no false-negative SLNs among patients with tumors smaller than 1.5 cm, and in 38% of node-positive cases the SLN was the only positive node.

In the final 107 patients of this series, we

Table 19.2 Radiation exposure during SLN biopsy: total absorbed dose in microsieverts (μSv) for clinical staff in 100 consecutive operations

	Total absorbed dose in 100 operations (μSv)	Annual dose limits for the general population recommended by ICRP (μSv)
Hands		
Surgeon, operating-room nurse	450 ± 20	50 000
Pathologist	75 + 3	
Lens of the eye		
Surgeon	110 + 30	15 000
Pathologist	15 + 5	
Effective dose		
Surgeon	90 + 25	1000
Pathologist	15 + 4	

Mean values and standard deviations were obtained from the air Kerma rate near patients or tissue specimens and the times required to carry out the different tasks. Approximately 50 SLN operations are performed per surgeon per year; for nurses, the figure is around 30. ICRP, International Commission on Radiological Protection.

performed an intraoperative frozen-section analysis of the SLN, finding that in 17% of patients with negative frozen sections (18/107), the SLN contained metastases on paraffin-section analysis. We have since developed a more exhaustive technique for intraoperative examination of the SLN, in which the *entire SLN* is sectioned at 50-μm intervals, with each section examined by both hematoxylin-and-eosin (H&E) stains and a rapid immunohisto-chemical stain for cytokeratins.[43] Although labor-intensive, this methodology has eliminated the problem of false-negative frozen sections.

In a larger cumulative series, we reported the results of SLN biopsy in 376 consecutive breast-cancer patients with results comparable to those of our earlier study (Tables 19.3 and 19.4).[22] We continue to observe a small proportion of false-negative procedures: 12 of 180 node-positive patients (6.7%). Based on these results, we began a randomized trial comparing SLN biopsy plus ALND (arm A) and SLN

biopsy followed by ALND only if the SLN was positive (arm B). From March 1998 to December 1999, a total of 649 patients aged 40–75 years with invasive breast cancers up to 2 cm in diameter were randomized, and 516 were

Table 19.3 Number of SLNs identified using Tc-99m-human colloidal albumin in 376 consecutive patients

No. of lymph nodes	No. of patients	%
1	249	66.2
2	97	25.8
3	24	6.4
4	1	0.3
None	5	1.3
Total	**376**	**100**

Identification rate 371/376 × 100 = 98.7%.

Table 19.4 Concordance between SLN evaluation and definitive status of all axillary nodes

SLN evaluation	Axillary node status	Number	% of total
Positive	Positive[a]	168	45.3
Negative	Negative	191	51.5
Negative	Positive	12	3.2
Total		**371**	**100**

Concordance 359/371 (96.8%).
[a]In 70 patients, the SLN was the only positive node.

evaluable. Patient and tumor characteristics were well balanced in both groups. The goals of the study are to compare:

1. the "staging power" of SLN biopsy as compared to conventional ALND—does SLN biopsy identify a proportion of node-positive cases comparable to ALND?
2. patient quality of life—is the morbidity of SLN biopsy really less than that of ALND?
3. the rate of axillary recurrence—is axillary recurrence after a negative SLN biopsy comparable to that after ALND?
4. the disease-free and overall survival between the two arms of the study.

FUTURE DIRECTIONS

We have performed more than 1200 SLN biopsy procedures in our institute under the standardized conditions described above. Isotope localization of the SLN results in a high rate of successful SLN localization and a finite but low incidence of false-negative results. Sentinel lymph-node biopsy is a multidisciplinary procedure and requires close cooperation among radiology, nuclear medicine, surgery, and pathology specialists. Further investigations, both randomized and observational, promise answers to many of the unresolved issues surrounding this exciting new technology.

REFERENCES

1. Gray JH, The relation of lymphatic vessels to the spread of cancer. *Br J Surg* 1938; **26**:462–95.
2. Turner-Warwick RT, The lymphatics of the breast. *Br J Surg* 1959; **46**:574–82.
3. Hultborn KA, Larsson LG, Ragnhult I, The lymph drainage of the breast to the axillary and parasternal lymph nodes: study with aid of colloidal Au[198]. *Acta Radiol* 1955; **43**:52–64.
4. Borgstein PJ, Meijer S, Pijpers R, van Diest PJ, Functional lymphatic anatomy for sentinel node biopsy in breast cancer. *Ann Surg* 2000; **232:** 81–9.
5. Gould EA, Winship T, Philbin PH, Hyland Kerr H, Observations on a "sentinel node" in cancer of the parotid. *Cancer* 1960; **13**:77–8.
6. Cope O, Surgery of the thyroid. In: Means JH, De Groot LJ, Stambury JB, eds, *The Thyroid and Its Diseases,* 561–98. McGraw-Hill: New York, 1963.
7. Weinberg J, Greaney EM, Identification of regional lymph nodes by means of vital staining dye during surgery of gastric cancer. *Surg Gynecol Obstet* 1950; **90**:561–7.
8. Cabanas RM, An approach for the treatment of penile cancer. *Cancer* 1977; **39**:1864–7.
9. Weinberg JA, Identification of regional lymph nodes in the treatment of bronchiogenic carcinoma. *J Thorac Surg* 1951; **22**:517–22.
10. Morton DL, Wen DR, Wong JH et al, Technical details of intraoperative lymphatic mapping for early stage melanoma. *Arch Surg* 1992; **127**:392–9.
11. Krag DN, Weaver DL, Alex JC, Fairbank JT, Surgical resection and radiolocalization of the sentinel node in breast cancer using a gamma probe. *Surg Oncol* 1993; **2**:335–9.

12. Giuliano AE, Kirgan DM, Guenther JM, Morton DL, Lymphatic mapping and sentinel lymphadenectomy for breast cancer. *Ann Surg* 1994; **220**:391–401.

13. Albertini JJ, Lyman GH, Cox C et al, Lymphatic mapping and sentinel node biopsy in the patient with breast cancer. *JAMA* 1996; **276**:1818–22.

14. Sandrucci S, Casalegno PS, Percivale P et al, Sentinel lymph node mapping and biopsy for breast cancer: a review of the literature relative to 4791 procedures. *Tumori* 1999; **85**:425–34.

15. Veronesi U, Paganelli G, Viale G et al, Sentinel-node biopsy to avoid axillary dissection in breast cancer with clinically negative lymph nodes. *Lancet* 1997; **349**:1864–7.

16. Borgstein PJ, Pijpers R, Comans EF et al, Sentinel lymph node biopsy in breast cancer: guidelines and pitfalls of lymphoscintigraphy and gamma probe detection. *J Am Coll Surg* 1998; **186**:275–83.

17. O'Hea BJ, Hill ADK, El-Shirbiny AM, Sentinel lymph node biopsy in breast cancer: initial experience at Memorial Sloan-Kettering Cancer Center. *J Am Coll Surg* 1998; **186**:423–7.

18. Bass SS, Cox CE, Ku NN et al, The role of sentinel lymph node biopsy in breast cancer. *J Am Coll Surg* 1999; **189**:183–94.

19. Cody HS, Hill AD, Tran KN et al, Credentialing for breast lymphatic mapping: how many cases are enough? *Ann Surg* 1999; **229**:723–8.

20. Pendas S, Dauway E, Cox CE et al, Sentinel node biopsy and cytokeratin staining for the accurate staging of 378 breast cancer patients. *Ann Surg* 1999; **65**:50–6.

21. Winchester DJ, Sener SF, Winchester DP et al, Sentinel lymphadenectomy for breast cancer: experience with 180 consecutive patients: efficacy of filtered technetium 99m sulfur colloid with overnight migration time. *J Am Coll Surg* 1999; **188**:597–603.

22. Veronesi U, Paganelli G, Viale G et al, Sentinel lymph node biopsy and axillary dissection in breast cancer: results in a large series. *J Natl Cancer Inst* 1999; **91**:368–73.

23. Wilhelm AJ, Mijnhout GS, Franssen EJ, Radiopharmaceuticals in sentinel lymph-node detection: an overview. *Eur J Nucl Med* 1999; 26(4 Suppl):36–42.

24. Pijpers R, Borgstein PJ, Meijers S et al, Transport and retention of colloidal tracers in regional lymphoscintigraphy in melanoma: influence on lymphatic mapping and sentinel node biopsy. *Melanoma Res* 1998; **8**:413–18.

25. Cody HS, Borgen IP, State-of-the-art approaches to sentinel node biopsy for breast cancer: study design, patient selection, technique, and quality control at Memorial Sloan-Kettering Cancer Center. *Surg Oncol* 1999; **8**:85–91.

26. Krag DN, Ashikaga T, Harlow SP, Weaver DL, Development of sentinel node targeting technique in breast cancer patients. *Breast J* 1998; **4**:67–74.

27. Doting MHE, Janden L, Nieweg OE et al, Lymphatic mapping with intralesional tracer administration in breast carcinoma patients. *Cancer* 2000; **88**:2546–52.

28. Hill ADK, Tran KN, Akhurst T et al, Lesson learned from 500 cases of lymphatic mapping for breast cancer. *Ann Surg* 1999; **229**:528–35.

29. Linehan DC, Hill AD, Akhurst T et al, Intradermal radiocolloid and intraparenchymal blue dye injection optimize sentinel node identification in breast cancer patients. *Ann Surg Oncol* 1999; **6**:450–4.

30. Roumen RM, Geuskens LM, Valkenburg JG, In search of the true sentinel node by different injection techniques in breast cancer patients. *Eur J Surg Oncol* 1999; **25**:347–51.

31. Valdés Olmos RA, Jansen L, Hoefnagel CA, Nieweg O, Contribution of nuclear medicine to lymphatic mapping and sentinel node identification in oncology. *Rev Esp Med Nucl* 1999; **18**:111–21.

32. Haigh PI, Hansen NM, Qi K, Giuliano AE, Biopsy method and excision volume do not affect success rate of subsequent sentinel lymph node dissection in breast cancer. *Ann Surg Oncol* 2000; **7**:21–7.

33. Miner TJ, Shrivers CD, Jaques DP et al, Sentinel lymph node biopsy for breast cancer: the role of previous biopsy on patients eligibility. *Am Surg* 1999; **65**:493–8.

34. Pendas S, Dauway, Giuliano R et al, Sentinel node biopsy in ductal carcinoma in situ patients. *Ann Surg Oncol* 2000; **7**:15–20.

35. Mertz L, Mathelin C, Marin C et al, Subareolar injection of 99m-Tc sulfur colloid for sentinel nodes identification in multifocal invasive breast cancer. *Bull Cancer* 1999; **86**:939–45.

36. Paganelli G, De Cicco C, Cremonesi M et al, Optimized sentinel node scintigraphy in breast cancer. *J Nucl Med* 1998; **42**: 49–53.

37. De Cicco C, Cremonesi M, Luini A et al, Lymphoscintigraphy and radioguided biopsy of the sentinel axillary node in breast cancer. *J Nucl Med* 1998; **39**:2080–4.

38. Schrenk P, Rieger R, Shamiyeh A, Wayand W,

Morbidity following sentinel lymph node biopsy versus axillary lymph node dissection for patients with breast cancer. *Cancer* 2000; **88:**608–14.

39. Liberman L, Cody HS, Hill AD et al, Sentinel lymph node biopsy after percutaneous diagnosis of nonpalpable breast cancer. *Radiology* 1999; **211:**835–44.

40. Luini A, Zurrida S, Paganelli G et al, Comparison of radioguided excision with wire localization of occult breast lesions. *Br J Surg* 1999; **86:**522–5.

41. Zurrida S, Galimberti V, Monti S, Luini A, Radioguided localization of occult breast lesions. *Breast* 1998; **7:**11–13.

42. Cremonesi M, Ferrari M, Sacco E et al, Radiation protection in radioguided surgery of breast cancer. *Nucl Med Commun* 1999; **20:**919–24.

43. Viale G, Bosari S, Mazzarol G et al, Intraoperative examination of axillary sentinel lymph nodes in breast carcinoma patients. *Cancer* 1999; **85:**2433–8.

20

The dye-plus-isotope technique

Charles E Cox, Christopher Salud and Douglas S Reintgen

The H Lee Moffitt Cancer Center technique for SLN Biopsy in breast cancer

Technique	Combination	**Isotope**	*Type*: Tc-99m-SC
Dye	*Type*: Isosulfan blue dye		*Filtered*: Yes (0.22-μm filter)
	Volume: 5.0 ml (cc)		*Dose*: 0.45 mCi (17 MBq)
			Volume: 6 ml (cc) in 1 ml portions
Injection site	*Isotope*: Peritumoral		
	Dye: Peritumoral		

In 1996, the authors of this chapter and their colleagues at the H Lee Moffitt Cancer Center were the first to report using a combination of radioisotope (technetium-99m-sulfur colloid) and blue dye (isosulfan blue) to map the sentinel lymph nodes (SLNs) in breast-cancer patients.[1] Based upon that initial experience with 62 patients and the subsequent results of more than 1700 SLN procedures,[2-4] we, and an increasing number of other investigators, strongly endorse this combined methodology.

Among our first 186 procedures (Phase I), in which SLN biopsy was validated by a complete axillary lymph-node dissection (ALND),[3] the SLN was found in 93% (173/186), and of 54 node-positive patients, there was only a single case in which the SLN was falsely negative, yielding an accuracy exceeding 99% (172/173), a sensitivity of 98% (53/54), a false-negative rate of 2% (1/54), and a negative predictive value (the proportion of SLN-negative patients

in whom the axilla was truly negative) greater than 99% (120/121). Among 809 subsequent SLN-negative patients (Phase II) in whom no ALND was performed (Figure 20.1), there have been no axillary recurrences at a mean follow-up of 20 months.

THE LEARNING CURVE

Sentinel lymph-node biopsy, like any new procedure, has a distinct learning curve. A major advantage of the combined technique is a significant shortening of this curve. Detailed reviews of the individual and cumulative learning curves of five surgeons at the H Lee Moffitt Cancer Center showed that an average of 23 cases was required to achieve a 90% success rate and 53 cases to achieve a 95% success rate (Figure 20.2).[4] We strongly recommend that institutions beginning to perform SLN biopsy

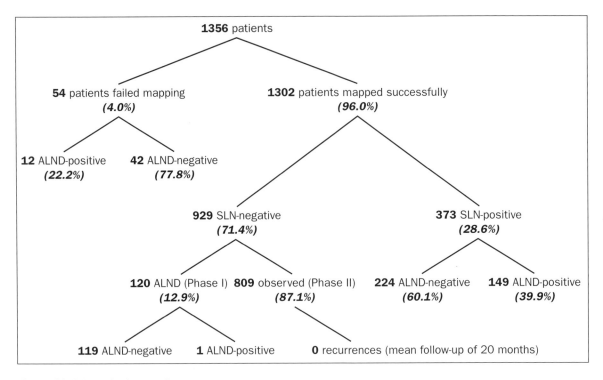

Figure 20.1 Lymphatic mapping summary.

do so under the aegis of a formal Institutional Review Board (IRB) protocol, in which SLN biopsy is performed with a planned backup ALND to validate the early experience of each surgeon.[2] Self-credentialing through a formal training course in the technique of SLN biopsy speeds the learning process, as does intraoperative proctoring by an experienced colleague. Each surgeon's (and institution's) rate of failed and false-negative results should be continuously monitored. Finally, long-term follow-up of all patients having SLN biopsy is essential. Neither the short-term nor the long-term morbidity of SLN biopsy has been directly compared with that of conventional ALND, and the rate of regional lymph-node recurrence following a negative SLN biopsy is unknown.

CASE SELECTION FOR SLN BIOPSY

In general, we have performed SLN biopsy in patients with T1–2 breast cancers and clinically negative axillary nodes. We have also included patients with ductal carcinoma in situ (DCIS), a group in whom 4 of 87 (5%) had positive SLN,[5] Paget's disease, and a small number of patients with T3 tumors.[2] Sentinel lymph-node biopsy has also been performed in patients prior to undergoing prophylactic mastectomy;[6] if an invasive cancer were unexpectedly found in the breast, it would be too late for SLN biopsy, and the patient would require conventional ALND.

Although our initial protocol required that patients had intact tumors (i.e., biopsy by either fine-needle aspiration or core needle),[1] we have subsequently demonstrated comparable results of SLN biopsy following tumor excision,[2] and now perform SLN biopsy regardless of biopsy technique.

ISOTOPE CONSIDERATIONS

Technetium-99m is the radioisotope of choice for lymphatic mapping procedures, but most

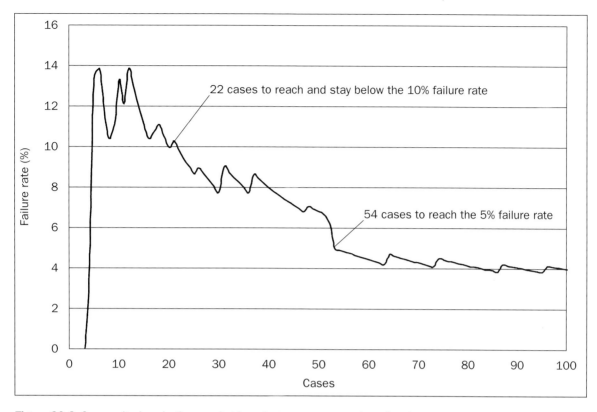

Figure 20.2 Composite lymphatic mapping learning curve: mean values for six surgeons.

nations have approved only a single carrier particle for medical use. Microcolloidal albumin is used widely in Europe, and antimony sulfide in Australia, both with excellent results. Technetium-99m-sulfur colloid (Tc-99m-SC) is the only preparation approved for use in the USA and Canada.

The reported isotope techniques vary widely regarding dose, filtration (particle size), route, volume, and timing of injection. The recommended dose of Tc-99m varies between 0.1 mCi and 1.0 mCi (4–37 MBq), with seemingly comparable results. We recommend 0.450-mCi (17-MBq) Tc-99m-SC preparations, which may be either filtered (resulting in a smaller particle size) or unfiltered (resulting in a mixture of particle sizes). We recommend a 0.22-μm filtered preparation, as used for lymphatic mapping in our patients with melanoma (see Chapter 10).[7] Isotope may be injected parenchymally (into the breast adjacent to the tumor), subdermally,[8]

intradermally,[9] or into the subareolar area.[10–12] We agree with Giuliano et al[13,14] in discouraging any of the latter approaches and continue to recommend peritumoral injection of isotope (and blue dye) into the breast parenchyma. The recommended volume of injectate and timing of injection vary as well. We recommend that the isotope be injected into the breast tissue surrounding the tumor or biopsy site in a total of six 1-ml aliquots, 1–6 hours preoperatively.

We have used three different models of gamma probe for SLN mapping, each of which has allowed accurate identification of the SLN.

BLUE-DYE CONSIDERATIONS

Immediately prior to the skin preparation in the operating room, we inject 5 ml (cc) of isosulfan blue dye into the breast tissue surrounding the tumor. In over 1700 mapping procedures, we have observed a 1% incidence of allergic reactions. The most common pattern includes an initial weal reaction followed by the development of blue hives scattered about the ipsilateral axilla, neck, groin, and other intertriginous areas. These allergic reactions have generally responded to intravenous antihistamine. Three of our patients experienced a dramatic drop in blood pressure about 30 minutes postinjection, all of whom responded to prompt intravenous administration of fluids, ephedrine, antihistamine, and (in one case) corticosteroids.

Isosulfan blue is excreted in the urine and bile, and patients should be told to expect transient discoloration of both urine and stool. Blue staining of the breast tissues usually disappears rapidly, but some residual discoloration may be present for up to 6 months.

Mapping agents and local anesthetic solutions should not be mixed with each other in the same syringe. Both isosulfan blue and sulfur-colloid solutions immediately precipitate when mixed with local anesthetic.

SURGICAL TECHNIQUE

In the ideal scenario, our patients are injected with isotope (0.450 mCi of filtered Tc-99m-SC, in 6 ml (cc) of isotonic saline, peritumorally in six 1-ml portions) 2 hours preoperatively. In the operating room, 5 ml of isosulfan blue dye is injected just prior to prepping and draping the patient.

To enhance lymphatic flow, Giuliano et al have recommended massaging the breast after injection,[13,14] and this is our recommendation as well. We perform a vigorous 5-minute massage of the breast immediately following the injection of both the isotope and the blue dye. To further study this phenomenon, we have accumulated data on 594 consecutive patients treated at our institution (Figure 20.3). To avoid

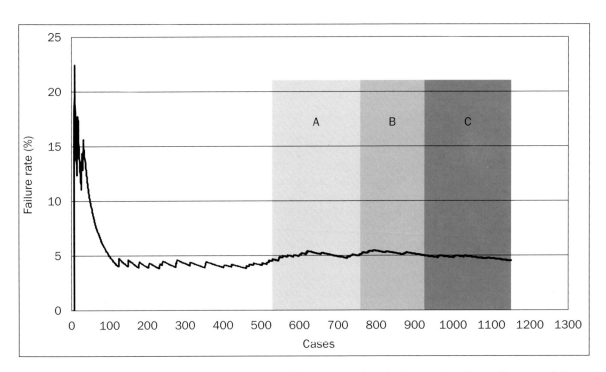

Figure 20.3 The effects of postinjection massage on failure rate in lymphatic mapping. The patient population consisted of 594 consecutive patients with breast cancer. Group A (*n* = 230): no massage; group B (*n* = 134): 5-minute massage following administration of blue dye *only*; group C (*n* = 230): 5-minute massage following administration of radiocolloid *and* 5-minute massage following blue dye.

any effects of mapping failure attributed to the learning curve, this study excluded our initial experience of 553 cases. The control group of 230 patients (group A) received no massage; 134 patients (group B) received a 5-minute massage following blue-dye injection; and 230 patients (group C) received a 5-minute massage following isotope injection in addition to the 5-minute massage following dye injection. Our current protocol is that of group C, to perform massage following the injection of both agents.

New operative techniques may take longer at first, and we recommend allocating ample operating time. This allows a calm environment and permits the operation to proceed without the pressure of time constraints. We recommend that the surgeon and assistant operate initially sitting down. Most surgeons will find that their first SLN biopsy procedures take longer to perform than a standard ALND. This can be frustrating and patience is required. Finally, lymphatic mapping is an interdisciplinary process requiring cooperation between surgeons, nuclear medicine physicians, and pathologists. The logistics of this multidisciplinary approach may add frustration to early efforts to perform SLN biopsy.

Prior to starting surgery, the gamma probe must be optimized to eliminate extraneous counts. This entails centering the photopeak of technetium-99m within the probe's range of detection by adjusting the threshold and window settings. The photopeak of Tc-99m is constant, but scatter around the peak varies dramatically, and this variation sometimes requires either narrowing or enlarging the detection window during the procedure. Count intervals in seconds must also be specified; we measure radioactivity in counts per second. Many of the above settings are fixed internally in some of the new probe designs, and do not require adjustment. Gamma probes may drift over time and require periodic calibration with a standard radiation source (see Chapter 4).

A vast majority of SLNs (94% in our experience) will be found at Level I in the axilla,[3] within a 5-cm circle centered at the apex of the axillary hair-line (Figure 20.4). The

remaining 6% are most often at axillary Level II. This 5-cm circle may be useful as a starting point for identifying the location of the SLN using the gamma probe. Counts are taken from the injection site in the breast, and from the axilla using the above landmarks. Once the SLN is localized, an accurate axillary incision can be made overlying the area of highest activity as determined by the gamma probe. The incision generally falls at or below the hair-line.

The visualization of small lymphatic channels and SLNs is optimized by good exposure and a bloodless operative field. If local anesthesia is being used, epinephrine (adrenaline) should be added. Electrocautery is very helpful for dissection. We use a Weitlander retractor in the incision to assist with exposure. Dissection should be very delicate, and the use of small, fine-tipped mosquito clamps can be extremely useful in this regard.

Care should be taken to extend the dissection toward the chest in a fashion perpendicular to the chest wall. This allows the identification of afferent blue lymphatics, which should then be traced cephalad toward the SLN. The tendency of many inexperienced surgeons is to make the incision and then immediately dissect in a cephalad direction. Internal landmarks useful in localizing the SLN include the lateral thoracic vein and the lateral branch of the third intercostal nerve (Figure 20.5). These anatomic structures are found beneath the clavipectoral fascia. The lateral thoracic vein can be found easily with careful dissection, as it courses toward the tail of the breast. The location at which the nerve crosses over the vein defines four quadrants, which collectively contain the vast majority of the SLNs found in breast lymphatic mapping ("Cox's pearl," Table 20.1).

Blue-stained lymphatic channels should be identified and traced to the SLN. Having identified the SLN, we recommend clipping the afferent lymphatic channels to prevent spillage of blue dye into the operative field when they are cut in removing the SLN. *It is crucial not to cut or clip a blue lymphatic channel until the SLN has been isolated.* Too-early ligation of a blue lymphatic may prevent dye from reaching the SLN, forc-

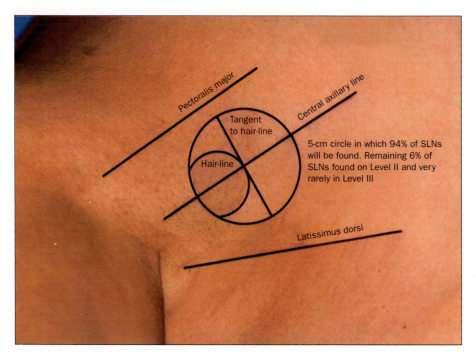

Figure 20.4 External anatomic localization of SLN.

ing the surgeon to rely on the gamma probe for localization.

For cases in which blue lymphatics or blue SLN are not immediately apparent, the gamma probe is indispensable in guiding the dissection, and can lead rapidly to the discovery of an SLN (often blue) that might not otherwise have been found. Identification of the SLN is certain when there is a zone of clearly diminished counts between the injection site and the axillary hot spot ("Reintgen's pearl," Table 20.1). In searching the axilla, one must be careful not to inadvertently aim the probe back toward the injection site in the breast. In this case, factitious counts will seem to be found in the axilla but actually be coming from the breast. We call this phenomenon "shine-through." One must always be sure that any hot spots in the axilla are identified *with the probe pointing away from the breast itself.* Remember where the "light bulbs" are, and "keep your eye on the ball." Shine-through is also a problem when the isotope has been injected very close to the axilla (as in the case of a high, upper outer quadrant

tumor). The radioactive shadow cast by the injection site overlaps the axilla, precluding radiolocalization of the SLN. In this setting, excision of the tumor site may remove enough of the injected isotope to allow the SLN to be identified with the probe. Otherwise the surgeon must rely on the blue dye to find the SLN.

For each of our SLN biopsy procedures, we record the type of gamma probe used, the probe size, the time of injection, and the dose of injected material. For each SLN removed we record the time of harvest and note whether it is "blue," "hot," or "blue and hot." We define a blue node as one that contains even the faintest blue discoloration. In taking isotope counts, the SLN should be exposed and the gamma probe placed directly on the SLN in situ. To obtain the ex vivo measurement, the SLN should be placed on a sterile towel located well away from the lymphatic basin and primary injection site. We record isotope counts of each SLN both in situ and ex vivo, and define a hot node as one with in situ counts greater than or equal to 3 times those of the axillary background, or

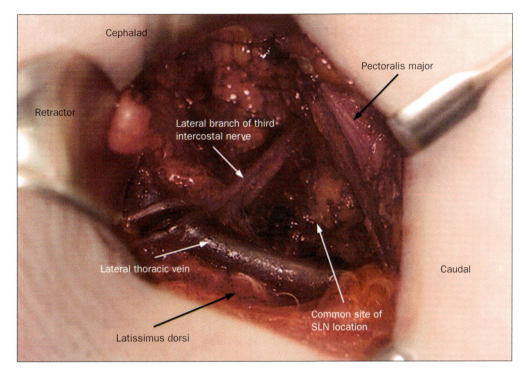

Figure 20.5 Landmarks useful in localizing the SLN.

with ex vivo counts greater than or equal to 10 times those of an excised non-SLN. We also take counts of any non-SLNs that have been removed. We check for radioactivity in the internal mammary region and document these counts whether proceeding with internal mammary node removal or not. Finally, we take counts of the postexcision axillary bed, by averaging counts taken from each of four quadrants within the axilla. This last step is particularly important to identify additional occult SLNs that may have been overlooked at the initial exploration.

Table 20.2 gives the overall results of the combined dye–isotope approach in our first 1356 cases. Isotope identified the SLN more often than blue dye, and the combination was superior to either method by itself. Neither method succeeded all the time. Twenty-two per cent of SLNs were found by isotope alone, and 12% by blue dye alone. Sentinel lymph nodes were successfully found in 95% of all patients.

CAVEATS

It is important in the face of these new mapping technologies not to abandon good clinical judgment. The identification of a positive lymph node is the primary goal of axillary surgery, and careful intraoperative palpation of the axilla is an important element of the SLN biopsy procedure. Any clinically suspicious nodes should be biopsied whether they contain dye/isotope or not. A dilated blue lymphatic channel ending abruptly in a palpable, firm lymph node indicates a clinically positive SLN which should be removed.

After an initial validation phase in which SLN biopsy is always followed by a confirmatory ALND, there are still circumstances in which the surgeon should not hesitate to abandon the SLN biopsy procedure and default to ALND. These include the identification of grossly positive SLNs or non-SLNs at surgery, borderline criteria (especially low node counts), and outright failure to locate the SLN. Even

Table 20.1 The H Lee Moffitt Cancer Center "pearls" of lymphatic mapping

- Do not mix isosulfan blue dye, Tc-99m-SC, or local anesthetic solutions in the same syringe for combined injection. A precipitate will form and neither dye nor colloid will migrate to the SLN, leading to mapping failure.
- Vigorously shake the Tc-99m-SC prior to injection to break up clumping of the particles. The optimal operating time is 2 hours postinjection.
- The photopeak of an isotope is constant, but scatter below the highest energy varies dramatically. Optimizing the window settings of the gamma probe minimizes extraneous counts.
- Isosulfan blue dye is excreted by the kidneys and liver. Patients should expect bluish-green discoloration of the urine and stool postoperatively.
- About 1% of patients have an allergic reaction to blue dye. Watch the injection site for weal reactions and monitor pulse and blood pressure during the procedure.
- Schedule ample operating time. Perform the procedure in a calm environment, and sit down to operate. Work in a bloodless field and use electrocautery. Use local anesthetic solutions with epinephrine (adrenaline). Have good retraction and good help. Do not divide a blue lymphatic until you have found the SLN, but clip the lymphatics when excising the SLN.
- "Shine-through" can be a problem. Keep in mind the isotope injection site and its position relative to the line of sight of the probe. Remember where the "light bulbs" are, and "keep your eye on the ball."
- Cox's pearl: 94% of all SLNs in breast cancer are found within a 5-cm circle; the center point is marked by the inferior border of the hair-line in the axilla and a line drawn through the center of the hair-bearing area, along the axis of the axilla. This point is situated where the lateral branch of the third intercostal nerve crosses the central axillary vein beneath the clavipectoral fascia.
- Reintgen's pearl: identification of the SLN is certain when there is an area of clearly diminished counts between the injection site and the hot spot in the nodal basin.

Table 20.2 Results of lymphatic mapping in 1356 patients

	No.	%
Method of SLN detection		
Blue dye	1105	81.5
Radiocolloid	1197	88.3
Blue dye and/or radiocolloid	1288	95.0
Node characteristics (N = 2927)		
Blue and hot	1848	63.1
Hot only	650	22.2
Blue only	364	12.4
All hot	2498	85.3
All blue	2212	75.6

Sentinel lymph nodes were identified in 1302 of 1356 patients (96%) and not found in 54 (4%). Data were incomplete in 12. One of 54 node-positive patients (2%) had a false-negative SLN.

with a mature technique and large experience with this procedure, we still fail to find the SLN in a few patients.

OUTCOMES MONITORING

The two crucial measures of the effectiveness of lymphatic mapping and SLN biopsy are first, a high rate of success in finding the SLN, and second, a low rate of false-negative results. For this new and highly multidisciplinary procedure, it is critical that all surgeons and institutions validate their results under the umbrella of a well-defined IRB protocol. We recommend that each surgeon complete a Phase I series of at least 30 SLN procedures followed by completion ALND. Surgeons with appropriate training should be able to find the SLN in 90% of cases, with at most one false-negative result in their first 10 *node-positive* cases. The surgeon meeting these goals may move on to a Phase II mapping protocol, in which SLN biopsy is performed and ALND done only if the SLN contains metastasis (or if the procedure fails to find the SLN). For surgeons or institutions not meeting this standard, we recommend either additional experience or on-site intraoperative mentoring to further evaluate the deficiencies of the surgeon or institution. Mapping failure does not simply represent a failure of the surgeon, but may involve procedural issues in the departments of nuclear medicine and pathology as well. All of these should be remediable through the review of an experienced mentor. The American Society of Breast Surgeons has now published guidelines similar to these,[15] recommending for each surgeon the documentation of at least 30 cases with a success rate in identifying an SLN of at least 85%, and 5% or fewer false-negatives.

CONCLUSION

The current standard of care for the patient with invasive breast cancer is either wide-local excision or mastectomy, followed by a complete ALND. Lymphatic mapping with SLN biopsy promises to be the next major advance in the treatment of breast cancer. Indeed, radioguided surgery and all of its potential applications (melanoma, vulvar cancer, Merkel-cell tumors, squamous-cell carcinoma, bone lesions, parathyroid mapping, radioguided seed biopsy and radioimmunoguided detection of colon cancer) may become the next revolution in general surgery.

Lymphatic mapping and SLN biopsy for breast-cancer diagnosis is rapid and accurate, enhancing the detection of lymphatic metastasis by about 10% when used with pathologic serial sections and cytokeratin stains. The procedure has a learning curve and carries a small risk of false-negative results, especially in the early experience of each surgeon. Sentinel lymph-node biopsy is a smaller operation than ALND, carries less morbidity, and allows the elimination of general anesthesia, surgical drains, and an overnight hospital stay in over 70% of the population treated.

Despite the keen interest of the media, institutions, and patients, we feel that this methodology is still investigational. Nevertheless, these concrete and significant advantages make it clear, to this author at least, that lymphatic mapping will soon become the standard of care for breast-cancer staging.

ACKNOWLEDGMENTS

This study was supported by grant 30079 from the H Lee Moffitt Cancer Center and Research Institute, Tampa, FL; grant R21 CA66553-01 from the National Institutes of Health, Bethesda, MD; the McDonnell Douglas Research Fund, Department of Defense grant DAMD 17-97-1-7209; and The Joy McCann Culverhouse Surgical Oncology Professorship of The University of South Florida Foundation, Tampa, FL.

REFERENCES

1. Albertini JJ, Lyman GH, Cox C et al, Lymphatic mapping and sentinel node biopsy in the

patient with breast cancer. *JAMA* 1996; **276:** 1818–22.

2. Cox CE, Pendas S, Cox JM et al, Guidelines for sentinel node biopsy and lymphatic mapping of patients with breast cancer. *Ann Surg* 1998; **5:**645–53.

3. Bass SS, Cox CE, Ku NN et al, The role of sentinel lymph node biopsy in breast cancer. *J Am Coll Surg* 1999; **189:**183–94.

4. Cox CE, Bass SS, Boulware D et al, Implementation of new surgical technology: outcome measures for lymphatic mapping of breast carcinoma. *Ann Surg Oncol* 1999; **6:**553–61.

5. Pendas S, Dauway E, Giuliano AE et al, Sentinel node biopsy in duct carcinoma in situ patients. *Ann Surg Oncol* 2000; **7:**15–20.

6. Dupont EL, McCann C, Shons AR et al, The role of sentinel lymph node biopsy in women undergoing prophylactic mastectomy. *Eur J Nucl Med* 1999; **26**(suppl):S72.

7. Reintgen D, Albertini J, Berman C et al, Accurate nodal staging of malignant melanoma. *Cancer Contr* 1995; **2:**405–14.

8. Veronesi U, Paganelli G, Galimberti V et al, Sentinel node biopsy to avoid axillary dissection in breast cancer with clinically negative lymphnodes. *Lancet* 1997; **349:**1864–7.

9. Linehan DC, Hill ADK, Akhurst T et al, Intradermal radiocolloid and intraparenchymal blue dye injection optimize sentinel node identification in breast cancer patients. *Ann Surg Oncol* 1999; **6:**450–4.

10. Klimberg VS, Rubio IT, Henry R et al, Subareolar versus peritumoral injection for location of the sentinel lymph node. *Ann Surg* 1999; **229:**860–5.

11. Kern KA, Sentinel lymph node mapping in breast cancer using subareolar injection of blue dye. *J Am Coll Surg* 1999; **189:**539–45.

12. Borgstein PJ, Meijer S, Pijpers R et al, Functional lymphatic anatomy for sentinel node biopsy in breast cancer; echoes from the past and the periareolar blue dye method. *Ann Surg* 2000; **232:**81–9.

13. Giuliano AE, Kirgan DM, Guenther JM, Morton DL, Lymphatic mapping and sentinel lymphadenectomy for breast cancer. *Ann Surg* 1994; **220:**391–401.

14. Giuliano AE, Jones RC, Brennan M, Statman R, Sentinel lymphadenectomy in breast cancer. *J Clin Oncol* 1997; **15:**2345–50.

15. American Society of Breast Surgeons consensus statement on guidelines for the performance of sentinel lymph node biopsy. *News Release*, 1998.

21

How we do it: the Cardiff University approach

Dayalan Clarke and Robert E Mansel

CONTENTS   The ALMANAC trial • Patient selection for SLN biopsy • Technique of SLN biopsy
• Conclusion

The University of Wales College of Medicine (ALMANAC) technique for SLN biopsy in breast cancer

Technique	Combination	Isotope	*Type*: Tc-99m-HSA
Dye	*Type*: Patent Blue-V dye		*Filtered*: N/A
	Volume: 4.0 ml (cc)		*Dose*: 0.5 mCi (20 MBq)
			or 1.1 mCi (40 MBq) prior afternoon
Injection site	*Isotope*: Peritumoral		*Volume*: 2.0 ml (cc)
	Dye: Peritumoral		

Sentinel lymph-node biopsy for breast cancer is a technically feasible procedure, as has been confirmed in many recent publications. The multidisciplinary approach required to successfully localize the sentinel lymph node (SLN) and obtain a pathological assessment is also well established: nuclear medicine personnel are needed to prepare the radiopharmaceutical, the radiologist to perform the lymphoscintigraphy (LSG) and mark the "hot" node on the skin, the surgeon to perform the SLN biopsy, and the pathologist to assess its histology. In this chapter, we describe our experience of setting up a program to perform SLN biopsy in breast cancer at the University Hospital of Wales, Cardiff, UK.

Our initial institutional protocol involved recruiting all patients with invasive breast cancer who would normally require axillary surgery as part of the management of their breast cancer. This was our practice during our pilot study of approximately 100 patients. We have subsequently designed the protocol for the ALMANAC trial based on our experience in this initial, pilot study.

THE ALMANAC TRIAL

The Axillary Lymphatic Mapping Against Nodal Axillary Clearance (ALMANAC) trial is a two-phase, multicenter, randomized clinical trial involving approximately 15 breast units in the United Kingdom, including university teaching hospitals and district general hospitals. It is coordinated from the University of Wales College of Medicine, with Professor RE Mansel serving as principal investigator.

Phase I: the audit phase

In Phase I, the audit phase, each surgeon is required to perform an SLN biopsy in 40 consecutive patients with invasive breast cancer, followed immediately by the standard axillary staging procedure of that center. All surgeons performing SLN biopsies in these centers are to have attended a training course on SLN biopsy, and they are to be proctored by a surgeon experienced in the procedure. The success rate of finding an SLN and the false-negative rate for the technique are determined in the audit phase in order to assess the learning curve of individual surgeons. Following the audit phase, which has now been completed in most centers, centers that have reached the set standard of successful localization (90%) and false-negative results (<5%) proceed to the second phase, the randomized phase.

Phase II: the randomized trial

In the randomized phase, all patients with an invasive breast cancer are randomized to either a control or a treatment arm (Figure 21.1). Patients in the control arm undergo conventional treatment, namely a wide excision or mastectomy as primary treatment of the breast cancer with axillary node sampling or clearance, whichever is the standard treatment of the axilla in that particular center. Patients in the treatment arm undergo a wide-local excision or mastectomy as primary treatment to the breast cancer along with an SLN biopsy. Patients with a positive SLN biopsy on paraffin-section histology have their axilla treated as a delayed procedure with either radiation therapy or a completion axillary clearance. Patients with a negative SLN biopsy have no further treatment to the axilla. Adjuvant treatment is given to patients in both groups depending on tumor and nodal characteristics.

The primary end-points in this randomized trial are axillary morbidity, health-care costs of SLN biopsy compared with those of conventional axillary procedures, and quality of life in patients who have an axillary procedure compared with that of patients who have an SLN biopsy. A secondary, longer-term goal of this trial is to measure the axillary recurrence rate in patients who have had a negative SLN biopsy and thus no treatment to the axilla.

PATIENT SELECTION FOR SLN BIOPSY

The patient selection criteria for performing SLN biopsy in breast cancer as part of the ALMANAC trial are outlined in Table 21.1.

TECHNIQUE OF SLN BIOPSY

It is obvious from a review of the literature that the best results for localizing the SLN in breast cancer are obtained using a combination of radioisotope and blue dye.[1] This has also been the experience at our institution, and we therefore use a combination of radioisotope and Patent Blue-V dye as our standard protocol for localizing the SLN.

Nuclear medicine

Various radiopharmaceuticals have been used in the localization of the SLN in breast cancer and in malignant melanoma. The major variations seem related to the size of the colloid used. The ideal radiopharmaceutical should have particles small enough to enter the lymphatic circulation, while at the same time being large enough to be trapped and retained by the draining lymph node. Australian studies have used antimony with a small particle size, 5–15 nm, as the radiopharmaceutical.[2] The advantage of a small particle size is the ease with which it enters the lymphatic circulation; however, it may not be retained in the SLN for any length of time, necessitating a dynamic lymphoscintigram to image the first draining

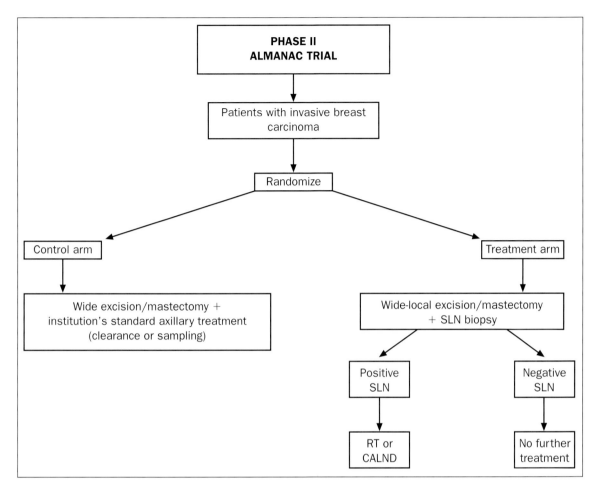

Figure 21.1 The Axillary Lymphatic Mapping Against Nodal Axillary Clearance (ALMANAC) trial, Phase II. The trial is a two-phase, multicenter, randomized clinical trial involving approximately 15 breast units in the United Kingdom, including university teaching hospitals and district general hospitals. CALND, completion axillary lymph-node dissection; RT, radiation therapy.

node or SLN. Most European countries have used technetium-99m-human serum albumin (Tc-99m-HSA)[3–5] with 95% of labeled particles having a size of less than 80 nm. The most common colloid used in the United States is Tc-99m-sulfur colloid (Tc-99m-SC), either filtered or unfiltered, with a particle size of 40 nm to 1000 nm.[6–8] Technetium-99m-human serum albumin is easily available in the UK, and we have used it in our study with reasonable success.

Dose
The dose of radioactivity used in localizing the SLN in breast cancer varies among studies, ranging from as little as 7 MBq (190 μCi) to as much as approximately 400 MBq (11 mCi).[3,9] We started out with a dose size of 40 MBq (1.1 mCi) of Tc-99m-HSA, regardless of the timing of the injection in relation to the timing of the surgery. We found that this dose worked well when the Tc-99m-HSA was injected the day before surgery. When 40 MBq

---

Table 21.1 ALMANAC Trial patient selection criteria

Inclusion criteria
- age 18–80 years
- Invasive breast cancer proved by cytology/histology
- Patient normally warranting an axillary procedure

Exclusion criteria
- In situ cancer only
- Multifocal invasive tumor
- Previous neoadjuvant therapy for same tumor
- Clinically involved nodes—where axillary treatment is deemed to be mandatory. If doubt remains about the significance of palpable nodes, fine-needle aspiration cytology to be done and suspicious node proved negative to allow inclusion
- Previous cancer in same breast
- Previous surgery for same tumor
- Established pregnancy (if in clinical doubt, a negative pregnancy test is required)
- Known allergy to human albumin or Patent Blue-V dye
- Pre-existing limb disease causing swelling or a history of previous axillary surgery
- Current or recent involvement in another interventional study

---

was injected on the day of surgery, however, and the patients were operated on only a few hours following the injection, the background counts were high in comparison with the SLN counts. We have since reduced the dose of radioactivity to 20 MBq (0.5 mCi) for patients receiving injection on the day of surgery, facilitating high SLN-to-background ratios.

Injection site
The site of injection of the radiopharmaceutical varies among studies. Some studies have injected around the tumor,[6] some into the tumor, some intradermally into the skin over the tumor,[10] and some subdermally at the site of the tumor.[3] Injection into the subareolar region has also been used, an approach based on the work of Sappey, who demonstrated that lymph from all parts of the breast flows into the subareolar plexus before reaching the axillary nodes.

The quantity of fluid in which the radioactiv-ity should be injected is another variable. One study reports that a small amount of fluid should be injected (0.4 ml) because the injection of a large amount of fluid causes increases in the interstitial pressure that may lead to collapse and blockage of the local lymph vessels.[11] On the other hand, another study reports that the highest rate of success in localizing the SLN involved the use of a large volume of radiopharmaceutical: 4–8 ml (cc).[12] We inject our patients peritumorally at four different sites around the tumor, using a volume of at least 2 ml, so that 0.5 ml can be injected at each site.

Our radiopharmaceutical guidelines are summarized in Table 21.2.

Lymphoscintigraphy
Most studies that have used radiopharmaceuticals to localize the SLN in breast cancer would agree that lymphoscintigraphy (LSG) gives valuable information on the anatomical site of

Table 21.2 Radiopharmaceutical guidelines
• Technetium-99m-labeled-human serum albumin colloid • 40 MBq (1.1 mCi), made up to 2 ml with saline, injected at four sites around tumor if injected day before surgery • 20 MBq (0.5 mCi), made up to 2 ml with saline, injected at four sites around tumor if injected on day of surgery • Spillage (or suspected spillage) will have to be monitored by methods agreed upon with the local radiation protection advisory committee

the SLN, including the level at which it is located, and that in some rare instances LSG will show other areas of lymphatic drainage, such as the internal mammary chain. There is no doubt that a dynamic scan followed by static images will provide the greatest amount of information; however, in our study, we have had to confine our LSG to static images for logistical reasons.

Timing of the static images
We set out doing static images immediately following injection of the Tc-99m-HSA, 3 hours after injection, and at 18 hours after injection, using a delayed film. With increasing experience, we realized that the immediate scan and the 18-hour delayed image offered no additional information to that obtained from the 3-hour film. We therefore now do a static scan at approximately 3 hours following injection of the Tc-99m-HSA using both an antero-oblique or lateral view, to reveal the presence of SLNs in the axilla, and an anterior view, to detect possible SLNs situated in the internal mammary chain.

Our LSG guidelines are summarized in Table 21.3.

Surgery

Dye technique
Isosulfan blue dye is commonly used in the USA, while European centers use Patent Blue-V dye. Isosulfan blue dye is available as a 1% solution, while Patent Blue-V dye is marketed as a 2.5% solution in 2 ml and is diluted before administration. In our study, Patent Blue-V dye is diluted to 4 ml and injected around the tumor following the induction of anesthesia. Here again, there has been some variation in the site of injection, with some centers injecting subdermally and others injecting into the periareolar region.[13]

We inject the blue dye peritumorally, as we do the radiopharmaceutical, and massage the breast following injection to facilitate the flow of the blue dye to the SLN. In our initial experience, we began the operation with a mastectomy or wide-local excision followed by SLN biopsy. We soon realized, however, that the SLN biopsy should be done first, in order to take full advantage of the use of the blue dye. When done in this order, with SLN biopsy preceding surgical removal of the breast cancer, optimal visualization of a blue-stained lymphatic occurs, and the lymphatic can be followed to a blue node, an SLN. When SLN biopsy follows surgical removal of the tumor, however, the blue dye has usually by then

Table 21.3 Lymphoscintigraphy guidelines
• Gamma camera imaging approximately 3 hours after Tc-99m-HSA-injection (2 hours—minimum time recommended) • Static lymphoscintigrams • Two views—anterior and oblique/lateral • Nuclear medicine staff to mark location of "hot" node on skin • Internal mammary node must be biopsied if seen on LSG

Table 21.4 Dye guidelines
• Patent Blue-V dye to be injected
• Inject immediately after induction and draping
• Inject around tumor
• Dilute 2 ml vial (2.5%) to 4 ml using isotonic saline
• SLN biopsy to be performed prior to lumpectomy/mastectomy unless proximity of tumor to SLN makes radiation "shine-through" a major problem. In this situation, excision of the tumor should be done first, thus removing the hottest area, which will facilitate accurate localization of the SLN
• Blue dye used to locate blue lymphatics leading to blue node

Table 21.5 Sentinel lymph node identification guidelines
Definition of SLN
• a hot node, defined as a node with a count of 10 times the background rate *or*
• a blue node *or*
• a hot and blue node
Background count
• ipsilateral upper arm to be recorded as 10-second count
• tumor count—highest count over tumor to be recorded as 10-second count prior to skin incision
• after the SLN is removed, check the rest of the axilla with the probe in order to identify other hot nodes that may not have shown up on the lymphoscintigram. If other hot nodes are found, they must be excised

already reached the SLN, rendering the lymphatics less visible. (Dye guidelines are summarized in Table 21.4.)

The blue node is then confirmed to be the "hot" node using a hand-held gamma probe, which detects radioactivity and converts the radioactivity trapped in a node to an audible sound signal. These probes are well shielded and well collimated, making them very effective for localizing the SLN. Once the SLN is identified, it is removed and sent separately for histology.

SLN identification

How hot must a node be to be labeled an SLN? What constitutes the background count if the radioactivity is to be measured as a ratio of SLN to background counts? In terms of radioactivity, we define an SLN as any node 10 or more times as hot as the background (Table 21.5). Initially, we used the counts of the operating-room air as the background count. Over time, however, we realized that there may be some radioactivity circulating in the patient and that the SLN should be 10 times as hot as this

radioactivity count. We now use the counts over the patient's upper arm, rather than that of the room air, as the background count (Table 21.5).

Pathology

Hematoxylin-and-eosin (H&E) staining of paraffin sections is still the "gold standard" in the UK for pathological assessment of the axillary lymph nodes in patients with breast cancer according to the National Health Service Breast Screening Programme (NHSBSP) guidelines. We use H&E staining as the method of assessment of the SLN in our study (Table 21.6). While this seems reasonable in the audit phase, when axillary treatment always follows the SLN biopsy, it does raise questions regarding the ideal method of evaluation of the SLN when axillary-treatment decisions are based fully on the results of the SLN biopsy.

Table 21.6 Pathology guidelines
• Each SLN should be identified by the surgeon and processed separately from other axillary nodes submitted • Currently, in routine practice, prognostic information is based on H&E-stained paraffin section of each axillary lymph node. This is the method we have used to assess the SLN. This will allow comparison of SLN-derived prognostic information with earlier, historical studies

Obviously, the SLN status would best be determined intraoperatively, if accurate and feasible, so that decisions about the management of the axilla could be made at the time of the primary operation on the breast. Frozen-section analysis, which can be performed while surgical excision of the breast tumor is being carried out, is as yet the only assessment method that will allow this. Unfortunately, however, frozen-section assessment of the SLN carries with it an unacceptably high false-negative rate.[3] Immunohistochemistry and frozen-section immunohistochemistry may provide the answer, and evaluation of these techniques is currently under way. Serial sections and polymerase chain reaction (PCR), two other more detailed pathological evaluation modalities, are also being evaluated. Initial results have shown that a more detailed pathological assessment of the SLNs does result in an upstaging of the disease, though the clinical relevance of this upstaging is unclear at the present time.

CONCLUSION

Early results show that all centers in the United Kingdom involved in the ALMANAC trial and using the above protocol have had a success rate of over 90% in localizing the SLN and a false-negative rate of less than 5%. The random-ized phase of the trial is now in progress. We hope that following the results of ongoing trials, SLN biopsy will become the staging procedure for the axilla in breast cancer based upon evidence rather than merely upon enthusiasm for the novelty value of this new technology.

REFERENCES

1. McIntosh SA, Purushotham AD, Lymphatic mapping and sentinel node biopsy in breast cancer. *Br J Surg* 1998; **85**:1347–56.
2. Uren RF, Howman-Giles RB, Thompson JF et al, Mammary lymphoscintigraphy in breast cancer. *J Nucl Med* 1995; **36**:1775–80.
3. Veronesi U, Paganelli G, Galimberti V et al, Sentinel-node biopsy to avoid axillary dissection in breast cancer with clinically negative lymph-nodes. *Lancet* 1997; **349**:1864–7.
4. Roumen RMH, Valkenburg JGM, Geuskens LM, Lymphoscintigraphy and feasibility of sentinel node biopsy in 83 patients with primary breast cancer. *Eur J Surg Oncol* 1997; **23**:495–502.
5. Borgstein PJ, Pijpers R, Comans EF et al, Sentinel lymph node in breast cancer: guidelines and pitfalls of lymphoscintigraphy and gamma probe detection. *J Am Coll Surg* 1998; **186**:275–83.
6. Krag D, Weaver D, Asikaga T et al, The sentinel node in breast cancer. *N Engl J Med* 1998; **339**:941–6.
7. Albertini JJ, Lyman GH, Cox C et al, Lymphatic mapping and sentinel node biopsy in the patient with breast cancer. *JAMA* 1996; **276**:1818–22.
8. Cox CE, Pendas S, Cox JM et al, Guidelines for sentinel node biopsy and lymphatic mapping of patients with breast cancer. *Ann Surg* 1998; **227**:645–53.
9. VanDer Ent FWC, Kengen RAM, Van der Pol HAG, Hoofwijk AGM, Sentinel node biopsy in 70 unselected patients with breast cancer: increased feasibility by using 10 mCi radiocolloid in combination with a blue dye tracer. *Eur J Surg Oncol* 1999; **25**:24–9.
10. Hill ADK, Tran KN, Akhurst T et al, Lessons learned from 500 cases of lymphatic mapping for breast cancer. *Ann Surg* 1999; **229**:528–35.
11. Cicco CD, Cremonesi M, Luini A et al, Lymphoscintigraphy and radioguided biopsy of the sentinel axillary node in breast cancer. *J Nucl Med* 1998; **39**:2080–4.

12. Krag DN, Harlow SP, Weaver DL, Asikaga T, Technique of selected resection of radiolabeled lymph nodes in breast cancer. *Sem Breast Dis* 1998; **1**:111–16.

13. Borgstein PJ, Meijer S, Pijpers R, Intradermal blue dye to identify the sentinel lymph node in breast cancer. *Lancet* 1997; **349**:1668–9.

22

How we do it: The Netherlands Cancer Institute approach

Emiel JT Rutgers and Omgo E Nieweg

CONTENTS   Technique of lymphoscintigraphy and SLN identification   •   Pathology   •   Results
•   **Current practice**

The Netherlands Cancer Institute/Antoni van Leeuwenhoek Hospital technique for SLN biopsy in breast cancer

Technique	Combination	**Isotope**	*Type*: Tc-99m-nanocolloid
Dye	*Type*: Patent Blue-V		*Filtered*: No
	Volume: 1.0 ml (cc)		*Dose*: 1.1–2.4 mCi (42–88 MBq);
			mean 1.7 mCi (61.6 MBq)
Injection site	*Isotope*: Intralesional		*Volume*: 0.2 ml (cc)
	Dye: Intralesional		

Lymphatic mapping with sentinel lymph-node biopsy was introduced at The Netherlands Cancer Institute in 1993. The combined technique with lymphoscintigraphy (LSG), an intraoperative gamma probe, and Patent Blue-V dye was used from the start in 1993.[1,2] After our initial positive experience in melanoma,[3] we turned our attention to breast cancer.

The notion that breast carcinoma spreads to the lymph nodes in a random manner rather than following an orderly pattern reigned at that time. Therefore, we decided to test first the hypothesis that breast cancer spreads in a sequential fashion, analogous to melanoma. A study was performed in 30 patients with clinically localized breast cancer.[4] Blue dye was injected into the breast tumor immediately before conventional mastectomy. The specimen was then taken to the pathology department where it was meticulously dissected. The blue channel was identified at the periphery of the tumor and then dissected until it was seen entering the sentinel lymph node (SLN). An SLN was found in 26 patients. In 10 patients, the SLN was found to contain metastatic disease. It was the only involved axillary node in 6 of these patients. More important were the findings in the remaining 16 patients, in whom the SLN was free of disease. All other axillary nodes in these patients were examined using immunohistochemistry (IHC) and were also shown to be free of disease. This could not be explained by chance and led to a Phase II study to determine our ability to find the SLN in vivo. Confirmatory axillary lymph-node dissection (ALND) was performed. This study was performed in cooperation with the University Hospital at Groningen and was initiated in 1996.

TECHNIQUE OF LYMPHOSCINTIGRAPHY AND SLN IDENTIFICATION

Our experience in melanoma (see Chapter 11) had led us to apply the combined technique in breast cancer as well: LSG after intralesional injection of a labeled colloid, intralesional blue dye, and the intraoperative use of a gamma probe.[2] As we were only interested in the lymphatic drainage of the tumor itself, we decided to inject both tracers intralesionally.

Lymphoscintigraphy was performed the day before surgery after administration of technetium-99m-labeled nanocolloid, which has a particle size of less than 80 nm. The tracer was administered into the tumor with a single slow injection of 0.2 ml (cc), using a fine needle (25 gauge). Syringes were measured after injection in order to calculate net administered doses. The mean injected dose was 61.6 MBq (1.7 mCi), range 42–88 MBq (1.1–2.4 mCi). Immediately after injection, simultaneous anterior and supine lateral dynamic LSG of the region was performed acquiring 20-second images over a period of 20 minutes, using a dual-head gamma camera with low-energy, high-resolution collimators. Subsequently, 5-minute anterior, supine, and prone lateral (hanging breast) planar images were obtained after 30 minutes, 2 hours, and 4 hours with simultaneous emission-transmission scanning using a cobalt-57 flood source. The location of the SLN was defined using Co-57 markers and marked on the skin with ink. Criteria to define the sentinel (first-echelon) node were the visualization of an afferent lymphatic vessel leading from the injection site to this node or, if no afferent vessels were seen, the first lymph node appearing in each basin.

Shortly before surgery, 1.0 ml of Patent Blue-V dye was injected into the tumor. Subsequently, measurements were made over the skin marks with a gamma probe to confirm the location of the SLN as seen on scintigraphy and to indicate the site for the incision. If no SLNs were seen on scintigraphy, the lower axilla was explored. Sites other than the lower axilla were explored only when scintigraphy revealed an SLN there. Following a small skin incision, the SLN was identified and removed after careful dissection of the afferent blue vessel and after confirmation with the probe that the blue node was radioactive.

PATHOLOGY

The SLNs up to 0.5 cm in size were completely embedded; larger nodes were dissected or lamellated in slides of 0.2 cm. All SLNs were step-sectioned with 500 μm intervals at three levels. At each level, both hematoxylin-and-eosin (H&E) and IHC staining were performed. Standard IHC procedures using an avidin-biotin detection system were used. A monoclonal antibody directed against cytokeratin was used (CAM 5.2). All other lymph nodes were examined with H&E and IHC staining at one level after complete embedding. The pathology result was described as positive when metastatic cells were found.

RESULTS

The two-institute Phase II study

For the Phase II validation studies, the selection criteria were palpable breast cancer, breast cancer proved by fine-needle aspiration (FNA) cytology or core biopsy, and a clinically unsuspected axilla. Patients with multifocal tumors, ductal carcinoma in situ, previous surgery, chemotherapy, or radiation therapy of the breast and axilla were excluded.

From 1996 to January 1999, the two institutes entered 136 patients in all. An SLN was visualized by LSG in 118 patients (87%). An SLN was localized intraoperatively in 126 patients (93%). A total of 224 SLNs were harvested (average 1.7; range 1–4 SLNs per patient). Of the total 224 SLNs, 37 were blue (17%), 68 were radioactive (30%), and 119 were both blue and radioactive (53%). The SLNs contained metastatic disease in 56 patients (41%). Three SLNB biopsies were falsely negative (sensitivity, 95%).[5]

The Netherlands Cancer Institute studies

An evaluation of our mammary scintigraphy technique by the intralesional injection of Tc-99m-nanocolloid in the first 150 breast cancer patients from our institute showed a learning experience.[6] A mean dose of 62 MBq (range 42–88 MBq) was used in the first 100 patients. The rate of visualization was 65% in the first 20 patients, 80% in the second 20, and increased to an average of 90% in the last three subgroups of 20 patients. Using multiple linear logistic regression analysis, age ($p = 0.01$), and tracer dose ($p = 0.04$), but not patient order number, were found to be significant factors for lymphnode visualization. Visualization was nearly 100% with doses above 65 MBq. It is clear that the retrieval of the SLN hardly ever fails when the SLN is visualized on scintigraphic images.

Another feature of our technique is the visualization of the SLN outside the axilla in 19% of the patients. In an evaluation of 113 consecutive patients, the SLN was identified in 100. Twenty-one (19%) of 113 patients had several lymph nodes outside Levels I–II of the axilla, mostly in the internal mammary chain. Twenty-two of the 30 SLNs at those sites (73%) were harvested. Three patients had only SLNs outside the axilla. Four patients had metastases outside the axilla; this changed postoperative treatment in three of them. No postoperative complications occurred.[7] Figures 22.1 and 22.2 illustrate the

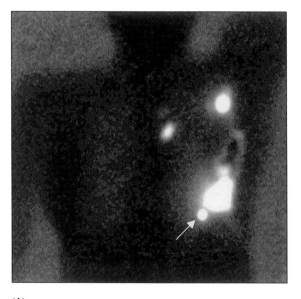

(A)

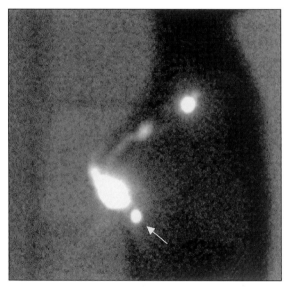

(B)

Figure 22.1 Lymphoscintigram of a 43-year-old woman with a 9-mm, grade I, estrogen and progesterone receptor-positive (ER+/PgR+) invasive ductal cancer in the lower outer quadrant of the left breast. Sentinel lymph nodes are seen in the axilla, the third intercostal space, and intramammary at the inframammary fold (arrowed). All SLNs were found and harvested. The first two SLNs were tumor-free. The third, 3–4 mm in size and located dorsally to the mammary gland on the pectoral muscle fascia, contained micrometastasis found after immunohistochemical staining. The patient was treated with a simple mastectomy (her wish, positive family history) and adjuvant bilateral oophorectomy followed by tamoxifen, 20 mg daily. Without knowledge of this SLN, she would not have been advised to undergo adjuvant systemic treatment.

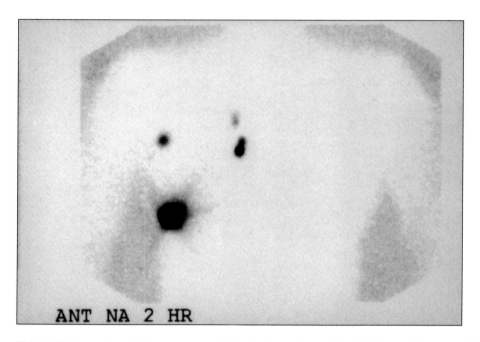

Figure 22.2 Lymphoscintigram showing SLNs in the axilla and fourth intercostal space. This 45-year-old patient had a 17-mm ductolobular (mixed type), grade II, PgR+/ER+ invasive cancer, located caudally from the nipple of the right breast. The SLN in the internal mammary chain (size 5 mm) was found to contain "macro" metastasis on H&E staining. The axillary SLN only had a micrometastasis on immunohistochemical staining after multiple slicing. The therapeutic axillary lymph-node clearance showed a further 11 nodes without metastasis. The patient received adjuvant systemic treatment and radiation therapy to the breast and the internal mammary chain nodes. The latter nodes would not have been given radiation therapy had the positive SLN not been found.

potential clinical value of lymphatic mapping by careful dynamic and static scanning after intralesional injection, followed by retrieval of all SLNs.

CURRENT PRACTICE

An SLN is identified in 97% of patients with our current approach, using all available diagnostic techniques: dynamic and static imaging, a gamma probe, and vital dye. Administration of the tracers into the tumor is part of this careful approach. Lymphatic drainage from the skin and the subareolar plexus is richer than drainage from the tumor. Administration of a tracer at these other sites is supposed to enhance the identification rate of an SLN;

however, injection of the tracer further away from the tumor increases the risk of crossing a lymphatic watershed and visualizing a node other than the node that drains the tumor. Depositing the tracer around the tumor is in theory virtually as accurate as injecting the tracer into the lesion, but it has several drawbacks. For instance, it is more difficult to distribute the tracer all around the tumor. A theoretical problem is that the needle tip may end up underneath the fascia in a deep-lying tumor since the resistance of the tumor is not felt after insertion of the needle. The danger of needle-track metastasis is real, as the needle may pass through one or more of the tumor protrusions. The risk of local recurrence is enhanced in patients who undergo mastectomy. A practical drawback is that excision of the tumor will not remove the entire injection site, as is desired when probe detection of a small amount of radioactivity in the SLN is prevented by the overwhelming scattered radiation surrounding the breast cancer.

Considering the results, we feel confident with our described technique. Thanks to our experience in melanoma, the learning phase in breast cancer was short, as no difference in SLN retrieval was seen in early versus recent patients. Nevertheless, the SLNB procedure in breast cancer is technically more demanding and requires a patient surgeon and a meticulous surgical technique. We find dynamic LSG helpful, acting "as a road map in a strange city."

As of January 1999, we offer patients with triple-diagnosis-proven (clinically overt) breast cancer or core-biopsy-proven occult invasive cancer the SLNB procedure for lymphatic staging. We inform the patients that there is a 3–5% chance of missing microscopic disease in the axilla. All patients will have an ultrasound scan of the axilla with an FNA cytology of lymph nodes larger than 7 mm in longest diameter. If the ultrasound scan and FNA cytology are negative, the SLNB procedure will follow. We aim to retrieve every SLN visible on the scan or traced by blue lymphatics. We are reluctant to offer SLNB to patients who have had a previous wide-local excision of the tumor, have proven multifocal invasive cancers, or have tumors larger than 4 cm.

In conclusion, based on our experience we believe in the adequacy of our concept of the lymphatic mapping technique by the intrale-sional injection of tracers and retrieval of all identified SLNs. We also believe that a careful workup of the SLNs by pathology, including multiple sections and IHC, is useful. The ultimate value of retrieving SLNs outside the axilla has still to be proven. This is subject of ongoing studies in our institute.

REFERENCES

1. Nieweg OE, Jansen L, Kroon BBR, Technique of lymphatic mapping and sentinel node biopsy for melanoma. *Eur J Surg Oncol* 1998; **24**:520–4.
2. Rutgers EJT, Jansen L, Nieweg OE et al, Technique of sentinel node biopsy in breast cancer. *Eur J Surg Oncol* 1998; **24**:316–19.
3. Kapteijn BAE, Nieweg OE, Liem IH et al, Localising the sentinel node in cutaneous melanoma: gamma probe detection versus blue dye. *Ann Surg Oncol* 1997; **4**:156–60.
4. Kapteijn BAE, Nieweg OE, Petersen JL et al, Identification and biopsy of the sentinel lymph node in breast cancer. *Eur J Surg Oncol* 1998; **24**:427–30.
5. Doting MHE, Jansen L, Nieweg OE et al, Lymphatic mapping with intralesional tracer administration in breast cancer patients. *Cancer* 2000; **88**:2546–52.
6. Valdés Olmes RA, Jansen L, Hoefnagel CA et al, Evaluation of mammary lymphoscintigraphy by single intratumoral injection for sentinel node identification. *J Nucl Med* 2000; **41**:1500–6.
7. Jansen L, Doting MH, Rutgers EJ et al, Clinical relevance of sentinel lymph nodes outside the axilla in patients with breast cancer. *Br J Surg* 2000; **87**:920–5.

23

How we do it: the Memorial Sloan-Kettering Cancer Center approach

Hiram S Cody III and Patrick I Borgen

The Memorial Sloan-Kettering Cancer Center technique for SLN biopsy in breast cancer

Technique	Combination	**Isotope**	*Type*: Tc-99m-SC
Dye	*Type*: Isosulfan blue dye		*Filtered*: No
	Volume: 4.0 ml (cc)		*Dose*: 0.1 mCi (3.7 MBq) *or* 0.5 mCi (18.5 MBq) prior afternoon
Injection site	*Isotope*: Intradermal		*Volume*: 0.05 ml (cc)
	Dye: Parenchymal		
		Gamma probe	*Detection threshold*: 120–130 keV
			Window: 40 keV

We began to perform sentinel lymph-node biopsy for breast cancer at Memorial Sloan-Kettering Cancer Center in September 1996, under a formal Institutional Review Board protocol in which we planned to perform a backup axillary lymph-node dissection (ALND) in our first 60 cases. Encouraged by the early experiences of Krag with isotope and Giuliano with blue dye,[1,2] we modeled our initial study on that of Reintgen and Cox at the H Lee Moffitt Cancer Center,[3] using a combination of isotope and blue dye in an effort to learn as much as possible about each method. Our hypothesis was that the two methods would prove complementary and would optimize results. Detailed reports of our first 60,[4] first 500,[5] and first 1000[6]

procedures support that hypothesis. While a large majority of sentinel lymph nodes (SLNs) were identified by both isotope and dye (Table 23.1), about 10% were found by isotope or dye alone. Among patients with *positive* SLNs, we observed comparable proportions (Table 23.2), suggesting that reliance on a single technique would not have succeeded as often, and might have missed positive nodes.

Our first 60 cases comprised the initial experience of two surgeons, our first 500 cases encompassed the learning phase for the remaining surgeons on our service, and our first 1000 cases reflect our mature technique of SLN biopsy. Throughout this period, the proportion of SLNs identified by isotope alone, dye alone,

Table 23.1 Relative success of isotope and blue dye in finding the SLN in 1000 patients at the Memorial Sloan-Kettering Cancer Center

	Dye failure	Dye success
Isotope failure	56/1000 (6%)[a]	80/1000 (8%)
Isotope success	136/1000 (14%)	728/1000 (73%)

Adapted from Cody and Borgen.[6]
[a]49 failed mappings, 4 missing data, and 3 noncancer diagnoses.

Table 23.2 Relative success of isotope and blue dye in finding the positive SLN in 253 patients at Memorial Sloan-Kettering Cancer Center

	Dye failure	Dye success
Isotope failure	—	27/253 (11%)
Isotope success	26/253 (10%)	200/253 (79%)

Adapted from Cody and Borgen.[6]

or by both methods did not significantly change. With an experience now exceeding 3500 cases, we continue to strongly endorse the combined technique.

PATIENT SELECTION FOR SLN BIOPSY

Patients eligible for SLN biopsy under our protocol have had T1–2 invasive breast cancers and clinically negative (N0–N1a) axillary nodes. We have performed SLN biopsy in patients with larger tumors (T3, or for T4 disease following neoadjuvant chemotherapy), but only on protocol with a planned backup ALND, as we have observed a disproportionate number of false-negative results in this setting. We have also occasionally performed SLN biopsy in patients with clinically positive axillary nodes (especially if thought to be reactive nodes following biopsy), but in this setting have had a low threshold for default to ALND on the grounds of intraoperative suspicion.

Most patients with ductal carcinoma in situ (DCIS) are not candidates for SLN biopsy, but we recommend it for a subset of DCIS patients (about 20% of the total) at high risk for occult invasion as evidenced by the presence of extensive disease, a palpable mass, or the need for mastectomy; 12% of this group have had nodal micrometastases in our experience.[7]

A previous surgical biopsy is not a contraindication to SLN biopsy (Figure 23.1A). Because of the referral pattern of our practice, more than half of patients have been diagnosed by open biopsy, and we have found the SLN as successfully (and the SLN has proved as predictive of axillary node status) in this group as in patients diagnosed by core biopsy or fine-needle aspiration (FNA).[5] Sentinel lymph-node biopsy should be undertaken cautiously in patients with a very large biopsy cavity high in the upper outer quadrant, where extensive lymphatic disruption may preclude SLN biopsy, and where injections of isotope and dye may spill directly into the operative field. Sentinel node biopsy is feasible in patients with two or more biopsy incisions concurrently in the same breast, as long as the lymphatics between the tumor site and the axilla are intact. Old, well-healed biopsy (or breast reduction) scars in the breast pose no problems.

While our initial protocol excluded patients requiring preoperative needle localization, SLN biopsy has succeeded as often in this group as in our experience overall. The localizing wire is placed first in the radiology department, and then used to guide the injections of isotope and blue dye.[8]

TECHNIQUE OF SLN BIOPSY

Nuclear medicine

Following Krag's isotope protocol,[1,9] we initially injected 1 mCi (37 MBq) of unfiltered technetium-99m-sulfur colloid (Tc-99m-SC) in 4–8 ml (cc) of isotonic saline into the breast parenchyma at four sites around the tumor (or biopsy cavity). We rapidly found that smaller doses were equally effective and settled on a dose of 0.3 mCi (11.1 MBq) for intraparenchymal injection. Inadvertent injection into a biopsy cavity or the retromammary fascial plane caused a few early failures. Isotope performance was frustratingly inconsistent in our early experience. In about 20% of cases, the isotope either failed to migrate from the injection site to the SLN, or spread so extensively that the axilla was diffusely "hot." While this may have been due to inconsistent colloid particle size, a brief trial using intramammary injection of 0.22-μm (220-nm) filtered isotope as used in SLN biopsy for melanoma at our institution was even less successful, with the axilla diffusely hot in one-fourth of patients.[10]

Most recently, a single *intradermal* injection of 0.1 mCi (3.7 MBq) of unfiltered Tc-99m-SC in 0.05 ml of isotonic saline, given directly over the tumor site (or just cephalad to the biopsy scar), has proven optimal for radioisotope localization of the SLN. The high interstitial pressure generated by the intradermal injection enhances lymphatic uptake, and the radioactive "blast zone" cast by the single injection site is much smaller. This facilitates SLN biopsy in general, especially for tumors in the extreme upper outer quadrant of the breast. In 200 consecutive operations by a single surgeon (HSC), all with parenchymal injection of blue dye, we compared parenchymal ($N = 100$) and intradermal ($N = 100$) injection of isotope (Table 23.3).[11] Successful isotope localization of the SLN increased from 78% to 97%, and with the addition of blue dye from 92% to 100%. The *same SLN* was both blue and hot in 97% of the parenchymal group and 95% of the intradermal group, strongly suggesting that intradermal and parenchymal injections of isotope in fact drain to the same SLN. Intradermal isotope injection has since become our standard technique.

Table 23.3 Comparison of intradermal and intraparenchymal injection of isotope		
SLN found by:	**Intraparenchymal injection ($N = 100$) (%)**	**Intradermal injection ($N = 100$) (%)**
Isotope	78	97
Blue dye	81	91
Isotope + blue dye	92	100
Isotope/dye concordance	97	95

Adapted from Linehan et al.[11]

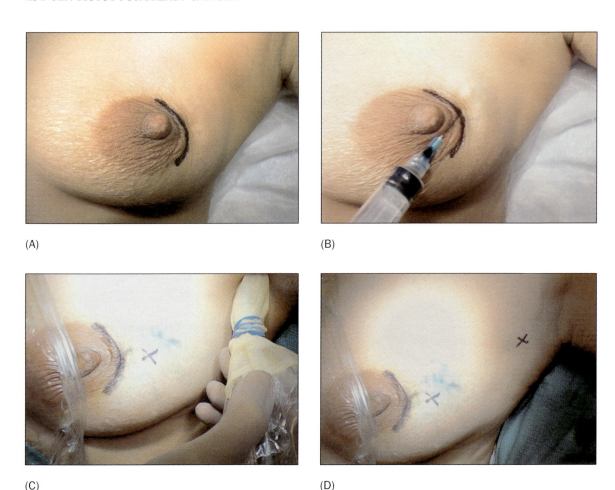

(A)

(B)

(C)

(D)

Figure 23.1 The patient is a 48-year-old woman who had previously undergone excision of a 2.0-cm invasive ductal carcinoma from the 2 o'clock subareolar aspect of the left breast, with a positive surgical margin. She elected breast conservation with SLN biopsy.

(A) The previous circumareolar biopsy scar is marked out.

(B) Isosulfan blue dye (4 ml) is injected superficially in the subcutaneous tissues just superolateral to the biopsy site.

(C) An adhesive drape pulls the breast inferomedially, facilitating exposure of the axilla. Counts are taken from the injection site in the breast and the axillary hot spot, and both are marked on the skin.

(D) A blush in the dermis confirms dye uptake by the lymphatics (and rules out inadvertent injection of the biopsy cavity).

(E) The axilla is explored through a transverse skin-line incision. Three-point countertraction facilitates dissection for the SLN. Here, three blue afferent lymphatics converge on a single blue SLN within Level I of the axilla. A second blue SLN was found adjacent to the first. Both contained high levels of isotope counts.

(F) Ex vivo counts are taken of each SLN, and both SLNs are submitted for frozen-section analysis.

(G) The postexcision axillary bed is checked for residual "hot spots," and the axilla is carefully palpated for suspicious non-SLNs (none was found).

(H) A re-excision of the biopsy cavity is done, and both the breast and axilla are closed routinely, without drainage. Frozen-section analysis of the SLN is benign. Striking blue discoloration of the skin overlying the injection site is common in the early postoperative period, and rapidly resolves; here, none was apparent 1 week later. The re-excision of the tumor site proved benign, and the serial sections (with IHC staining) of the SLN were negative as well.

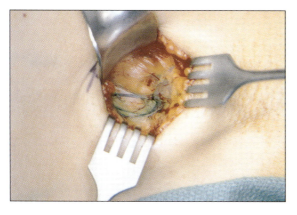

(E)

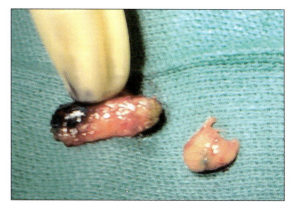

(F)

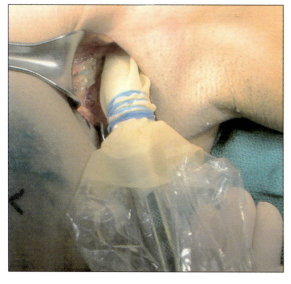

(G)

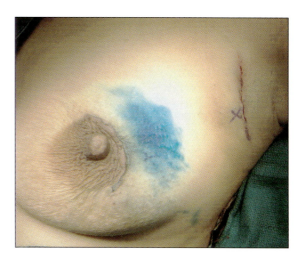

(H)

Routine lymphoscintigraphy (LSG) after iso-tope injection plays a less important role in breast lymphatic mapping than in melanoma, where it is indispensable for defining unex-pected patterns of lymphatic drainage. We have performed LSG in all patients having SLN biopsy for breast cancer, and 11% in our initial study demonstrated internal mammary uptake.[4] This is primarily significant for patients with tumors smaller than 1.0 cm and negative axillary nodes, a group to whom sys-temic adjuvant therapy is not normally given.

In this subgroup, 10–20% have internal mam-mary node metastases,[12–14] are at increased risk of distant relapse, and yet will be unrecognized as candidates for systemic adjuvant therapy. In this small minority of patients, an internal mammary SLN biopsy should be considered.

Most of our patients have had isotope injected on the day of surgery, and the opera-tion at least 1 hour later (following LSG), with successful SLN localization in more than 90% of cases. We have begun a program of isotope injection the afternoon before, allowing surgery early the following morning; here we inject a larger dose of isotope (0.5 mCi, 18.5 MBq) to allow for radioactive decay over the 6-hour half-life of technetium. Successful localizations and the mean number of SLNs obtained at surgery are comparable with the 1- and 2-day programs.

As the dosages involved are trivial, we use no special radiation precautions during surgery, or for the handling of surgical specimens (see Chapter 4).

Surgery

General anesthesia is given to all patients having mastectomy, and to conservation patients having SLN biopsy with ALND, whether planned in advance or done on the basis of a positive frozen section. Except for obese patients for whom airway management under sedation is of concern, all others have local anesthesia with monitored intravenous sedation. Tilting the table away from the operative side, raising the back, and pulling the breast inferomedially away from the axilla with an adhesive drape (see Figure 23.1C) all help to straighten the lymphatics and pull the isotope/dye injection site further from the axilla, facilitating exploration for the SLN.

We initially followed Giuliano's method of blue-dye mapping,[2] injecting a total of 4 ml of isosulfan blue dye into the breast parenchyma at four points around the tumor or biopsy site. Injection of the entire volume of dye at one or two sites just superolateral to the tumor site (in the direction of the axilla) has subsequently proved at least as effective (Figure 23.1B). As with the isotope injection, care is taken not to inject into either the biopsy cavity or the retro-mammary fascial plane. We have avoided intradermal injection of dye in an effort to avoid tattooing of the skin, although this concern may be unfounded. We do not routinely massage the breast postinjection. Axillary exploration is begun within 5–10 minutes of dye injection, but should be delayed if the dye has farther to travel (as in a very obese patient with a medially placed tumor).

The hand-held gamma probe (if adjustable) should be set for a detection threshold of 120–130 keV and a window of 40 keV. This centers the 144 keV photopeak of Tc-99m within the detection window. Gamma counters drift over time and should be recalibrated periodically using a standard radiation source. After injection of the blue dye, 10-second counts are taken from the injection site in the breast and the axilla, placing a skin mark over the axillary hot spot (Figure 23.1D). For axillary scanning, the probe should always be pointed away from the injection site in the breast (Figure 23.1C); inadvertently "looking back" toward the injection site will falsely elevate the counts, a phenomenon less likely with the use of a collimator. Ideally, there will be an area devoid of counts between the injection site and the axilla, although this is not always the case, particularly for upper outer quadrant tumors where the shadow of the isotope injection site may overlap the axilla.

The axillary operation is almost always done prior to further surgical procedures (excision, re-excision, or mastectomy) on the breast. If the patient has required as the first step a tumor excision to confirm the diagnosis of cancer, then the blue dye can be injected into the breast tissue through the wall of the biopsy cavity (taking care to inject deeply enough that the dye does not simply flow back into the operative defect).

Five to ten minutes following the dye injection and after taking counts, a transverse axillary skin line incision is made, placed as usual for a normal ALND and about half as long. For patients needing mastectomy, SLN biopsy is easily done either through a small parallel counterincision or through the lateral portion of the usual oblique/elliptical mastectomy incision. The latter approach has the advantage that lymphatics can be identified well down in the breast and traced cephalad into the axilla. Adequate exposure is required, and we perform SLN biopsy under direct vision. Adequate two- or three-point retraction for exposure is essential throughout, and dramatically facilitates the search for the SLN (Figure 23.1E). The field of dissection is deepened toward the axillary fascia, and the axillary fascia is incised transversely. The lymphatics exiting the breast usually run just deep to this layer. During the search for blue lymphatic vessels, the dissection should be meticulous and proceed layer by layer in a transverse direction to avoid sensory-nerve injury. Any blue lymphatics found should be traced first toward the breast, searching for SLNs in the axillary tail, and then higher into the axilla, taking care to preserve the lymphatics intact until their nodes are identified (Figure 23.1E). Sentinel lymph nodes are usually found low in Level I of the axilla, but in about 20% of cases, they may lie far posteriorly along the latissimus muscle, unexpectedly high in the axilla near the axillary vein, beneath the pectoralis minor in Level II, in the Rotter's node area, or within the breast as intramammary nodes. The gamma probe is very useful throughout this dissection, and for patients with a very large or fatty axilla, it can be invaluable in directing the dissection when blue lymphatics/nodes are not readily apparent.

All blue and/or hot SLNs are removed after taking counts in vivo. Counts are taken again of each node ex vivo (Figure 23.1F). Most often, the blue node and the hot node are the same. We have found a median of two SLNs per patient (range 1–11), and the SLNs have been localized to a single site in 42% of cases, to two sites in 44%, and to more than two sites in 14%, with a similar site distribution of *positive* SLNs.[5] In one-fourth of patients with at least one positive SLN and multiple SLN sites, the first SLN site was benign. Putative SLNs that prove after excision to be neither blue nor hot are submitted routinely as non-SLNs. Additional hot spots in the axillary bed are sought (Figure 23.1G) until the level of axillary background counts is less than one-fourth that of the least-hot SLN ex vivo (we arbitrarily defined successful radiolocalization as at least a fourfold reduction in axillary bed counts relative to the ex vivo counts of the SLN). In patients with a diffusely hot axilla, this process is not needlessly prolonged, and more reliance is placed on the blue dye for localization.

Careful intraoperative palpation of the axilla is essential, and any suspicious non-SLNs should be submitted as well. *In three of our five patients with a false-negative SLN, the positive non-SLNs were discovered in this fashion* (among the 104 patients in our first 500 procedures who had a planned axillary dissection).[5] Sentinel node localization does not succeed 100% of the time, and if the search for SLNs *after a reasonable effort* is unsatisfactory in any way, or if suspicious non-SLNs are found, the safest and most reasonable course is for the surgeon to default to a conventional ALND.

While the morbidity of SLN biopsy is substantially less than that of a conventional ALND, it remains a real operation, and a small minority of patients have developed sensory loss, pain, seroma, hematoma, or infection. All patients have had transient bluish-green discoloration of the skin and urine by the blue dye (Figure 23.1H). Striking blue urticaria has occurred in 1% of patients (Figure 23.2), and hypotensive allergic reactions occurred in 0.5%. A faint blue stain may persist at the breast injection site for as long as 1 year postoperatively. The long-term risk of lymphedema or cellulitis

Figure 23.2 Blue urticaria noted on the abdomen of a patient 30 minutes after injection of 4 ml of isosulfan blue dye prior to SLN biopsy. Following antihistamine treatment (diphenhydramine) the urticaria resolved within 1 hour. The patient felt otherwise well and was not hypotensive; she was discharged home 3 hours postoperatively.

after SLN biopsy, while presumed to be minimal, is unknown. With admittedly short follow-up, we have observed none.

Pathology

During our initial trial of SLN biopsy, in which all patients had a formal ALND, the SLNs were examined by routine pathologic technique with a single hematoxylin-and-eosin (H&E) section taken through each node.[4] Of the three patients in that trial whose SLN proved to be falsely negative, one (with a T2 tumor) proved to be SLN-positive on retrospective pathologic analysis by serial sections and immunohistochemistry (IHC). Under our current algorithm, intraoperative frozen-section analysis is done on the SLN. If the node is positive, a conventional ALND is done immediately. If it is negative, the remainder of each SLN is fixed; three additional paraffin sections are taken and stained by both H&E and IHC (using cytokeratin preparations).

In our first 500 procedures, the sensitivity of frozen-section analysis in detecting positive SLNs was excellent: 68 of 78 node-positive patients (88%) were identified intraoperatively and thereby spared a second trip to the operating room.[5] In our first 1000 cases, frozen-section analysis proved less accurate: overall sensitivity was 58% and ranged from 40% for T1a lesions to 76% for T2 tumors.[15] Our current policy is to perform intraoperative frozen-section analysis for all patients with T1b or larger invasive cancers. Too few T1a (or microinvasive) patients have metastatic disease detected by frozen-section analysis (4%) to justify its routine use in this group.

Follow-up issues

In general, we have recommended that patients with positive SLNs undergo ALND, as 40% overall have had residual axillary disease.[5] Even among patients whose SLNs were positive only on IHC, completion ALND found residual metastases in 10% of cases. Among our first 1000 SLN procedures, we have defined a small subgroup of 25 SLN-positive patients in whom a completion ALND was always negative: those with T1a,b (≤1.0 cm) tumors, micrometastatic disease (≤2 mm) in the SLN, and no lymphovascular invasion by the primary tumor.[16] Pending further experience, we continue to recommend ALND for most SLN-positive patients.

Enhanced pathologic examination of axillary lymph nodes by serial sections and/or IHC demonstrates micrometastatic disease in 10–20% of patients deemed "node-negative" by conventional analysis, and six of seven large retrospective studies demonstrate significantly worse disease-free (and/or overall) survival among this group.[17] Strikingly similar results appear in two German studies of node-negative breast-cancer patients in whom bone-marrow micrometastases were strongly predictive of outcome.[18,19] We and our medical oncologists find this evidence persuasive, believe that SLN micrometastases are prognostically significant, and recommend systemic adjuvant chemotherapy for these patients. Nevertheless, "node-negative" patients found by enhanced pathologic techniques to have nodal metastases may represent as broad a spectrum of disease as does breast cancer in general. Some of them have missed macrometastases, some have micrometastases, some have tiny clusters of a few cells, and some have single tumor cells. It is quite unlikely that the last group has the same prognosis as the first, and current clinical trials (by masking both patient and clinician to the results of lymph-node IHC) have the potential to answer this compelling question.

REFERENCES

1. Krag DN, Weaver DL, Alex JC, Fairbank JT, Surgical resection and radiolocalization of the sentinel lymph node in breast cancer using a gamma probe. *Surg Oncol* 1993; **2**:335–40.
2. Giuliano AE, Kirgan DM, Guenther JM, Morton DL, Lymphatic mapping and sentinel lymphadenectomy for breast cancer. *Ann Surg* 1994; **220**:391–401.

3. Albertini JJ, Lyman GH, Cox C et al, Lymphatic mapping and sentinel node biopsy in the patient with breast cancer. *JAMA* 1996; **276:**1818–22.

4. O'Hea BJ, Hill ADK, El-Shirbiny A et al, Sentinel lymph node biopsy in breast cancer: initial experience at Memorial Sloan-Kettering Cancer Center. *J Am Coll Surg* 1998; **186:**423–7.

5. Hill ADK, Tran KN, Akhurst T et al, Lessons learned from 500 cases of lymphatic mapping for breast cancer. *Ann Surg* 1999; **229:**528–35.

6. Cody HS, Borgen PI, State-of-the-art approaches to sentinel node biopsy for breast cancer: study design, patient selection, technique, and quality control at Memorial Sloan-Kettering Cancer Center. *Surg Oncol* 1999; **8:**85–91.

7. Klauber-DeMore N, Tan LK, Liberman L et al, Sentinel lymph node biopsy: is it indicated in patients with high-risk ductal carcinoma-in-situ and ductal carcinoma-in-situ with microinvasion? *Ann Surg Oncol* 2000; **7:**636–42.

8. Liberman L, Cody HS, Hill ADK et al, Sentinel lymph node biopsy after percutaneous diagnosis of nonpalpable breast cancer. *Radiology* 1999; **211:**835–44.

9. Krag DN, Ashikaga T, Harlow SP, Weaver DL, Development of sentinel node targeting technique in breast cancer patients. *Breast J* 1998; **4:**67–74.

10. Linehan DC, Hill ADK, Tran KN et al, Sentinel lymph node biopsy in breast cancer: unfiltered radioisotope is superior to filtered. *J Am Coll Surg* 1999; **188:**377–81.

11. Linehan DC, Hill ADK, Akhurst T et al, Intradermal radiocolloid and intraparenchymal blue dye injection optimize sentinel node identification in breast cancer patients. *Ann Surg Oncol* 1999; **6:**450–4.

12. Cody HS, Urban JA, Is the major prognosticator in axillary node-negative breast cancer being overlooked? The importance of internal mammary node status in 195 extended radical mastectomy patients followed 10 years. *Breast Cancer Res Treat* 1993; **27:**141 (Abstract).

13. Veronesi U, Cascinelli N, Bufalino R, Risk of internal mammary lymph node metastases and its relevance on prognosis of breast cancer patients. *Ann Surg* 1983; **198:**681–4.

14. Veronesi U, Cascinelli N, Greco M, Prognosis of breast cancer patients after mastectomy and dissection of internal mammary nodes. *Ann Surg* 1985; **202:**702–7.

15. Weiser MR, Montgomery LL, Susnik B et al, Is routine intraoperative frozen-section examination of sentinel lymph nodes in breast cancer worthwhile? *Ann Surg Oncol* 2000; **7:**651–5.

16. Weiser MR, Montgomery LL, Tan LK et al, Lymphovascular invasion enhances the prediction of non-sentinel node metastases in breast cancer patients with positive sentinel nodes. *Ann Surg Oncol* 2000; **8:**145–9.

17. Dowlatshahi K, Fan M, Snider HC, Habib FA, Lymph node micrometastases from breast carcinoma: reviewing the dilemma. *Cancer* 1997; **80:**1188–97.

18. Diel IJ, Kaufmann M, Costa SD et al, Micrometastatic breast cancer cells in bone marrow at primary surgery: prognostic value in comparison with nodal status. *J Nat Cancer Inst* 1996; **88:**1652–64.

19. Braun S, Pantel K, Muller P et al, Cytokeratin-positive cells in the bone marrow and survival of patients with stage I, II, or III breast cancer. *New Engl J Med* 2000; **342:**525–33.

24

How we do it: the University of Louisville approach

Sandra L Wong, William R Wrightson and Kelly M McMasters

CONTENTS Dermal injection of radioactive colloid • Intraoperative SLN localization • Pathologic evaluation of the SLN • Conclusion

---

The University of Louisville James Graham Brown Cancer Center technique for SLN biopsy in breast cancer

Technique	Combination	Isotope	*Type*: Tc-99m-SC
Dye	*Type*: Isosulfan blue dye (1%)		*Filtered*: Yes (0.2-μm filter)
	Volume: 5.0 ml (cc)		*Dose*: 0.5 mCi (18.5 MBq)
			Volume: 0.2–0.5 ml (cc)
Injection site	*Isotope*: Intradermal		
	Dye: Peritumoral		

Numerous studies have demonstrated that sentinel lymph-node (SLN) biopsy provides accurate nodal staging information for patients with breast cancer.[1–6] As the procedure is becoming more widely accepted, attention is focused on optimizing the technique for SLN biopsy, which is performed by mapping the lymphatic drainage of the tumor using injection of blue dye, radioactive colloid, or both. Although excellent results have been reported in single-institution studies using a variety of techniques, the best technique is not clear from analysis of the literature.

Data from the University of Louisville Breast Cancer Sentinel Lymph Node Study demonstrate that, in widespread multi-institutional practice, the use of blue dye in combination with radioactive colloid gives superior results.[7] As with any surgical technique, there are always minor technical differences from institution to institution and from surgeon to surgeon. Significant controversy persists regarding the optimal type of radioactive colloid (filtered versus unfiltered technetium-99m-sulfur colloid), timing of injection, volume of injection, location of injection (peritumoral, subdermal, dermal, subareolar), use of routine preoperative lymphoscintigraphy (LSG), the site, timing and volume of blue-dye injection, and use of massage following injection. Our technique has in part developed from personal experience, preferences, and biases. We describe our current approach to SLN biopsy, which we believe is simple, reliable, and accurate.

Patients with T1 and T2 breast cancers (tumor size less than 5 cm) without palpable nodal metastases (N0) are eligible for SLN biopsy. Patients may choose either breast-conservation surgery or mastectomy. Contraindications include palpable axillary nodes, preoperative chemotherapy or radiation therapy, multifocal cancers, hypersensitivity to either blue dye or radiocolloid, and prior major breast or axillary surgeries, which could interfere with lymphatic drainage.

DERMAL INJECTION OF RADIOACTIVE COLLOID

Following approved nuclear medicine guidelines, injection of 0.5 mCi (18.5 MBq) of 0.2-μm filtered Tc-99m-SC in a volume of 0.2–0.5 ml (cc) is made at least 30 minutes but not more than 6 hours prior to planned operation. The skin overlying the tumor is injected in five separate locations, each time raising a weal in the injection site (Figure 24.1A). Using a tuberculin syringe with a 30-gauge needle assists in assuring that the injection is dermal and not subcutaneous. Intradermal injection appears to reflect

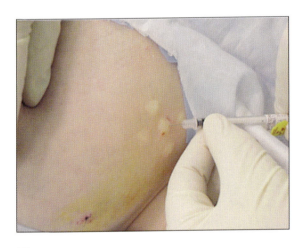

(A)

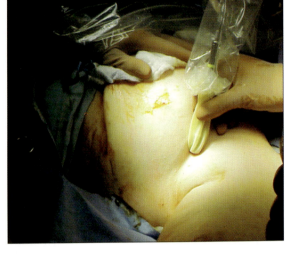

(C)

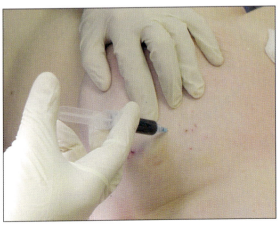

(B)

Figure 24.1 Sentinel lymph-node biopsy: the University of Louisville approach. (A) Dermal injection of Tc-99m-sulfur colloid. (B) Peritumoral injection of isosulfan blue dye. (C) Transcutaneous localization of the SLN using the hand-held gamma probe. (D) Using the gamma probe to pinpoint the location of the SLN. (E) Axillary incision for SLN biopsy. (F) Dissection is guided by the gamma probe. (G) Identification of a blue, radioactive SLN. (H) Dissection and removal of SLN. (I) Example of SLN with blue-stained afferent lymphatic channels.

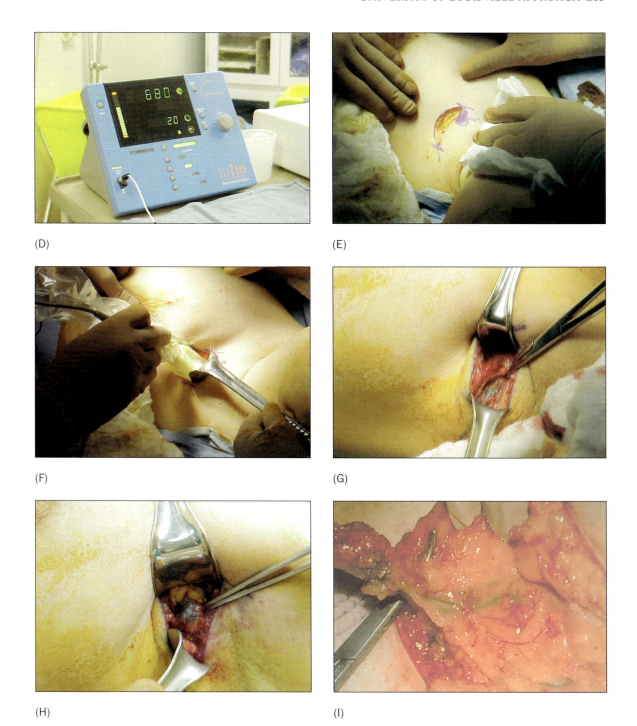

(D)

(E)

(F)

(G)

(H)

(I)

accurately the lymphatic drainage of the breast tissue beneath it and results in much more radioactivity reaching the SLNs. We have found that peritumoral injection of radioactive colloid results in a large zone of diffusion that has the potential to obscure the SLN, especially in upper outer quadrant tumors.[7]

Choosing the injection site is easy in the case of palpable tumors, but in cases of nonpalpable tumors or tumors that have previously been biopsied, the technique is not as straightforward. Patients with nonpalpable tumors undergo placement of a localization wire under mammographic or ultrasound guidance prior to radioactive-colloid injection. The radiologist is asked to mark the skin overlying the tumor with an indelible marker, but it is also a simple matter to judge the location of the tumor by inspection of the direction of the wire and by assessment of the depth of imbedded wire on the localization mammogram. For tumor locations in which it is not possible to identify the area of skin overlying the tumor, peritumoral injection is recommended. It is important to use a larger volume (6 ml) for peritumoral injection; however, the smaller volume for skin injection is preferable. If a patient presents following an excisional biopsy, the injection is given into the skin around the scar (provided the prior surgery did not involve a long tunnel in the breast to reach the tumor), avoiding injecting into the scar itself.

Because of the predictable axillary nodal drainage in breast cancer, it is not clear that LSG (nuclear medicine scan) is necessary for localization of the SLN. Our data indicate that routine preoperative LSG is neither necessary nor helpful in the identification of axillary SLNs.[8] Others have reported success with the dermal injection technique.[9] We recently updated a multi-institutional experience of 511 patients using dermal injection of radioactive colloid with concomitant peritumoral injection of blue dye. In this study, the sentinel node identification rate was 98%, and the false negative rate was 6.5% using this technique. The identification rate is significantly higher than that seen with use of peritumoral blue dye alone or peritumoral radioactive colloid injection.[10]

Blue-dye injection

The patient is transported from the nuclear medicine suite to the operating room, and the blue-dye injection is given following induction of general anesthesia but before standard prepping and draping of the patient for surgery. We prefer not to have the patient paralyzed. We inject 5 ml of 1% isosulfan dye into the normal breast parenchyma surrounding the tumor (peritumoral injection) (Figure 24.1B). For palpable tumors, the dye may be injected directly using 1 ml in each of the four quadrants around the tumor and 1 ml just superficial to the tumor (between the tumor and the skin). The injection is started at the level of the tumor and the needle is withdrawn as the injection takes place. Care must be taken to avoid injection into the skin, which can result in tattooing for several months. We have found that a 1.5-inch 25-gauge needle works best for this injection. Ultrasound guidance may be used to inject the dye around, but not into, the biopsy cavity if prior excisional biopsy was performed. In nonpalpable lesions for which needle localization has been performed, we specifically advise against injecting the entire volume of blue dye down the needle, as this concentrates the dye deep within the breast and usually does not result in efficient lymphatic uptake. The dye should instead be well dispersed around the tumor, including the superficial breast tissue beneath the skin.

Following blue-dye injection, brief massage over the tumor site is performed. The patient is then prepped and draped to include the arm circumferentially. Prior to the incision in the axilla, the primary tumor site is massaged for a full 5 minutes to facilitate the flow of dye through the afferent lymphatics.

INTRAOPERATIVE SLN LOCALIZATION

The location of the SLN is initially determined by transcutaneous scanning using a hand-held gamma counter. A "hot spot" in the axilla indicates the location of the SLN (Figure 24.1C,D). An incision 3–4 cm in length is made in the axilla over the suspected location of the SLN. The incision should be made along the line of a classic axillary lymph-node dissection (ALND) incision (Figure 24.1E). If no hot spot is identified, a curved transverse (anterior-to-posterior) incision in the lower axilla provides excellent exposure. With dermal injection of the radioactive colloid, however, an axillary hot spot is always evident transcutaneously. Blue lymphatic channels are sought and, if found, traced into the axilla. After incising the clavipectoral fascia to gain access to the axillary contents, the gamma probe is once again used to guide the dissection toward the SLN (Figure 24.1F). Sometimes we find it helpful to retract the skin overlying the tumor medially (away from the axilla) to facilitate gamma-probe detection. Adjusting the position of the arm can also help in pinpointing the SLN.

The radioactive signal increases in intensity as the dissection proceeds closer to the SLN. Electrocautery should be used for the dissection in order to maintain a hemostatic field. Lymphatic channels and small blood vessels are ligated with clips to decrease the incidence of seroma or hematoma formation. Frequently, it is helpful to place a figure-of-eight suture using 3–0 silk through the node once it is identified to provide traction without fragmenting the node while it is removed.

Inspection of the axilla for blue-stained afferent lymphatic channels should also be made during the course of dissection (Figure 24.1G–I). The stained channels can be traced to the SLN. Blue nodes usually have concomitant high radioactive counts as well, although it is possible to have radioactive lymph nodes that are not blue or blue nodes that are not radioactive. All blue nodes should be removed, since blue-dye staining is indicative of direct lymphatic drainage from the tumor and is considered to be the "gold standard" for identification of an SLN.

The number of counts per second should be recorded for each SLN in situ (in the nodal basin) and ex vivo (after removal from the patient). The latter is best performed by placing the node on top of the gamma probe pointed toward the ceiling (Figure 24.2). After the

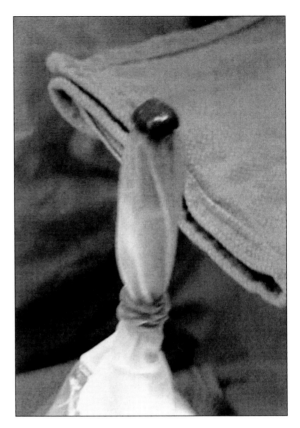

Figure 24.2 Gamma probe positioned pointing towards the ceiling.

removal of each SLN, the background activity in the axilla also should be recorded. To minimize the false-negative rate, all nodes with counts greater than or equal to 10% of the ex vivo count of the hottest node should be harvested as part of the SLN biopsy procedure.[11] Sentinel lymph-node biopsy is followed by either breast-conservation therapy or mastectomy. If no SLN is identified, Levels I and II ALND should be carried out in the standard fashion.

PATHOLOGIC EVALUATION OF THE SLN

Based on our institutional experience, we have accepted SLN biopsy as an alternative to ALND. We therefore perform frozen-section analysis of the SLN intraoperatively. If the SLN is positive for metastatic disease, completion ALND is performed. Patients must be informed preoperatively that frozen-section analysis will not detect some positive nodes and that final analysis may be different. Patients also should be informed of the small but real risk of a false-negative result when completion ALND is not carried out.

Each SLN is placed in formalin and labeled separately, numbered sequentially in the order harvested, with the dye-staining and radioactive-count information to be listed on the pathology report. Sentinel lymph nodes are examined more intensely than nodes from routine ALND; thus, the SLN biopsy has an increased sensitivity for detection of nodal metastases and micrometastatic disease. Each SLN should be processed by cutting the lymph node at 2-mm intervals ("bread loafing") for paraffin embedding of each piece. At least one section should be taken from each piece (about five sections for a 1.0-cm lymph node). For smaller lymph nodes, multiple pieces can be embedded in a single block. Routine hematoxylin-and-eosin (H&E) stains are performed. Immunohistochemistry using antibodies for cytokeratin is performed for at least two sections from each block. If completion ALND is performed, the Level I and II nodes are submitted for routine pathologic examination.

CONCLUSION

We believe that peritumoral blue dye remains the "gold standard" in showing direct lymphatic drainage from the tumor, and we recommend using it in combination with intradermal radiocolloid injection for optimal results in SLN biopsy for breast cancer. These are complementary techniques that allow rapid and reliable detection of the SLN when a hand-held gamma probe is used intraoperatively. We continue to study the many variations in surgical technique as part of the ongoing University of Louisville Breast Cancer Sentinel Lymph Node Study.

REFERENCES

1. Giuliano AE, Jones RC, Brennan M, Statman R, Sentinel lymphadenectomy in breast cancer. *J Clin Oncol* 1997; **15:**2345–50.
2. Ollila DW, Brennan MB, Giuliano AE, The role of intraoperative lymphatic mapping and sentinel lymphadenectomy in the management of patients with breast cancer. *Adv Surg* 1999; **32:**349–64.
3. Veronesi U, Paganelli G, Viale G et al, Sentinel lymph node biopsy and axillary dissection in breast cancer: results in a large series. *J Natl Cancer Inst* 1999; **91:**368–73.
4. Cody HS, Sentinel lymph node mapping in breast cancer. *Oncology* 1999; **13:**25–34.
5. Cox CE, Haddad F, Bass S et al, Lymphatic mapping in the treatment of breast cancer. *Oncology* 1998; **12:**1283–92.
6. Krag D, Weaver D, Ashikaga T et al, The sentinel node in breast cancer—a multicenter validation study. *N Engl J Med* 1998; **339:**941–6.
7. McMasters KM, Tuttle TM, Carlson DJ et al, Sentinel lymph node biopsy for breast cancer: a suitable alternative for routine axillary dissection in multi-institutional practice when optimal technique is used. *J Clin Oncol* 2000; **18:**2560–6.
8. McMasters KM, Wong SL, Tuttle TM et al, Preoperative lymphoscintigraphy for breast cancer does not improve the ability to accurately identify axillary sentinel lymph nodes. *Ann Surg* 2000; **231:**724–31.
9. Linehan DC, Hill ADK, Akhurst T et al, Intradermal radiocolloid and intraparenchymal blue dye injection optimize sentinel node identification in breast cancer patients. *Ann Surg Oncol* 1999; **6:**450–4.
10. McMasters KM, Wong SL, Martin RCG et al, Dermal injection of radioactive colloid is superior to peritumoral injection for breast cancer sentinel lymph node biopsy: Results of a multi-institutional study. *Ann Surg* 2001; **233:**676–87.
11. Martin RCG, Edwards MJ, Wong SL et al, Practical guidelines for optimal gamma probe detection of sentinel lymph nodes in breast cancer: results of a multi-institutional study. *Surgery* 2000; **128:**139–44.

25

Clinical trials

Mathew H Chung and Armando E Giuliano

A National Institutes of Health (NIH) consensus conference on treatment of breast cancer recommended routine Level I and II axillary lymph-node dissection (ALND) as the "gold standard" for axillary staging.[1] This procedure's false-negative rate of less than 2% has clearly stood the test of time. In addition, ALND offers excellent regional control with a low risk of axillary recurrence. The role of ALND for patients with clinically negative axillae has recently become controversial, however. Because only about one-third of these patients have histopathologic evidence of nodal metastases, routine ALND may subject many patients to potential operative morbidity without likely benefit. On the other hand, one-third of patients with clinically occult axillary metastases, many of whom have primary tumors less than 1 cm in diameter, cannot receive appropriate chemotherapy until the tumor status of the axillary basin has been established.

The recent trend toward aggressive adjuvant systemic therapy for both node-positive and node-negative breast cancer, the increasingly frequent detection of small invasive carcinomas with mammography, the use of axillary radiation as a potential therapeutic alternative to ALND in clinically node-negative patients, and increased public awareness of the potential morbidity of ALND, have prompted many clinicians to question the need for routine axillary dissection. This debate has been fueled by the recent emergence of sentinel lymph-node (SLN) biopsy as an accurate but less invasive means of staging the regional lymph nodes draining a primary tumor.

DEVELOPMENT OF SLN BIOPSY

The historical background to the development of SLN biopsy is described in Chapter 1. The success of this technique in melanoma stirred interest in its application to breast cancer, where identification of nodal metastases has prognostic and therapeutic significance. In 1991, our group at the John Wayne Cancer Institute modified the dye-directed SLN biopsy technique for use in primary breast cancer and began a feasibility trial.[2] In the last 107 SLN biopsy cases performed with concurrent ALND, the SLN was 100% predictive of axillary node status.[3] To further determine the accuracy of SLN biopsy, we used multiple sections and immunohistochemical (IHC) staining to evaluate all nonsentinel axillary nodes from patients whose SLNs were free of tumor by hematoxylin-and-eosin (H&E) and IHC. Review of 1087 nonsentinel nodes from 60 patients with tumor-free SLNs identified only one tumor-positive node.[4] This validated our initial hypothesis that the histopathologic status of the SLN accurately reflects the status of the remaining axillary nodes in women with breast cancer. The validity of SLN biopsy for staging breast cancer has been confirmed in many other studies and this technique has become a significant modification in the management of patients with breast cancer.

SLN BIOPSY IN BREAST CANCER

We have shown the safety and feasibility of SLN biopsy without further axillary dissection when this procedure is performed by a surgeon who has demonstrated a high success rate and a low false-negative rate. Our more recently reported results suggest that ALND may not be required in patients whose SLNs are tumor-free by both H&E and IHC.[5] In this study of 125 patients who underwent SLN biopsy, 67 had tumor-free SLNs by H&E and IHC and therefore received no further surgical or nonsurgical axillary intervention. Their rate of complications was only 3%, compared with 35% in patients undergoing ALND after SLN biopsy ($p = 0.001$), and none of the 67 patients had developed local or axillary recurrence at a median follow-up of 39 months. These data suggest that routine ALND may be eliminated for patients with histopathologically negative SLNs; however, our study was small, and its results remain to be confirmed at other centers.

Any patient with invasive breast cancer and clinically normal axillary nodes is a potential candidate for SLN biopsy. The absolute contraindications for SLN biopsy include a history of hypersensitivity reaction to the lymphatic-mapping agents, and pregnancy. Patients with known axillary metastases should undergo ALND instead of SLN biopsy. Relative contraindications include multicentric disease, a large primary tumor, a large biopsy cavity, and recent prior breast and/or axillary surgery.

No uniform technique of SLN biopsy has yet been defined, and there is unlikely to be a single standard way to perform the procedure. Because all the reported mapping techniques can identify the SLN with comparable accuracy and false-negative rates, the SLN biopsy team at each institution must determine the technique that best suits its expertise and allows it to achieve a consistently high rate of accuracy with minimal false negatives. Therefore, SLN biopsy for breast cancer should be conducted in a protocol or clinical trial setting.

TRIALS OF SLN BIOPSY IN BREAST CANCER

Sentinel lymph-node biopsy can accurately determine axillary nodal status,[2,6,7] and widespread enthusiasm for this technique has inevitably fostered various modifications. These technical variations reflect differences in mapping agent, site and timing of injection, and in the case of radiopharmaceutical-directed mapping, the definition of a "hot" SLN. In general, the reported accuracy of SLN identification exceeds 90% using blue dye and/or radiopharmaceutical, and the reported rate of false-negatives is less than 10% (Table 25.1).

Dye-directed SLN biopsy studies

The use of vital blue dye to map the lymphatic pathway to the SLN(s) from a primary breast carcinoma was first reported by Giuliano et al in 1994.[2] Using 1% isosulfan blue dye as the mapping agent, the authors included 174 consecutive SLN biopsy procedures in their initial feasibility study. All patients subsequently underwent completion ALND. Sentinel lymph-node biopsy was successful in 114 patients (65.5%) and accurately reflected axillary tumor status in 109 of 114 SLN biopsy procedures (95.6%). In 1997, Guenther et al reported a feasibility trial of SLN biopsy in a health-maintenance organization (HMO) setting.[6] An SLN was identified in 71% of 145 patients and accu-

Table 25.1 Clinical trials of SLN biopsy in patients with breast cancer

Series by mapping agent	Year	N	Rate of SLN identification (%)	Accuracy (%)	False-negative rate (%)
Blue dye alone					
Giuliano et al[2]	1994	174	66	96	12
Guenther et al[6]	1997	145	71	97	10
Giuliano et al[3]	1997	107	94	100	0
Koller et al[7]	1998	98	98	97	3
Morgan et al[8]	1999	44	73	94	6
Morrow et al[9]	1999	50	88	95	—
Radiopharmaceutical alone					
Krag et al[10]	1993	22	82	100	0
Veronesi et al[12]	1997	163	98	98	5
Pijpers et al[11]	1997	37	92	100	0
Krag et al[13]	1998	443	93	97	11
Crossin et al[14]	1998	50	84	98	2
Miner et al[15]	1998	41	98	98	2
Blue dye + radiopharmaceutical					
Albertini et al[16]	1996	62	92	100	0
O'Hea et al[20]	1998	59	93	95	15
Linehan et al[19]	1999	200	93	98	4
Hill et al[18]	1999	500	93	—	11[a]

[a]Only 104 patients underwent complete axillary lymph-node dissection (ALND) following SLN biopsy.

rately predicted axillary status in 97% of these patients; the false-negative rate of SLN biopsy was 10%. Results of both feasibility studies are impressive because in each case the technique was being developed in a protocol setting (SLN biopsy followed by ALND), and the absence of a previous description of lymphatic mapping for breast cancer meant that the technique was being altered and the protocol modified as each study progressed. Moreover, selection criteria had not been established to exclude patients in whom SLN biopsy was unlikely to be successful (i.e., patients with previous breast and/or axillary surgery, palpable nodal disease, and multifocality). With technical refinements and

optimal patient selection, our group has since achieved a 100% success rate for SLN biopsy.

The SLN concept has rapidly gained acceptance by the surgical community, and SLN biopsy is now being performed in a community hospital setting. Morgan et al reported results for 44 patients who underwent SLN biopsy followed by ALND during 1996 and 1997.[8] An SLN was successfully identified in 32 patients (73%) and was falsely negative in two patients, yielding an accuracy of 93.8%, sensitivity of 83.3%, and negative predictive value of 91%.

Morrow et al published an interesting study of SLN biopsy using blue dye with and without a radiopharmaceutical.[9] The purpose of this study was to determine which technique resulted in a higher rate of SLN identification and whether the learning curve for SLN identification varied when mapping was performed with dye alone versus dye plus radiopharmaceutical. Fifty patients were randomized to dye-directed mapping and 42 patients to combined-agent mapping. The SLN identification rate did not differ for dye alone (88%) versus combined agents (86%), and the authors did not identify any advantage for the combination, even for surgeons learning the techniques. The surgeons' success rate for finding the SLN was 73% (range 60–90%) during the first 10 cases; this rate increased to 91% after 30 cases when all patients in the study were considered as a group. The surgeons' learning curves for procedures on the randomized patients undergoing dye-directed mapping and those undergoing combined-agent mapping did not, however, reveal a significant advantage for either technique at any point. Although this study was small, it remains important as the only prospective, randomized trial comparing learning curves for different techniques of identifying the SLN.

Radioguided SLN biopsy studies

Other investigators have successfully performed SLN biopsy with a radiopharmaceutical as the primary mapping agent.[10–15] With this technique, radioactive SLNs are identified intraoperatively using a hand-held gamma probe. Depending on the agent used, the radiopharmaceutical is injected 1 hour to 24 hours before the procedure. Usually, a technetium-99m-labeled colloid, most commonly sulfur colloid or albumin, is injected peritumorally, in the perimeter of the wall of the biopsy cavity, or even subdermally, and radioactive SLNs are removed until the surrounding counts drop to background levels. Krag et al were the first to report radioguided SLN identification in breast cancer.[10] In their 1993 pilot study of radiopharmaceutical-directed lymphatic mapping, 22 patients received an injection of unfiltered Tc-99m-sulfur colloid (Tc-99m-SC) 1–4 hours

before surgery. A hand-held gamma probe was used to follow the lymphatic path of the radiopharmaceutical. An SLN was identified in 18 patients (82%) and predicted the status of the axilla in each case. There were no false-negatives. Subsequently, Pijpers and colleagues reported their experience with radiopharmaceutical-directed SLN biopsy in 37 patients undergoing peritumoral injection of Tc-99m-colloidal albumin.[11] Sentinel lymph-node biopsy was successful in 34 patients (92%) and there were no false-negatives. In 1997, Veronesi et al published their consecutive series of 163 women with breast cancer who underwent SLN biopsy using a subdermal injection of Tc-99m-human serum albumin (Tc-99m-HSA).[12] All patients subsequently underwent ALND. An SLN was successfully identified in 160 patients (98%) and accurately predicted axillary lymph-node status in 156 (97.5%) of these patients, with a false-negative rate of 5%.

In 1998, a multicenter study to evaluate radiopharmaceutical-directed SLN biopsy was reported by Krag and colleagues.[13] Surgeons in various practice settings from 11 centers participated in this study. The overall rate of SLN identification was 91% (405 of 443 patients). The accuracy of the SLN as a predictor of axillary status was 97% (392 of 405), with a false-negative rate of 11%. Critics of this study have noted its variable rate of successful SLN identification (79.1% to 98%) among different surgeons, and its high rate of false-negatives. In the same year, Crossin and coworkers reported their SLN biopsy experience in 50 clinically node-negative breast cancer patients who underwent peritumoral injection of Tc-99m-SC.[14] The SLN biopsy success rate was 84% and the false-negative rate was 13%. This false-negative rate seems extremely high when compared with those of the initial feasibility trials.

SLN biopsy studies using blue dye plus radiopharmaceutical

A number of reports advocate the combined use of blue dye and radiopharmaceutical for lymphatic mapping.[16–20] These authors contend that the combination of two lymphatic-mapping agents increases the success rate of identifying the SLN and lowers the false-negative rate. Albertini and associates first reported breast SLN biopsy using both mapping agents in 62 patients with primary breast cancer.[16] Sentinel nodes were identified in 92% of the patients, and there were no false-negatives. Cox and coauthors compiled results from three breast SLN biopsy protocols that used the combined-agent technique.[17] The overall SLN biopsy success rate among 466 patients was 94%, with one false-negative SLN. Because not all patients in this study underwent completion ALND, the false-negative rate cannot be accurately determined. Hill and colleagues reported 500 cases of SLN biopsy performed using a combination of isosulfan blue dye and Tc-99m-SC.[18] An SLN was identified in 458 of 492 evaluable cases (93%), and the false-negative rate was 10.6%. Linehan and others evaluated intradermal radiopharmaceutical and intraparenchymal blue dye to identify the SLN in 200 consecutive breast-cancer patients undergoing SLN biopsy: they discovered that dermal and parenchymal lymphatics of the breast drained to the same SLNs in most patients.[19]

No agreement on mapping agents or injection sites is likely in the near future; however, the only prospective randomized trial of SLN biopsy that compared the learning curve for blue dye alone with that for blue dye plus radiopharmaceutical found both techniques to be virtually equivalent.[3] If both lymphatic-mapping agents are used, intradermal injection of the radiopharmaceutical may be preferable because the smaller dose of radioactivity decreases the shine-through effect, thereby simplifying SLN localization.

CURRENT US NATIONAL PROTOCOLS

Several multicenter, prospective, randomized trials in the United States are examining the role of SLN biopsy in the care of patients with breast cancer. In the National Surgical Adjuvant Breast and Bowel Project (NSABP) B-32 trial, all patients undergo SLN biopsy. If the SLN contains metastases or is not found, ALND is performed. Patients with pathologically negative SLNs are randomly assigned to observation or to ALND, with 2000 patients in each group (Figure 25.1). This study will have 90% power to detect a 2% difference in 5-year survival, local control, and overall morbidity in the two groups of patients. It will determine whether ALND can be safely omitted in breast-cancer patients who have pathologically negative SLNs.

The American College of Surgeons Oncology Group (ACSOG) is accruing patients for their multicenter Z0010 and Z0011 trials. The former is a prognostic study of SLN and bone-marrow micrometastases in women with clinical T1 or T2 N0M0 breast cancer. Patients undergo segmental mastectomy, SLN biopsy, and bilateral iliac-crest bone-marrow aspirations (Figure 25.2). If SLNs are tumor-negative by H&E, no specific axillary treatment is offered but IHC is performed on the SLNs and on bone-marrow aspirate. Clinicians are masked to the results of IHC analysis of the SLN, which is performed at a central site. This study will evaluate the prevalence and prognostic significance of SLN micrometastases detected by IHC, and will determine the risk of regional recurrence in women whose SLNs are negative by H&E. The target accrual is 7600 patients over the next 4 years.

The Z0011 protocol is for Z0010 patients whose SLNs contain tumor identified by H&E. Patients in the Z0011 trial are randomly assigned to ALND or to observation (Figure 25.3). This trial will clarify the role of ALND in patients with histologically involved axillae. Its short-term objective is to quantify and compare the surgical morbidities associated with SLN biopsy plus ALND versus SLN biopsy alone. The long-term goal is to determine whether immediate ALND has a significant impact on overall survival.

The US Department of Defense (DOD) is funding a national effort to determine the broad applicability of the SLN biopsy technique and its accuracy in patients who have undergone a previous biopsy. Additionally, this trial will evaluate new methods of detecting occult metastases using IHC staining and a reverse

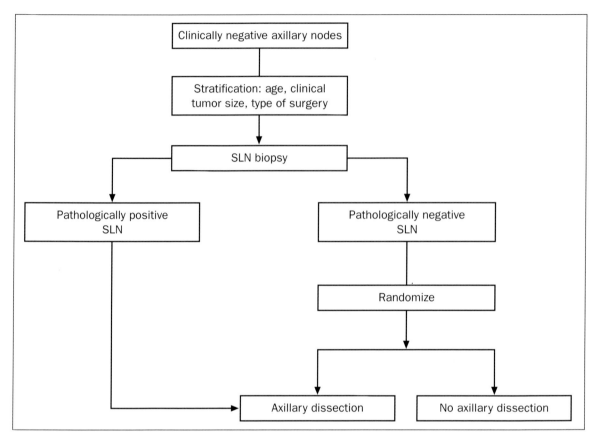

Figure 25.1 National Surgical Adjuvant Breast and Bowel Project (NSABP) B-32 trial. Axillary lymph-node dissection is performed if no SLN is identified.

transcriptase–polymerase chain reaction (RT-PCR) assay based on a keratin probe. To participate in this trial, teams of surgeons and nuclear medicine physicians from each participating center must attend a formal training session conducted at the primary investigational center.

CONTROVERSIES

Biopsy technique

No standard technique of SLN biopsy in breast cancer has been adopted by all surgeons. Various materials have been used for intraoperative lymphatic mapping. Additionally, various methods of injecting the lymphatic-mapping agent have been used. It is unlikely that a standard technique will be described and adopted in the near future. Therefore, surgeons performing SLN biopsy for breast cancer should identify and use the technique with which they can *consistently* achieve a high accuracy rate (>90%) and a low false-negative rate (<10%).

The role of preoperative lymphoscintigraphy

The role of preoperative lymphoscintigraphy (LSG) is controversial. Many authors advocate its routine use, but others do not.[17,21] At the John Wayne Cancer Institute, we have selectively

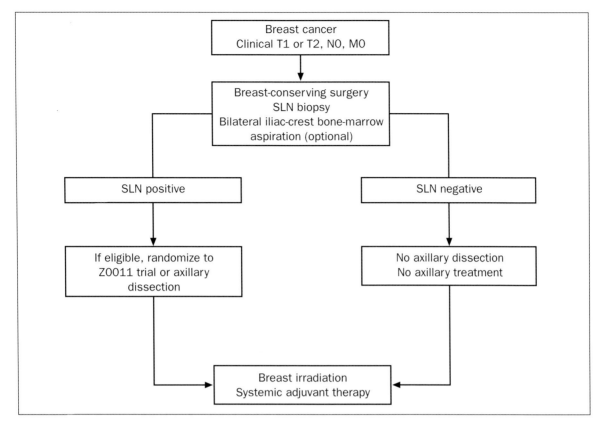

Figure 25.2 American College of Surgeons Oncology Group (ACSOG) Z0010 trial. Bone-marrow aspirates and SLNs are examined by H&E only; IHC staining is performed at a central site, and results masked to clinicians. If no SLN can be identified, ALND is performed.

employed LSG for those patients with medial breast cancers because of the increased propensity for medial lesions to drain to internal mammary nodes in addition to the axilla. Approximately 5% of medial lesions drain exclusively into the internal mammary chain; in these cases, preoperative LSG can avoid operative exploration of the axillary nodal basin. We do not use preoperative LSG for patients with outer quadrant tumors because peritumoral injection of radiopharmaceutical in the outer quadrant can cause a shine-through effect that impairs recognition of the SLN. Additionally, we employ preoperative LSG whenever previous breast and/or axillary surgery might have disrupted lymphatic drainage (see Chapter 18).

The role of immunohistochemical staining

Another area of controversy is the clinical impact of SLN analysis. Micrometastases (tumor deposits <2 mm in diameter) missed by standard H&E examination of an ALND specimen will often be revealed by IHC staining of the SLN. There is some evidence that micrometastases in the SLN are associated with a low risk of further axillary nodal metastases beyond this node,[22] but the clinical significance of micrometastases is not yet known. Numerous studies have demonstrated that micrometastasis is a negative prognosticator, but many others have found that it is not. To resolve this controversy, in May 1999 ACSOG

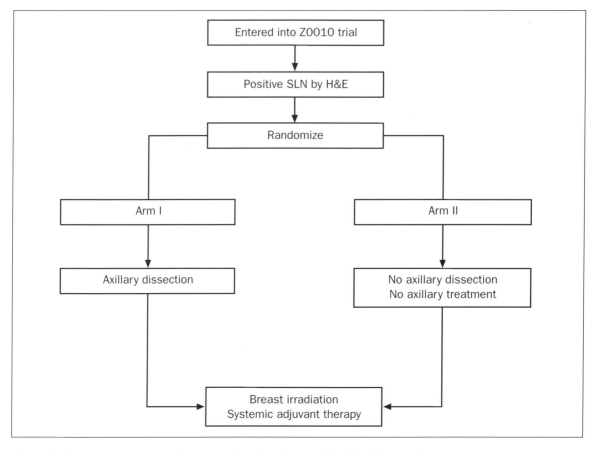

Figure 25.3 American College of Surgeons Oncology Group (ACSOG) Z0011 trial.

began its multicenter, masked, prospective Z0010 and Z0011 trials as described above. Continued refinements in technique will identify patients with increasingly smaller nodal deposits, including nonviable cells and cell fragments. Reverse transcriptase–polymerase chain reaction to identify tumor messenger RNA within lymph nodes is now identifying new populations of patients with "mRNA micrometastases." It is hoped that, through the ACSOG studies and other ongoing investigations, an analysis of carefully defined and prospectively acquired data will bring us closer to resolving the dilemma of micrometastatic nodal disease.

CONCLUSION

Axillary lymph-node dissection will remain the "gold standard" for staging breast cancer until results of prospective, randomized trials of SLN biopsy are available. In the interim, however, SLN biopsy offers many advantages for patients with small tumors and clinically negative axillae. This procedure can accurately determine the regional nodal status with less morbidity; it allows more focused examination of the node, thereby potentially upstaging more cancers; and it is done in an ambulatory surgical setting with rapid recovery. Until more definitive data on this innovative technique are available, SLN biopsy should be performed as part of one of the previously mentioned trials or in a protocol setting approved by the local institutional review board. In all cases, SLN biopsy should be undertaken only by a qualified team of physicians (surgeons, nuclear medicine physicians, and pathologists) who have documented their own accuracy rates of SLN biopsy. The development and clinical assessment of SLN biopsy is an important step that will help to make the management of breast cancer less invasive.

REFERENCES

1. National Institutes of Health, NIH consensus conference on the treatment of early stage breast cancer. *JAMA* 1991; **265**:391–5.
2. Giuliano AE, Kirgan DM, Guenther JM et al, Lymphatic mapping and sentinel lymphadenectomy for breast cancer. *Ann Surg* 1994; **220**: 391–401.
3. Giuliano AE, Jones RC, Brennan M et al, Sentinel lymphadenectomy in breast cancer. *J Clin Oncol* 1997; **15**:2345–50.
4. Turner RR, Ollila DW, Krasne DL et al, Histopathological validation of the sentinel node hypothesis in breast cancer. *Ann Surg* 1997; **226**:271–8.
5. Giuliano AE, Haigh PI, Brennan MB et al, Prospective observational study of sentinel lymphadenectomy without further axillary dissection in patients with sentinel node-negative breast cancer. *J Clin Oncol* 2000; **18**: 2553–9.
6. Guenther JM, Krishnamoorthy M, Tan LR, Sentinel lymphadenectomy for breast cancer in a community managed care setting. *Cancer J Sci Am* 1997; **3**:336–40.
7. Koller M, Barsuk D, Zippel D et al, Sentinel lymph node involvement—a predictor for axillary node status with breast cancer—has the time come? *Eur J Surg Oncol* 1998; **24**:166–8.
8. Morgan A, Howisey RI, Aldape HC et al, Initial experience in a community hospital with sentinel lymph node mapping and biopsy for evaluation of axillary lymph node status in palpable invasive breast cancer. *J Surg Oncol* 1999; **72**: 24–31.
9. Morrow M, Rademaker AW, Bethke KP et al, Learning sentinel node biopsy: results of a prospective randomized trial of two techniques. *Surgery* 1999; **126**:714–22.
10. Krag DN, Weaver DL, Alex JC et al, Surgical resection and radiolocalization of the sentinel lymph node in breast cancer using a gamma probe. *Surg Oncol* 1993; **2**:335–9.
11. Pijpers R, Meijer S, Hoekstra OS et al, Impact of lymphoscintigraphy on sentinel node identification with technetium-99m-colloidal albumin in breast cancer. *J Nucl Med* 1997; **38**:366–8.
12. Veronesi U, Paganelli G, Galimberti V et al, Sentinel-node biopsy to avoid axillary dissection in breast cancer with clinically negative lymph-nodes. *Lancet* 1997; **349**:1864–7.
13. Krag D, Weaver D, Ashikaga T et al, The sentinel node in breast cancer: a multicenter validation study. *N Engl J Med* 1998; **339**:941–6.
14. Crossin JA, Johnson AC, Stewart PB et al, Gamma-probe-guided resection of the sentinel lymph node in breast cancer. *Am Surg* 1998; **64**:666–9.
15. Miner TJ, Shriver CD, Jaques DP et al, Ultrasonographically guided injection improves localization of the radiolabeled sentinel lymph node in breast cancer. *Ann Surg Oncol* 1998; **5**: 315–21.
16. Albertini JJ, Lyman GH, Cox C et al, Lymphatic mapping and sentinel node biopsy in the patient with breast cancer. *JAMA* 1996; **276**:1818–22.
17. Cox CE, Pendas S, Cox JM et al, Guidelines for sentinel node biopsy and lymphatic mapping of patients with breast cancer. *Ann Surg* 1998; **227**:645–53.
18. Hill AD, Tran KN, Akhurst T et al, Lessons learned from 500 cases of lymphatic mapping for breast cancer. *Ann Surg* 1999; **229**:528–35.
19. Linehan DC, Hill AD, Akhurst T et al, Intradermal radiocolloid and intraparenchymal blue dye injection optimize sentinel node identification in breast cancer patients. *Ann Surg Oncol* 1999; **6**:450–4.
20. O'Hea BJ, Hill ADK, El-Shirbiny AM et al, Sentinel lymph node biopsy in breast cancer: initial experience at Memorial Sloan-Kettering Cancer Center. *J Am Coll Surg* 1998; **186**:423–7.
21. Burak WE, Walker MJ, Yee LD et al, Routine preoperative lymphoscintigraphy is not necessary prior to sentinel node biopsy for breast cancer. *Am J Surg* 1999; **177**:445–9.
22. Chu KU, Turner RR, Hansen NM et al, Do all patients with sentinel node metastasis from breast carcinoma need complete axillary node dissection? *Ann Surg* 1999; **229**:536–54.

26

The University of Louisville study

Sandra L Wong, William R Wrightson and Kelly M McMasters

CONTENTS   **SLN biopsy technique**   •   **Overview of results**   •   **Future investigations**

The University of Louisville Breast Sentinel Lymph Node Biopsy Study was initiated in November 1997 with the goal of determining the accuracy of sentinel lymph-node (SLN) biopsy in a multicenter setting. Since its induction, the study has accrued over 1800 patients from 166 surgeons. The vast majority of participating surgeons are from community general surgery practices with minimal previous experience in SLN biopsy.

This ongoing study is approved by the Institutional Review Board (IRB) of each participating institution, and informed consent is obtained in writing from all patients after discussion of risks and benefits with the operating surgeon. Importantly, all patients have undergone attempted SLN biopsy followed by completion Level I/II axillary lymph-node dissection (ALND). Clinicopathologic data and biopsy results are recorded on case-report forms, which are submitted along with pathology reports to a central data-management site for inclusion in this nationwide study. Eligibility criteria are as follows: age 18 years or older; tumor size less than 5.0 cm (T1 or T2); no palpable axillary lymph nodes (clinical N0); invasive breast cancer documented by fine-needle aspiration (FNA),

core needle, incisional, or excisional biopsy. Patients are excluded on the following criteria: hypersensitivity to isosulfan blue dye or technetium-99m-sulfur colloid (Tc-99m-SC); preoperative chemotherapy or radiation therapy; locally advanced breast cancer (T3 or T4); recurrent breast cancer; or multifocal/multicentric disease.

The primary end-points of the study include the sensitivity, specificity, negative predictive value, overall accuracy, and false-negative rate of SLN biopsy for breast cancer using single-agent injection (blue dye alone or radioactive colloid alone) versus dual-agent injection (blue dye in combination with radioactive colloid). The influence of patient and tumor characteristics, as well as surgeon experience, on identification and false-negative rates are also examined. The major hypothesis of the study is that SLN biopsy can be performed with acceptable SLN-identification and false-negative rates across a wide spectrum of surgical practices and hospital environments. Other major objectives of the study are to determine the technical factors that are associated with optimal SLN identification and false-negative rates; and to establish the learning curve for the technique, developing practical guidelines for the number of cases that must be performed prior to abandoning completion ALND.

SLN BIOPSY TECHNIQUE

Surgeons were allowed flexibility in performing SLN biopsy, using techniques with which they had been trained. Recommended guidelines for performance of SLN biopsy were provided in the protocol, but the decision to perform SLN biopsy using blue dye alone, radioactive colloid alone, or a combination of the two agents was left to the discretion of the individual surgeon. Radioisotope variations are allowed; type of particle used, particle size, timing of injection, volume of injection, technique of injection, and type of hand-held gamma probe used differ among participating surgeons. The decision whether or not to use preoperative lymphoscintigraphy (LSG) is made by the individual surgeon. We required that radioactive counts be recorded for SLNs harvested, including transcutaneous counts over the SLN, in situ, ex vivo, and final background counts.

An SLN was defined as any blue node, or any node that could be identified as substantially more radioactive than background levels. A specific node/background ratio was not specified in the protocol for defining an SLN, as the background count varies depending on the location of the primary tumor and the placement of the probe. After the first radioactive SLN was removed, any node that contained radioactive counts that were at least 10% of the ex vivo count of the "hottest" SLN (the most radioactive node) was considered to be an additional SLN. Each SLN was examined by routine hematoxylin-and-eosin (H&E) staining at a minimum of 2-mm intervals. In addition, immunohistochemical analysis using antibodies for cytokeratin was performed in some institutions. The axillary non-SLNs were evaluated by routine H&E staining of bivalved nodes. The study protocol did not mandate removal of nonaxillary (internal mammary, supraclavicular) nodes, as the primary objective is to determine whether SLN biopsy could replace Level I/II ALND as the method of nodal staging.

OVERVIEW OF RESULTS

To date, we have performed several analyses of the University of Louisville Breast Sentinel Lymph Node Study database to answer many fundamental questions regarding SLN biopsy.

Is blue dye plus radiocolloid better than either agent alone?

There has been considerable controversy regarding the optimal technique for SLN biopsy, with variable false-negative rates among multiple studies.[1–8] Sentinel lymph-node biopsy is performed by mapping lymphatic drainage after injection of blue dye, radioactive colloid, or both around the breast tumor. Results of our multi-institutional study indicate that injection of blue dye plus radioactive colloid injection provide more accurate nodal staging than the use of either agent alone.[9] We found a 90% identification rate with the dual-agent technique as opposed to 86% with use of a single agent. The false-negative rates were likewise better with dual-agent localization (5.8%) compared with either agent alone (5.8% versus 11.8%, $p < 0.05$). Although this is not a randomized study, the data support the use of radioactive colloid in combination with blue-dye injection as the method of choice to minimize false-negative results (Table 26.1). These results do not, however, negate the excellent results obtained in some centers with single-agent injection, but rather suggest that when SLN biopsy is performed across a wide range of surgical practices and hospital environments, the combination of blue dye plus radioactive-colloid injection produces more uniformly accurate nodal staging.

What factors are associated with improved SLN identification and false-negative rates?

We examined clinicopathologic characteristics to determine if any were related to increased false-negative results or decreased SLN identification rates (Table 26.2).[9] Patient age (≥50

Table 26.1 Results of SLN biopsy by injection technique

	Single agent	Dual agent	All techniques
No. of patients	244	562	806
No. of surgeons	38	96	99[a]
SLN identified (%)	86	90	88
Mean no. of SLN removed	1.50	2.10[b]	1.95
Sensitivity (%)	89.1	94.2	92.2
Specificity (%)	100	100	100
Positive predictive value (%)	100	100	100
Negative predictive value (%)	93.7	97.5	96.4
Overall accuracy (%)	95.7	98.2	97.5
False-negative rate (%)	11.8	5.8[c]	7.2

[a]Number of surgeons in each group does not equal 99 because some surgeons used both techniques.
[b]$p < 0.0001$ vs single-agent injection, analysis of variance.
[c]$p < 0.05$ vs single-agent injection, Fisher's exact test.

years) was inversely correlated with the ability to identify the SLN. This may be related to the decreased ability of the lymphatic system in older women to take up the injected blue dye and radioactive colloid because of the fatty nature of the postmenopausal breast. Tumor in the upper outer quadrant was associated with a greater probability of a false-negative result, which may be related to difficulty in discriminating signal from background when peritumoral injection of radioactive colloid is performed near the axilla. Prior excisional biopsy has previously been shown to be associated with failure to identify an SLN,[5] but our results do not confirm such a correlation.

Does preoperative lymphoscintigraphy improve either SLN identification or false-negative rate?

Although preoperative LSG frequently is performed prior to SLN biopsy for breast cancer, little information exists regarding the utility of this nuclear medicine scan. Lymphoscinti-

graphy is routinely employed for localization of SLNs in malignant melanoma because anatomic predictions of lymphatic drainage are often unreliable, especially for lesions of the trunk or head and neck. Axillary nodal drainage for breast cancer is, however, predictable. This analysis was performed to determine whether preoperative LSG added diagnostic accuracy to offset the additional time and cost required.

In our study,[10] preoperative LSG did not improve the ability to identify axillary SLNs, nor did it improve the false-negative rate. The SLN was identified in 92.1% of patients who had no preoperative lymphoscintigram performed, with a false-negative rate of 1.6%. The patients who underwent preoperative LSG had an SLN-identification rate of 89.1%, with a false-negative rate of 8.7%. There were no statistically significant differences in the SLN identification rates or the false-negative rates (Table 26.3). Furthermore, there was no difference in the mean number of SLNs removed per patient. Therefore, we concluded that routine preoperative LSG is neither necessary nor helpful for identification of axillary SLNs for patients with

Table 26.2 Factors affecting SLN-identification and false-negative rates

Variable	No. of patients	SLN identification rate (%)	Odds ratio (95% CI)	p	False-negative rate (%)	Odds ratio (95% CI)	p
Age (yr)							
<50	216	92.6	1.99 (1.10–3.88)	0.03	5.8	1.61 (0.53–6.02)	0.43
≥50	590	87.6			8.7		
Location of tumor							
Upper outer quadrant	421	89.8	0.82 (0.51–1.31)	0.40	11.2	3.10 (1.09–11.09)	0.05
All other locations	381	87.9			3.9		
Size of primary tumor							
T1	553	87.7	0.76 (0.42–1.32)	0.34	10.7	0.51 (0.16–1.47)	0.39
T2 or T3	215	91.6			5.5		
Previous biopsy							
FNA or core needle	265	89.0	1.01 (0.61–1.71)	0.98	7.0	0.60 (0.19–2.01)	0.39
Excisional	530	88.7			10.2		
Surgeon experience[a]							
<10 cases	456	87.9	0.73 (0.44–1.20)	0.22	7.6	1.29 (0.43–3.97)	0.65
≥10 cases	350	90.0			9.3		

[a]Number of SLN biopsy cases performed by the surgeon prior to enrolling patients in the study.

Table 26.3 Results of SLN biopsy

Preoperative LSG	SLN identified	False-negative rate (%)	Mean no. of SLNs removed
Yes	310/348 (89.1%)	8.7	2.00
No	221/240 (92.1%)	1.6	2.16
Total	531/588 (90.3%)	6.1	2.07

breast cancer. Preoperative LSG does add time and cost to the procedure, however. In one representative institution, preoperative LSG increased patient charges by $545 per patient.

How many radioactive SLNs should be removed?

Of critical importance is the definition of a sentinel node. While most would agree in principle that an SLN can be defined as the first node or nodes to receive afferent lymphatic drainage from a tumor, there is actually considerable controversy over the practical definition of an SLN. Some believe that the only true way to define an SLN is to visualize a blue lymphatic channel leading to a blue lymph node, yet one can have a positive node with no blue staining. We agree that all blue nodes should be harvested; however, multiple radioactive lymph nodes are often identified using the gamma probe, and these nodes may not always be blue. In practice, one often finds the first and hottest SLN, which is usually blue as well. Inspection of the axilla may reveal no other evidence of blue nodes or channels. When the gamma probe is used, however, focal areas of increased radioactivity are often identified that may be found, upon dissection, to contain blue staining. Furthermore, some positive SLNs are not blue. Although many guidelines have been proposed for defining the nodes that should be removed, none of them are based on empiric data related to the likelihood of a false-negative

result. Therefore, there has been no clear consensus to indicate which radioactive nodes should be removed and considered true SLNs.

We sought to provide practical guidelines for removal of SLNs based on degree of radioactivity of the nodes.[11] We wanted to determine whether harvesting radioactive nodes in addition to the most radioactive node improved the false-negative rate. In 11.5% of those patients with multiple SLNs removed, the hottest SLN was negative while a less radioactive node was positive for tumor. All of these less radioactively positive SLNs had radioactive counts greater than 10% of that of the hottest lymph node (Table 26.4). By harvesting all nodes with counts greater than or equal to 10% of that of the hottest node, the false-negative rate for the study was 5.8%, which is statistically different from the 13.0% false-negative rate that would have resulted had only the hottest node been removed ($p = 0.01$) (Table 26.5). Removal of all blue nodes and all nodes with counts 10% or more of that of the hottest node will ensure optimal detection of nodal metastases.

Is unfiltered Tc-99m-sulfur colloid better than filtered?

Variations in the materials used may contribute to difficulty in localization. One such area in question was the difference between filtered and unfiltered radioactive colloid. The prevailing theory is that unfiltered colloid, with a greater proportion of larger particle sizes, will

Patient (n = 24)	Ex vivo radioactive count (hottest node)	Ex vivo radioactive count (positive node)	Percentage of hottest node (mean 42.2%)	Was the node blue?
1	121	50	41.3	No
2	811	386	47.6	No
3	11 399	7000	61.4	Faint blue
4	800	500	62.5	Obvious blue
5	89	24	27	Faint blue
6	2300	900	39.1	Faint blue
7	10 721	5391	50.3	Obvious blue
8	569	359	63.1	No
9	68	29	42.6	Obvious blue
10	465	39	8.4	No
11	36	29	80.6	Obvious blue
12	1323	220	16.6	No
13	89	24	27	Faint blue
14	78	58	74.4	No
15	1695	551	32.5	Obvious blue
16	1215	188	15.5	Obvious blue
17	8348	1273	15.2	Obvious blue
18	196	68	34.7	No
19	100	19	19	No
20	159	64	40.3	Obvious blue
21	75	6	8	Obvious blue
22	312	275	88.1	No
23	145	119	82.1	Faint blue
24	27	3	11.1	No

Table 26.4 Results of SLN biopsy when the hottest node was falsely negative for metastatic disease

be more likely to "stick" in the true SLN and not pass through to second-tier nodes. This would lead to fewer radioactive nodes in the axilla. We found no significant difference, however, in the SLN identification rate (90.9% vs 92.3%), false-negative rate (10.0% vs 6.8%), or mean number of SLNs removed (1.97 vs 1.96) whether unfiltered and filtered colloid was used, respectively (authors' unpublished data).

FUTURE INVESTIGATIONS

Despite the decline in false-negative rates since the introduction of SLN biopsy, much remains to be learned about the optimal techniques, learning curves, clinicopathologic predictors of nodal status, rate of non-nodal metastases based on tumor size and other characteristics, and the significance of micrometastasis. In particular, this study will provide valuable

Table 26.5 Effect of criteria for SLN removal on the false-negative rate

SLN removal criteria	False-negatives/patients with positive nodes in whom an SLN was identified	False-negative rate (%)
Only hottest node removed	27/207	13.0
Hottest node and all obviously blue nodes removed[a]	24/207	11.6
Hottest node and all blue nodes removed[a]	18/207	8.7
All blue nodes and all nodes with counts ≥10% of that of the hottest node	12/207	5.8[b]

[a]This assumes that the faintly blue and/or obviously blue nodes would have been identified without the gamma probe, or that blue-dye staining could be established prior to removing the node.
[b]Statistically significant vs only hottest node removed, $p = 0.01$.

information regarding the optimal injection technique for radioactive colloid, including peritumoral, subdermal, dermal, periareolar, and subareolar injection. The University of Louisville Sentinel Lymph Node Study is an ongoing study with an accrual of approximately 100 patients per month. It is by far the largest study of its kind, in which all patients undergo SLN biopsy followed by completion ALND. As such, it should continue to provide important information that will be helpful in refining the SLN biopsy technique, and in identifying factors that assure optimal SLN identification and minimize the false-negative rate.

REFERENCES

1. Ollila DW, Brennan MB, Giuliano AE, The role of intraoperative lymphatic mapping and sentinel lymphadenectomy in the management of patients with breast cancer. *Adv Surg* 1999; **32**:349–64.
2. Veronesi U, Paganelli G, Viale G et al, Sentinel lymph node biopsy and axillary dissection in breast cancer: results in a large series. *J Natl Cancer Inst* 1999; **91**:368–73.
3. Cody HS, Sentinel lymph node mapping in breast cancer. *Oncology* 1999; **13**:25–34.
4. Cox CE, Haddad F, Bass S et al, Lymphatic mapping in the treatment of breast cancer. *Oncology* 1998; **12**:1283–92.
5. Krag D, Weaver D, Ashikaga T et al, The sentinel node in breast cancer—a multicenter validation study. *N Engl J Med* 1998; **339**:941–6.
6. McMasters KM, Giuliano AE, Ross MI et al, Sentinel-lymph-node biopsy for breast cancer—not yet the standard of care. *N Engl J Med* 1998; **339**:990–5.
7. Hill AD, Mann GB, Borgen PI et al, Sentinel lymphatic mapping in breast cancer. *J Am Coll Surg* 1999; **188**:545–9.
8. Cox CE, Pendas S, Cox JM et al, Guidelines for sentinel node biopsy and lymphatic mapping of patients with breast cancer. *Ann Surg* 1998; **227**:645–51.
9. McMasters KM, Tuttle TM, Carlson DJ et al, Sentinel lymph node biopsy for breast cancer: a suitable alternative to routine axillary dissection in multi-institutional practice when optimal technique is used. *J Clin Oncol* 2000; **18**:2560–6.
10. McMasters KM, Wong SL, Tuttle TM et al, Preoperative lymphoscintigraphy for breast cancer does not improve the ability to identify axillary sentinel lymph nodes. *Ann Surg* 2000; **231**:724–31.
11. Martin RCG, Edwards MJ, Wong SL et al, Practical guidelines for optimal gamma probe detection of sentinel lymph nodes in breast cancer: results of a multi-institutional study. *Surgery* 2000; **128**:139–44.

27

Review of published experience

Laura Liberman and Lisa Schneider

CONTENTS Validation studies • Technique • SLN biopsy findings • Pathologic analysis of SLNs • Other issues in SLN biopsy • Conclusion

Axillary lymph-node dissection (ALND) has traditionally been part of the surgical treatment for infiltrating breast carcinoma.[1] The information obtained from ALND is an important prognostic indicator, is used to guide treatment decisions, and may provide regional control for women with axillary metastases.[1] It remains controversial, however, whether or not ALND improves survival. Also, ALND has associated morbidity, including numbness, scarring, and lymphedema. Women with small breast carcinomas, such as those detected by screening mammography, are least likely to have axillary metastases and therefore are least likely to benefit from ALND (Table 27.1).[2–9]

Sentinel lymph-node biopsy has recently

Table 27.1 Frequency of metastases (%) at conventional ALND versus tumor size

| Investigator/year | Tumor size | | | | | |
	T1a	T1b	T1c	T1	T2	T3
Carter/1989[5]				31	49	70
Cody/1991[6]				28	48	65
Silverstein/1994[7]	3	7	32	24	44	60
Mustafa/1997[8]	11	17				
Port/1998[9]	10	15				

Adapted from Liberman et al,[2] with permission. Values are all percentages. Tumor size is classified by the TNM system of the American Joint Committee on Cancer[4] according to the size of invasive carcinoma: T1a, ≤0.5 cm; T1b, >0.5–1.0 cm; T1c, >1.0–<2 cm; T2, 2–5 cm; T3, >5 cm.

been introduced into the management of women with breast carcinoma.[10-66] The sentinel lymph node (SLN) hypothesis states that the SLNs are the first nodes draining a tumor, and that the histologic status of the SLNs predicts the status of the regional nodes. The SLNs can be identified with blue dye, radioisotope, or a combination of methods, excised, and analyzed. If the SLN is correct, women with infiltrating breast carcinoma and negative SLNs may be spared the morbidity of an ALND.

VALIDATION STUDIES

The SLN biopsy procedure has been validated in over 3000 women who underwent SLN biopsy followed by ALND reported in published peer-reviewed literature (Table 27.2). In these studies, the SLNs were identified in 88% (range 69–100%) of patients. The status of the SLN accurately predicted the status of the axilla in 97% (range 94–100%) of all patients and in 93% (range 78–100%) of node-positive patients. In light of these excellent results, some surgeons have begun to offer SLN biopsy as an alternative to ALND for women with small infiltrating breast carcinomas.

TECHNIQUE

Technical parameters for SLN biopsy are not standardized. Studies differ with respect to many parameters, including labeling agent (radioisotope, blue dye, or both), volume and site of injection, and interval between injection and surgery (Tables 27.3 and 27.4). In many published series, some of these parameters are not reported.

The labeling agent: success is highest when radioisotope and blue dye are used in combination

The literature suggests that the technical success rate (i.e., frequency of identifying SLNs) is higher if radioisotope and blue dye are used in combination. Radioisotope injection allows the surgeon to localize the site of the SLN prior to making an incision, and blue dye enables the surgeon to visually identify the SLN; the combination of methods may be complementary (Table 27.5). The reported technical success rates of SLN biopsy are 91% (range 69–99%) for radioisotope alone, 80% (range 66–98%) for blue dye alone, and 91% (range 81–100%) for the combined method (see Table 27.2). In a large series using the combined method, Cody et al reported that the SLNs were identified by radioisotope only in 14% (137/966), by blue dye only in 8% (78/966), and by both methods in 707/966 (73%).[60]

There is evidence that the combination of radioisotope and blue dye can increase the sensitivity as well as the technical success of the SLN biopsy procedure. Of 126 women with tumor-containing SLNs in the study of Hill et al, the positive SLNs were identified by blue dye only in 11% (14/126), by radioisotope only in 12% (15/126), and by both blue dye and isotope in 77% (97/126).[57] Of 255 patients with tumor-containing SLNs reported by Cody et al, the positive SLNs were found by radioisotope only in 11% (28/255), by blue dye only in 11% (27/255), and by both methods in 200/255 (78%).[60] These data indicate that some positive SLNs may be either hot or blue but not both, and suggest that the combined method reduces the risk of a false-negative SLN biopsy.

Particle size: unfiltered is better than filtered technetium-99m-sulfur colloid

For methods that use radioisotope, the particle size is important: ideally, the particles must be small enough to gain access to the lymphatics but large enough to be trapped in the first draining (i.e., sentinel) node. Krag et al reported that the highest technical success was achieved with unfiltered technetium-99m-sulfur colloid (Tc-99m-SC) rather than other radioisotopes,[23] but their experience with other agents was limited: unfiltered Tc-99m-SC was used in 120 (76%) of 157 cases. Linehan et al showed that the SLN was identified in 65 (88%)

of 74 cases using unfiltered Tc-99m-SC versus 27 (66%) of 41 cases using filtered Tc-99m-SC.[62] The higher success rate with unfiltered Tc-99m-SC is probably due to most of the colloid being injected as large particles that are trapped in the SLNs. The smaller particles that are injected after filtering tend to pass through the SLNs and cause diffuse axillary activity.

Volume, site, and guidance of injection

The volume of injection may affect technical success. In a study using radioisotope methods, Krag et al found that an intraparenchymal injection volume of 8 ml (cc) or greater was significantly associated with a higher success rate,[23] and postulated that the acute expansion of the interstitial space associated with a large injection volume led to increased tracer uptake into the lymphatics.

The site of injection in the breast may also affect outcome. Blue dye is usually injected into the parenchyma (injection into the skin may cause a long-lasting blue stain), but radioisotope can be injected into the parenchyma, intradermally, or subdermally. Some investigators have suggested that the lymphatic drainage of the skin and the breast parenchyma may differ: for example, internal mammary node drainage is more frequently encountered after injection into the parenchyma rather than the skin.[61] Most existing data, however, show high concordance between SLNs identified after intraparenchymal versus intradermal injection and suggest that the intradermal method is highly accurate. It has been suggested that the high interstitial pressure of intradermal injection enhances lymphatic uptake. Furthermore, the smaller dose required for intradermal injection decreases the "blast" zone of the tumor, facilitating radioisotope localization of the SLN.

Borgstein et al reported 100% concordance in delineation of the SLN with intradermal blue dye and intramammary radioisotope in a series of 33 women.[13] Then Linehan et al compared parenchymal ($n = 100$) and intradermal ($n = 100$) injection of radioisotope.[63] Successful radioisotope localization of the SLN increased from 78% (intraparenchymal radioisotope) to 97% (intradermal radioisotope). With the addition of intraparenchymal blue dye, successful localization of the SLN increased from 92% (intraparenchymal isotope and intraparenchymal blue dye) to 100% (intradermal isotope and intraparenchymal blue dye). The same SLN was both blue and hot in 97% of the intraparenchymal radioisotope group and in 95% of the intradermal radioisotope group. In a validation study, Boolbol et al reported accuracy of 96% in 100 patients who had SLN biopsy after intradermal injection of radioisotope (0.1 mCi, 3.7 MBq) and intraparenchymal blue dye, including 46 patients with axillary metastases; among patients with T1 or T2 tumors and clinically negative nodes, the accuracy of the procedure was 100%.[64]

In previous studies, injection of labeling agent has been performed using a variety of methods, including the guidance of palpation or imaging, along a localizing wire, or beneath the skin. Krag et al found that the method of guiding radioisotope injection (palpation, mammography, or ultrasound) did not affect the technical success rate.[23] The high concordance in delineation of the SLN regardless of whether injection was intradermal or intraparenchymal suggests that there may be considerable latitude with respect to the precise site of injection of the labeling agent. Further work is necessary to clarify this issue.

Learning curve

The technical success of SLN biopsy is also affected by other factors. The success rate is higher with experience.[11,14,16,65–67] Giuliano et al reported a technical success rate for the blue-dye method of 66% in 1994 (59% in the first half and 72% in the last half),[11] which rose to 94% in a subsequent study in 1997.[14] Guenther et al, also using blue dye, identified the SLN in 12 (48%) of the first 25 cases and in 48 (80%) of the last 60 cases.[16]

Cody et al reviewed 500 consecutive SLN biopsies at Memorial Sloan-Kettering Cancer Center performed by eight surgeons.[65] They

Table 27.2 Validation studies of SLN biopsy in breast cancer

Investigator/year [ref]	Technical success rate	No. of SLNs mean [range]	Sensitivity	Specificity	PPV	NPV	Accuracy	SLN is only site of disease[a]
Radioisotope series								
Krag/1993[10]	18/22 (82)	3.4 [NS]	7/7 (100)	11/11 (100)	7/7 (100)	11/11 (100)	18/18 (100)	3/7 (43)
Pijpers/1997[17]	30/37 (81)	NS [1–3]	11/11 (100)	19/19 (100)	11/11 (100)	19/19 (100)	30/30 (100)	7/11 (64)
Roumen/1997[18]	57/83 (69)	2 [1–4]	22/23 (96)	34/34 (100)	22/22 (100)	34/35 (97)	56/57 (98)	12/23 (52)
Galimberti/1998[19]	238/241 (99)	1.4 [1–4]	109/115 (95)	123/123 (100)	109/109 (100)	123/129 (95)	232/238 (97)	39/115 (34)
Borgstein/1998[20]	122/130 (94)	1.2 [1–3]	44/45 (98)	59/59 (100)	44/44 (100)	59/60 (98)	103/104 (99)[b]	26/45 (58)
Krag/1998[23]	119/157 (76)	3.0 ± 2.0 [NS]	39/41 (95)	78/78 (100)	39/39 (100)	78/80 (98)	117/119 (98)	23/41 (56)
Offodile/1998[25]	40/41 (98)	3.0 [1–7]	18/18 (100)	22/22 (100)	18/18 (100)	22/22 (100)	40/40 (100)	NS
Crossin/1998[27]	42/50 (84)	2.0 [1–7]	7/8 (88)	34/34 (100)	7/7 (100)	34/35 (97)	41/42 (98)	NS
Krag/1998[28]	405/443 (91)	1.1 [1–3][c]	101/114 (89)	291/291 (100)	101/101 (100)	291/304 (96)	392/405 (97)	60/114 (53)
Snider/1998[29]	70/80 (88)	2.2 [1–5]	13/14 (93)	56/56 (100)	13/13 (100)	56/57 (98)	69/70 (99)	7/14 (50)
Miner/1998[24]	41/42 (98)	3 [NS]	7/8 (88)	33/33 (100)	7/7 (100)	33/34 (97)	40/41 (98)	4/8 (50)
Rubio/1998[31]	53/55 (96)	NS [1–4]	15/17 (88)	36/36 (100)	15/15 (100)	36/38 (95)	51/53 (96)	9/17 (53)
Gulec/1998[38]	30/32 (94)	2.5 (1–6)	8/8 (100)	22/22 (100)	8/8 (100)	22/22 (100)	30/30 (100)	5/8 (63)
Veronesi/1999[44]	371/376 (99)	1.4 [1–4]	168/180 (93)	191/191 (100)	168/168 (100)	191/203 (94)	359/371 (97)	70/180 (39)
Feldman/1999[43]	70/75 (93)	2.2 ±1.5	17/21 (81)	49/49 (100)	17/17 (100)	49/53 (92)	66/70 (94)	7/21 (33)
Moffat/1999[46]	62/70 (89)	4.1 ± 2.9 [1–12]	18/20 (90)	42/42 (100)	18/18 (100)	42/44 (95)	60/62 (97)	14/20 (70)
SUBTOTAL	*1768/1934 (91)*	*1.7 [1–7]*	*604/650 (93)*	*1100/1100 (100)*	*604/604 (100)*	*1100/1146 (96)*	*1704/1750 (97)*	*286/624 (46)*
Blue-dye series								
Giuliano/1994[11]	114/174 (66)	1.7 [NS]	37/42 (88)	72/72 (100)	37/37 (100)	72/77 (94)	109/114 (96)	16/42 (38)
Giuliano/1997[14]	100/107 (93)	1.8 [1–8]	42/42 (100)	58/58 (100)	42/42 (100)	58/58 (100)	100/100 (100)	28/42 (67)
Guenther/1997[16]	103/145 (71)	1.6 [NS][d]	28/31 (90)	72/72 (100)	28/28 (100)	72/75 (96)	100/103 (97)	12/31 (39)
Flett/1998[26]	56/68 (82)	1.2 [NS]	15/18 (83)	38/38 (100)	15/15 (100)	38/41 (93)	53/56 (95)	5/18 (28)
Koller/1998[30]	96/98 (98)	2.7 ± 1.2	48/51 (94)	45/45 (100)	48/48 (100)	45/48 (94)	93/96 (97)	13/51 (25)
Kapteijn/1998[34]	26/30 (87)	1.4 [1–3]	10/10 (100)	16/16 (100)	10/10 (100)	16/16 (100)	26/26 (100)	6/10 (60)
Imoto/1999[41]	65/88 (74)	2.0 [1–7]	25/29 (86)	36/36 (100)	25/25 (100)	36/40 (90)	61/65 (94)	9/29 (31)
Ratanawichitrasin/1998[40]	35/40 (88)	1.6 ± 0.8	7/9 (78)	26/26 (100)	7/7 (100)	26/28 (93)	33/35 (94)	3/9 (33)
Dale/1998[39]	14/20 (70)	1.2 [NS]	5/5 (100)	9/9 (100)	5/5 (100)	9/9 (100)	14/14 (100)	3/5 (60)
Kern/1999[47]	39/40 (98)	2 ± 1.5 [1–7]	15/15 (100)	24/24 (100)	15/15 (100)	24/24 (100)	39/39 (100)	7/15 (47)
Morgan/1999[48]	32/44 (73)	1.1 [1–2]	10/12 (83)	20/20 (100)	10/10 (100)	20/22 (91)	30/32 (94)	6/12 (50)
Morrow/1999[49]	110/139 (79)	1.8 [1–6]	28/32 (88)	78/78 (100)	28/28 (100)	78/82 (95)	106/110 (96)	12/32 (38)
SUBTOTAL	*790/993 (80)*	*1.8 [1–8]*	*270/296 (91)*	*494/494 (100)*	*270/270 (100)*	*494/520 (95)*	*764/790 (97)*	*120/296 (41)*

Radioisotope + blue-dye series

Study	Technical success rate	No. of SLNs	Sensitivity	Specificity	PPV	NPV	Accuracy	[a]
Albertini/1996[12]	57/62 (92)	2.2 [NS]	18/18 (100)	39/39 (100)	18/18 (100)	39/39 (100)	57/57 (100)	12/18 (67)
Borgstein/1997[13]	33/33 (100)	NS	14/14 (100)	11/11 (100)	14/14 (100)	11/11 (100)	25/25 (100)	9/14 (64)
O'Hea/1998[21]	55/59 (93)	2.2 [1-8]	17/20 (85)	35/35 (100)	17/17 (100)	35/38 (92)	52/55 (95)	7/20 (35)
Barnwell/1998[22]	38/42 (90)	1 [1-3][e]	15/15 (100)	23/23 (100)	15/15 (100)	23/23 (100)	38/38 (100)	5/15 (33)
Nwariaku/1998[36]	96/119 (81)	1.8 ± 0.9	26/27 (96)	69/69 (100)	26/26 (100)	69/70 (99)	95/96 (99)	18/27 (67)
Schneebaum/1998[35]	28/30 (93)	NS	11/13 (85)	15/15 (100)	11/11 (100)	15/17 (88)	26/28 (93)	1/13 (8)
Canavese/1998[37]	96/100 (96)	1.3 [NS]	28/33 (85)	63/63 (100)	28/28 (100)	63/68 (93)	91/96 (95)	8/23 (35)[f]
Czerniecki/1999[45]	41/43 (95)	2.6 [1-7]	15/15 (100)	26/26 (100)	15/15 (100)	26/26 (100)	41/41 (100)	7/15 (47)
van der Ent/1999[42]	70/70 (100)	2.6 [NS]	26/27 (96)	43/43 (100)	26/26 (100)	43/44 (98)	69/70 (99)	14/27 (52)
Bass/1999[50]	173/186 (93)	NS	53/54 (98)	119/119 (100)	53/53 (100)	119/120 (99)	172/173 (99)	NS
Burak/1999[51]	45/50 (90)	1.7 [1-5]	14/14 (100)	31/31 (100)	14/14 (100)	31/31 (100)	45/45 (100)	8/14 (57)
Jaderborg/1999[52]	64/79 (81)	1.9 ± 1.2 [1-6]	19/20 (95)	44/44 (100)	19/19 (100)	44/45 (98)	63/64 (98)	14/20 (70)
SUBTOTAL	*796/873 (91)*	*2.0 [1-8]*	*256/270 (95)*	*518/518 (100)*	*256/256 (100)*	*518/532 (97)*	*774/788 (98)*	*103/206 (50)*
TOTAL	**3354/3800 (88)**	**1.8 [1-8]**	**1130/1216 (93)**	**2112/2112 (100)**	**1130/1130 (100)**	**2111/2198 (96)**	**3242/3328 (97)**	**509/1126 (45)**

Adapted from Liberman et al,[2] with permission. Numbers in parentheses are percentages.
Technical success rate: proportion of patients in whom SLNs were found at surgery.
Sensitivity: proportion of patients with axillary metastases in whom the SLNs contain tumor (true positive/[true positive + false negative]).
Specificity: proportion of patients without axillary metastases in whom the SLNs are free of tumor (true negative/[true negative + false positive]).
Positive predictive value (PPV): proportion of patients with tumor in SLNs in whom the axilla contains tumor (true positive/[true positive + false positive]).
Negative predictive value (NPV): proportion of patients without tumor in SLNs in whom the axilla is free of tumor (true negative/[true negative + false negative]).
Accuracy: proportion of patients with successful SLNB in whom the status of the SLN correlated with the status of the axilla ([true positive] + true negative/[true positive + true negative + false positive + false negative]).
[a]Indicates the proportion of women with axillary metastases in whom the SLNs were the only nodes containing tumor.
[b]Data refer to women who had successful SLNB and consented to undergo ALND.
[c]Refers to number of hot spots (mean and range); an SLN was found underneath the hot spot in 405/413 (98%) women.
[d]Mean number of SLNs in women with histologically positive axillae. The mean number of SLNs in women with negative axillae was not reported.
[e]Median number of SLNs (mean not reported).
SLN, sentinel lymph node; NS, not stated.

Table 27.3 Nuclear medicine protocols for SLN biopsy

Investigator/year	Agent	Particle size	Isotope injection site	Counts (mCi)	Volume (ml)	Interval to surgery	Definition of SLN
Radioisotope series							
Krag/1993[10]	Tc-99m-SC	NS	Peritumoral[a]	0.4	0.5	NS	Counts per 10 s ≥30 prior to incision or ≥25 ex vivo in resected specimen
Veronesi/1997[15]	Tc-99m-CA	50–200 nm	Subdermal	0.1–0.3	0.2	1 d	Guided by acoustic signal
Pijpers/1997[17]	Tc-99m-CA	3–80 nm; 77 ± 12% <30 nm	Peritumoral[b]	1.1	4	22 ± 2 h	All radioactive lymph nodes
Roumen/1997[18]	Tc-99m-CA	NS	Peritumoral	1.6	2	>4 or >18 h	Guided by acoustic signal
Galimberti/1998[19]	Tc-99m	NS	Subdermal	0.14–0.3	NS	1 d	NS; 10–2000 counts/s
Borgstein/1998[20]	Tc-99m-CA	NS	Peritumoral[c]	1.1	4	23 ± 2 h	Lymph nodes with highest tracer content were considered SLNs; nodes with <50% of maximum count rate were non-SLNs
Krag/1998[23]	Tc-99m-SC (n = 133) Other (n = 24)[d]	Tc-99m-SC filtered in 120, unfiltered in 13	Peritumoral[e]	≥1 (n = 119) <1 (n = 38)	≥8 (n = 29) 3–8 (n = 85) ≤3 (n = 43)	<1 h (n = 11) 1–3 h (n = 44) >3 h (n = 63)	Discrete area of radiolocalization separate from the injection site with a count of at least 25 per 10 s (preincision)
Offodile/1998[25]	Tc-99m-Dextran	NS	Peritumoral[f]	1	0.5	NS	Used gamma detector probe
Crossin/1998[27]	Tc-99m-SC	NS	Peritumoral[g]	1	4	1–4 h	Areas separate from injection sites with >25 counts per 10 s

Study/Year	Radiocolloid	Size/Filter	Injection site			Time	Definition of sentinel lymph node
Krag/1998[28]	Tc-99m-SC	NS	Peritumoral[g]	1	4	30 min–8 h	Area of localized radioactivity separate from injection site with counts ≥25 per 10 s
Snider/1998[29]	Tc-99m-SC	Filtered	Peritumoral	1	4	45–310 min (mean, 97 min)	The count in the bed of the resected hot spot was <10% of sum of activity in excised SLNs
De Cicco/1998[32]	Tc-99m-HSA (n = 182) Other (n = 100)[h]	0.2–1 μm	Peritumoral or subdermal	0.3	0.3	1 d	Node with highest radioactivity
Miner/1998[24]	Tc-99m-SC	Unfiltered	Peritumoral	1	4	1–9 h (median, 3.5 h)	"Hot spots": >25 counts per 10 s and target/background ratio >3:1
Gulec/1998[38]	Tc-99m-SC	Unfiltered	Peritumoral	1	4	NS	Focus of increased radioactivity with a 10-s count of ≥25, and >3 times counts of adjacent normal skin
Veronesi/1999[44]	Tc-99m-CA[i]	200–1000 nm	Peritumoral or subdermal	0.14–0.27	0.2	1 d (usually 14–20 h)	The radioactive lymph node
Feldman/1999[43]	Tc-99m-SC	NS	Peritumoral	1	4	0.5–7.25 h	Discrete area of radioisotope uptake separate from injection site, counts per 10 s >25 and clearly higher than background counts
Rubio/1998[31]	Tc-99m-SC	NS	Peritumoral	1	4	0.5–6 h	Areas of radiolocalization separate from injection site with ≥25 counts per 10 s

Table 27.3 (continued)

Investigator/year	Agent	Particle size	Isotope injection site	Counts (mCi)	Volume (ml)	Interval to surgery	Definition of SLN
Moffat/1999[46]	Tc-99m-SC	Unfiltered	Peritumoral	1	4 (n = 61) 8 (n = 9)	≤8 h	All specimens with at least 10% of ex vivo count of hottest specimen
Radioisotope and blue-dye series							
Albertini/1996[12]	Tc-99m-SC	Filtered	Peritumoral	0.43	NS	2–4 h	Nodes that had SLN/non-SLN ratios >10
Borgstein/1997[13]	Tc-99m-CA	NS	Peritumoral	1.1	NS	NS	Scintigraphic foci
O'Hea/1998[21]	Tc-99m-SC	Unfiltered	Peritumoral[g]	0.3	4	NS	Counts taken of node in situ and ex vivo, seeking >4-fold reduction in axillary counts
Barnwell/1998[22]	Tc-99m-SC	Filtered (0.22 μm)	Peritumoral[g]	1	4[e]	60–90 min	Areas of colloid concentration using the gamma detector
Nwariaku/1998[36]	Tc-99m-SC	NS	Peritumoral	NS	NS	NS	NS
Schneebaum/1998[35]	Tc-99m-rhenium colloid	NS	NS	1.6	NS	Usually 24 h	Counts taken in vivo and ex vivo to verify that the right node had been removed
Canavese/1998[37]	Tc-99m-MS or HSA	MS <50 nm; HSA 200–1000 nm	Peritumoral	0.3	0.2	6–18 h	Node with node/background ratio >5 in vivo and >10 ex vivo
Czerniecki/1999[45]	Tc-99m-SC or -CA	Tc-99m-SC filtered (0.22 μm)	Peritumoral	2	6–8	3–14 h	In vivo counts ≥3 times counts of negative lymph nodes or fat

Study/year	Radioisotope	Filter	Injection site	Dose (mCi)	No. of injections	Time to surgery	Comments
van der Ent/1999[42]	Tc-99m-nanocolloid	NS	Peritumoral	10	4	<1 d (injected late afternoon the d before surgery)	Gamma probe was used; if remaining activity was <10% of most active SN, no additional SLNs were believed to exist
Bass/1999[50]	Tc-99m-SC	Filtered (0.22 μm)	Peritumoral	0.45	6	2 h	NS
Burak/1999[51]	Tc-99m-SC	Filtered (0.22 μm)	Peritumoral	0.1	4	>2 h	Ex vivo counts of excised node were ≥twice that of surrounding fat
Jaderborg/1999[52]	Tc-99m-SC	NS	Peritumoral	0.25–0.4	2–6	>2 h	Gamma probe was used.

Adapted from Liberman et al,[2] with permission.

NS, not stated; SC, sulfur colloid; CA, colloidal albumin; HSA, human serum albumin; MS, microcolloid sulfide; SLN, sentinel lymph node; Tc, technetium.

[a]5 0.1-cc injections along a 180-degree perimeter on axillary side of tumor.

[b]In 2–4 aliquots in axillary peritumoral hemisphere.

[q]In 2–4 aliquots around tumor.

[d]Other radioisotopes included Microlite ($n = 11$), Cardiolite ($n = 7$), Dextran 40 ($n = 40$), and HSA ($n = 2$).

[e]In 4 equal aliquots around tumor; for nonpalpable lesions, injection performed under mammographic or sonographic guidance.

[f]For nonpalpable lesions, solution was injected during localization under stereotactic guidance.

[g]In 4 aliquots at 12, 3, 6, and 9 o'clock positions around tumor.

[r]Tc-99m-antimony sulfide colloids, <50 nm ($n = 50$); colloidal particles of HSA <80 nm ($n = 50$); 54 patients also had 3 ml isosulfan blue dye injected immediately after excision of primary tumor.

[s]54 of 376 patients also had blue dye injected 5 min before surgery, subdermally or peritumorally.

Table 27.4 Blue-dye protocols for SLN biopsy

Investigator/year	Agent	Volume (ml)	Blue-dye injection site	No. of injection sites	Compression/massage	Interval to surgery
Blue-dye series						
Giuliano/1994[11]	Isosulfan blue	0.5–10 (first 20 cases) 3–5 (subsequent 154 cases)	Into/surrounding mass or in biopsy cavity wall)	Several	NS	1–20 min (first 20 cases) 5 min (subsequent 154 cases)
Giuliano/1997[14]	Isosulfan blue	3–5	Peritumoral or biopsy cavity wall and surrounding tissue	Same as above	NS	5 min
Guenther/1997[16]	Isosulfan blue	3–5	Peritumoral (tumor-breast interface) or in biopsy cavity wall	NS	Yes, 3–5 min	3–5 min; if no node seen, waited up to 10 min
Flett/1998[26]	Patent Blue-V	2–4	Peritumoral	NS	NS	5–10 min
Koller/1998[30]	Methylene blue or Patent Blue-V	3–5	Subcutaneous	NS	NS	10 min
Kaptejn/1998[34]	Patent blue	1	Into the tumor	3 injections from different angles	NS	"Immediately afterwards"
Imoto/1999[41]	Indigocarmine blue	4–5	Subcutaneous	2–3 sites	"the breast lesions were rubbed well"	15 min
Ratanawichitrasin/1998[40]	Isosulfan blue	3–5	Peritumoral	6–10 (in 0.5 quantities)	"injection site was gently compressed for a few minutes"	Within 20 min
Dale/1998[39]	Isosulfan blue	3–5	Peritumoral	4 sites	NS	Within 15 min
Kern/1999[47]	Isosulfan blue	5	Subareolar	NS	Yes, 1–2 min	1–2 min
Morgan/1999[48]	Isosulfan blue	4–6	Peritumoral	NS	NS	5 min
Morrow/1999[49]	Isosulfan blue[a]	5	Peritumoral	NS	Yes, 5 min	5 min
Radioisotope and blue-dye series						
Albertini/1996[12]	Isosulfan blue	NS	Peritumoral (palpable) Around localizing wire (nonpalpable)	NS	NS	10–15 min
Borgstein/1997[13]	Patent Blue-V	0.5	Intradermal	NS	NS	"Directly before surgery"
O'Hea/1998[21]	Isosulfan blue	4	Peritumoral	4 sites	NS	5–10 min
Barnwell/1998[22]	Isosulfan blue	4 (3 cc dye, 1 cc isotope)	Peritumoral	4 sites	NS	60–90 min
Nwariaku/1998[36]	Isosulfan blue	3–4	Subcutaneous	NS	NS	"Intraoperative"
Schneebaum/1998[35]	Patent Blue-V	2	NS	NS	NS	10 min
Canavese/1998[37]	Patent Blue-V	1–2	Subdermal (n = 76), peritumoral (n = 11)	NS	NS	Intraoperative
Czerniecki/1999[45]	Isosulfan blue	4–8	Peritumoral	NS	NS	Intraoperative
van der Ent/1999[42]	Patent Blue-V	0.5–0.8	Intradermal[b]	NS	NS	Intraoperative
Bass/1999[50]	Isosulfan blue	5	NS	NS	Yes, 5 min	5 min
Burak/1999[51]	Isosulfan blue	4–5	Peritumoral	4 sites or 1 (through localization needle)	NS	5–10 min
Jaderborg/1999[52]	Isosulfan blue	2–5	Peritumoral	NS	NS	Intraoperative

Adapted from Liberman et al,[2] with permission.

NS, not stated.

[a]42 of 139 patients also received intraparenchymal injection of radioisotope 1.4–7.8 h before surgery.

[b]Protocol was injection of 1–2 cc Patent Blue-V dye peritumorally in first 12 cases, but SLNs were found in only 2; protocol was then modified as shown here.

Table 27.5 Complementarity of radioisotope and blue dye in studies using combined method

Investigator/year	Technical success rate		
	Radioisotope	Blue dye	Radioisotope + blue dye
Albertini/1996[12]	NS	45/62 (73)	57/62 (92)
Borgstein/1997[13]	33/33 (100)	33/33 (100)	33/33 (100)
O'Hea/1998[21]	52/59 (88)	44/59 (75)	55/59 (93)
Barnwell/1998[22]	37/42 (88)	9/42 (21)	38/42 (90)
Van der Ent/1999[42]	68/70 (97)	2/70 (3)	70/70 (100)
Hill/1999[57]	393/492 (80)	419/492 (85)	458/492 (93)
Bass/1999[50]	631/700 (90)	533/700 (76)	665/700 (95)
Cody/2001[60]	844/966 (87)	785/966 (81)	922/966 (95)

Adapted from Liberman et al,[2] with permission. Numbers in parentheses are percentages.
NS, not stated.

found that the procedures performed by the more experienced surgeons were associated with a higher success rate (94%) than those performed by less experienced surgeons (86%). There were 10 failed mapping procedures in the first 100 cases. For each of the ensuing 100 cases, there were 8, 6, 6, and 4 failed mapping procedures, suggesting that experience diminishes but does not eradicate the likelihood of technical failure. Experience can also lower the false-negative rate. Among the 104 patients who had SLN biopsy with planned "backup" ALND, the false-negative rate was 10.6%. When the first 6 cases of every surgeon were eliminated, the false-negative rate fell to 5.2%; eliminating the first 15 cases of each surgeon reduced the false-negative rate to 2%.

The largest learning curve experience with SLN biopsy was reported by Cox et al.[66] In 1355 cases performed by six surgeons at one center, an average of 22 cases was needed to achieve at least a 90% success rate for finding an axillary SLN, and 54 cases were needed to achieve a 96% success rate. Success rates as a function of number of cases performed were: 1 or 2 per month, success 81.8 ± 0.1%; 2 to 6 per month, success 89.8 ± 0.1%; more than 6 per month,

97.4 ± 0.004%. These findings support the importance of using "backup" ALND early in one's experience with SLN biopsy.

Prior surgical biopsy and other factors

In order to identify the SLNs, the lymphatic pathways that drain the tumor must take up the labeling agent. Lymphatic drainage pathways can be disrupted by surgical biopsy. It has therefore been suggested that prior surgical excision may lower the success rate and accuracy of SLN biopsy,[12,20] and some studies of SLN biopsy have excluded women with prior surgical biopsy.[12,15,17,19] Krag et al reported a significantly higher frequency of failure to identify a "hot spot" in women who had prior surgical biopsy when compared with women who had percutaneous breast biopsy or no previous biopsy (odds ratio 7.1; 95% confidence interval, 2.17–23.3).[28] Borgstein et al also noted a statistically lower likelihood of successful SLN biopsy in women who had prior surgical excision.[20] Most investigators, however, have found no significant difference in the technical success rate of SLN mapping in women who did or

Table 27.6 Impact of prior biopsy technique on success of SLN biopsy		
Investigator/year	**Success rate after excisional biopsy**	**Success rate without prior excisional biopsy**
Radioisotope series		
Krag/1993[10]	7/8 (88)	11/14 (79)*
Veronesi/1997[15]	NA	160/163 (98)
Pijpers/1997[17]	NA	30/37 (81)
Galimberti/1998[19]	NA	238/241 (99)
Borgstein/1998[20]	16/22 (73)	106/108 (98)**
Krag/1998[28]	40/54 (74)	79/103 (77)*
Feldman/1999[43]	43/48 (90)	9/9 (100)*
Blue-dye series		
Imoto/1999[41]	8/12 (67)	57/76 (75)*
Kern/1999[47]	8/9 (89)	31/31 (100)*
Radioisotope + blue dye		
Albertini/1996[12]	NA	57/62 (92)
O'Hea/1998[21]	33/35 (94)	22/24 (92)*
Barnwell/1998[22]	20/21 (95)	18/21 (86)*
Cox/1998[a][56]	216/227 (95)	180/195 (92)*
Czerniecki/1999[45]	18/19 (95)	23/24 (96)*
van der Ent/1999[42]	35/36 (97)	33/34 (97)*

Adapted from Liberman et al,[2] with permission. Numbers in parentheses are percentages.
*p value was not significant.
**$p < 0.001$.
[a]A clinical study with 422 evaluable patients, not all of whom had correlative ALND.
NA, not applicable; women who had prior excisional biopsy were excluded.

did not have prior surgical biopsy (Table 27.6).[10,22,23,25,46]

Other factors suggested to be associated with technical failure of SLN biopsy included age greater than 50 years[28] or 60 years,[60] medial tumor location,[28] and negative lymphoscintigram.[60]

Lymphoscintigraphic imaging

Published studies that have used lymphoscintigraphic (LSG) imaging have reported LSG visualization of SLNs in 69–99% of cases (Table 27.7).[13,15,17–21] The wide variability in results probably reflects the different protocols used, including the radioisotope employed, the site of injection, and the interval between injection and imaging.

Although SLNs can be identified by the gamma probe after radioisotope injection even without obtaining LSG images, LSG has several potential advantages. First, visualization of SLNs on the lymphoscintigram is strongly predictive of a successful SLN biopsy: Cody et al found that a positive lymphoscintigram was statistically significantly ($p < 0.0005$) associated with technical success in both univariate and

Table 27.7 Lymphoscintigraphic imaging of the SLN		
Investigator/year	Interval to LSG	Success of LSG
Veronesi/1997[15]	15, 30, 180 min	160/163 (98)
Pijpers/1997[17]	2 h	33/37 (89)
	18 h	34/37 (92)
Roumen/1997[18]	4 h or 18 h	57/83 (69)
Galimberti/1998[19]	NS	238/241 (99)
Borgstein/1998[20]	2 h and 18 h	116/130 (89)
De Cicco/1998[32]	15–30 min, 3 h, and immediately before surgery (if no activity seen)	245/250 (98)
Veronesi/1999[44]	NS	371/376 (99)
Borgstein/1997[13]	NS	30/33 (91)
O'Hea/1998[21]	50–60 min	42/56 (75)
Nwariaku/1998[36]	NS	NS
Schneebaum/1998[35]	20 min, 2 h, 6 h, and 24 h	28/30 (93)
Canavese/1998[37]	10 min, then q15 min to maximum 2 h	NS
Czerniecki/1999[45]	1–2 h	31/44 (70)
van der Ent/1999[42]	16 h	68/70 (97)
Burak/1999[51]	30 min, ≥2 h	17/24 (71)
Jaderborg/1999[52]	Immediately after, then 2 h	NS

Adapted from Liberman et al,[2] with permission. Numbers in parentheses are percentages.
NS, not stated.

multivariate models.[60] In addition, LSG can alert the surgeon preoperatively to the presence of multiple SLNs and/or less common lymphatic pathways, such as drainage to the internal mammary region. The optimal protocol for and the role of preoperative LSG in SLN biopsy deserves further investigation.

SENTINEL LYMPH-NODE BIOPSY FINDINGS

Number of SLNs

Sentinel lymph-node biopsy often results in the removal of more than one SLN (see Table 27.2). The mean number of SLNs removed is 1.7 (range 1–7) for studies using radioisotope, 1.8 (range 1–8) for studies using blue dye, and 2.0 (range 1–8) for studies using a combination of both methods. Some investigators who have used a combination of radioisotope and blue dye suggest that more nodes are found with the combination technique than with either method individually: Albertini et al reported that use of the gamma probe compared with using just the blue-dye technique increased the mean number of SLNs removed from 1.2 to 2.2 per patient.[12]

Location of SLNs

Although most SLNs are found in Level I of the axilla, investigators have reported SLNs outside of Level I in 6% to 37% of women (Table 27.8).[12–14,25] In a multi-institutional study of SLN biopsy using radioisotope with correlative ALND, Krag et al reported that 89% of 445 "hot spots" in women who had SLN biopsy were in

Table 27.8 Location of SLNs

Investigator/year	No. of women with SLNs in Level I only	No. of women with SLNs outside of Level I only	No. of women with SLNs in and outside of Level I
Krag/1993[10]	22/22 (100)	0 (0)	0 (0)
Roumen/1997[18]	40/57 (70)	10/57 (18)[a]	7/57 (12)[b]
Krag/1998[28]	112/119 (94)	7/119 (6)[c]	0 (0)
Giuliano/1994[11]	27/43 (63)	10/43 (23)[a]	6/43 (14)[d]
Imoto/1999[41]	65/65 (100)	0 (0)	0 (0)
Albertini/1996[12]	50/57 (88)	7/57 (12)[a]	0 (0)
Borgstein/1998[20]	122/122 (100)[e]	NS[e]	NS[e]
Jaderborg/1999[52]	57/64 (89)	3/64 (5)[a]	4/64 (6)[d]

Adapted from Liberman et al,[2] with permission. Numbers in parentheses are percentages. NS, not stated.
[a]Level II.
[b]Axillary and internal mammary nodes.
[c]Internal mammary nodes, excised through small (<2 cm) incision.
[d]Level I & II.
[e]Lymphoscintigraphy showed internal mammary nodes in 21/130 (16%) patients, not considered SLNs and not excised; in two of these, drainage was exclusively to internal mammary nodes.

Level I; the rest were in the internal mammary region (4%), Level II (4%), or elsewhere.[28] Published literature prior to the advent of SLN biopsy indicated the frequency of "skip" metastases (axillary metastases in Level II or elsewhere with no evidence of metastases in Level I) to be 10–12%;[54] in fact, these "skip" metastases are likely to represent SLNs outside of Level I. Sentinel lymph-node mapping can identify these variations of lymphatic drainage and is therefore preferable to axillary "sampling" or Level I ALND for assessment of the axilla. If radioisotope methods are used, the gamma probe (with or without LSG) can alert the surgeon to the possibility of an unusual location for the SLN (i.e., Level II or the internal mammary chain) prior to making an incision.

Few data address the issue of internal mammary lymph nodes at SLN biopsy. While Albertini et al stated that internal mammary SLNs could not be localized adequately because of interference from the activity around the site of the primary tumor,[12] Krag et al found and excised internal mammary SLNs in 6 (5%) of 119 patients.[23] Cody and Urban reported internal mammary metastases in 20% of T1N0 lesions in a highly selected group of women (many with medial lesions) who underwent radical mastectomy and internal mammary dissection in the period 1965–1978; internal mammary node metastases were associated with worse disease-free and overall survival rates.[68] Although internal mammary node status is a prognostic indicator, it rarely affects treatment. At our institution, chemotherapy is given to women with tumors measuring over 1 cm and for women with tumor in axillary nodes. Therefore, a positive internal mammary node would only affect the treatment decision for women with subcentimeter carcinomas and negative axillary nodes. The assessment of internal mammary nodes at SLN biopsy should be addressed in future work.

Frequency of carcinoma in sentinel versus nonsentinel lymph nodes

The SLNs are the nodes most likely to contain metastases. Weaver et al reported the results of final pathology review from 431 patients enrolled in a multicenter validation study of SLN biopsy.[54] Metastases were identified in 15.9% of SLNs and in 4.2% of non-SLNs (odds ratio 4.3, $p < 0.001$; 95% CI, 3.5–5.4). Occult metastases (all measuring 1 mm or less) were found in 4.1% of SLNs and in 0.4% of non-SLNs (odds ratio 12.3, $p < 0.001$; 95% CI, 5.6–28.6). The likelihood (odds ratio) of metastases in non-SLNs was 13.4 times higher for SLN-positive than for SLN-negative patients.

Validation studies have reported that in approximately 45% of women with tumor in SLNs, ALND revealed tumor in non-SLNs (see Table 27.2). For women with tumor in sentinel nodes, the likelihood of finding tumor in non-SLNs is greater in tumors that are larger (e.g., T3 as opposed to T1 or T2 tumors),[23] have a greater tumor burden in the SLNs,[23,28] or have lymphovascular invasion.[69]

There has been interest in identifying a subgroup of women with SLN metastases in whom the likelihood of non-SLN metastases is low enough that ALND can be safely avoided. Among 206 patients with SLN metastases who had ALND, Weiser et al reported that the frequency of non-SLN metastases was dependent on

1. tumor size: 8% (1/12) for T1a, 21% (9/43) for T1b, 31% (30/97) for T1c, and 48% (26/54) for T2 tumors ($p = 0.007$)
2. SLN metastasis size: 18% (17/93) for micrometastasis ≤ 2 mm and 45% (48/107) for macrometastasis >2 mm ($p < 0.001$)
3. lymphovascular invasion: 26% (32/124) if absent and 41% (33/80) if present ($p = 0.021$).[69]

No metastasis was observed in the non-SLNs in 24 T1a,b patients with SLN micrometastasis and no lymphovascular invasion: this may represent a subgroup in whom ALND can be avoided.[69] Further work is necessary to confirm these findings.

PATHOLOGIC ANALYSIS OF SLNs

Standard ALND involves removal of as many as 20 or more lymph nodes, with conventional histologic analysis limited to one or a small number of paraffin hematoxylin-and-eosin (H&E) sections obtained per lymph node. Because SLN biopsy identifies the nodes most likely to be involved with tumor, the procedure allows the pathologist to focus intensive scrutiny on the few nodes with the highest yield.[70–73] Although protocols for pathologic analysis of SLNs vary, the data suggest that frozen-section analysis and immunohistochemistry (IHC) may be useful. Because fewer nodes are removed at SLN biopsy, the cost of frozen-section analysis and IHC is less than it would be if these techniques were applied to the larger number of nodes removed at conventional ALND.

Intraoperative frozen-section analysis of SLNs

Frozen-section analysis, rarely used in ALND, may be valuable in SLN biopsy because the results influence intraoperative management: a positive frozen-section finding in an SLN may lead to immediate ALND, sparing the need for a separate procedure at a later date. In the published literature, the sensitivity of frozen-section analysis of SLNs ranges from 42% to 100% (Table 27.9).

The largest experience with intraoperative frozen-section analysis of SLNs was reported by Weiser et al in a study of 890 patients with invasive breast cancer.[74] Sentinel lymph-node metastases were present in 231 of 890 (26%) lesions, including 15 of 143 (10%) T1a, 50 of 249 (20%) T1b, 108 of 379 (28%) T1c, and 58 of 119 (49%) T2 lesions. Frozen-section analysis identified 135 of 231 (58%) women with SLN metastases, including 6 of 15 (40%) with T1a, 25 of 50 (50%) with T1b, 59 of 108 (55%) with T1c, and 45 of 58 (78%) with T2 carcinomas. By identifying tumor in SLNs on the day of the SLN biopsy, frozen-section analysis spared reoperation in 135 of 890 (15%) women in the study, including 6 of 143 (4%) with T1a, 25 of 249 (10%) with T1b, 59 of 379 (16%) with T1c, and 45 of 119 (38%) with T2 carcinomas.

More extensive intraoperative evaluation can

Table 27.9 Frozen-section analysis of SLNs: published experience

Investigator/year	Frozen-section sensitivity	Frozen-section specificity	Frozen-section accuracy
Radioisotope series			
Veronesi/1997[15]	32/50 (64)[a]	57/57 (100)	89/107 (83)
Galimberti/1998[19]	53/76 (70)	105/105 (100)	158/181 (87)
Veronesi/1999[44]	55/81 (68)[a]	111/111 (100)	166/192 (86)
Veronesi/1999[44]	52/52 (100)[b]	67/67 (100)	119/119 (100)
Blue-dye series			
Flett/1998[26]	12/15 (80)[c]	41/41 (100)	53/56 (95)
Imoto/1999[41]	8/11 (73)	24/24 (100)	32/35 (91)
Morgan/1999[48]	5/12 (42)	20/20 (100)	25/32 (78)
Radioisotope + blue-dye series			
Schneebaum/1998[35]	10/11 (91)	36/36 (100)	46/47 (98)
Canavese/1998[37]	24/28 (86)	68/68 (100)	92/96 (96)
Weiser/2001[69]	135/231 (58)	659/659 (100)	794/890 (89)

Numbers in parentheses are percentages. Except for the study of Schneebaum et al, sensitivity is defined as the proportion of women with SLN metastases in whom frozen-section analysis revealed tumor in SLNs; specificity is defined as the proportion of women without SLN metastases in whom the SLNs were free of tumor; and accuracy is the proportion of women in whom frozen-section analysis diagnosis of SLNs accurately predicted final SLN histology. In the study of Schneebaum et al, the sensitivity, specificity, and accuracy reflect proportions of SLNs, not women.
[a]Frozen-section protocol was to bisect the node, freeze half, and obtain at least three serial sections.
[b]"Exhaustive intraoperative frozen section": 15 pairs of frozen sections (4 μm thick cut at 50 μm intervals) from each half node: i.e., 30 sections/half node, or 60/node. One section of each pair was stained with H&E; if this was negative or doubtful, the other was examined with a rapid staining method for cytokeratins.
[c]In three women with positive SLNs at final analysis, frozen section was interpreted as "suspicious" in two and "negative" in one.

increase the sensitivity of frozen-section analysis. Veronesi et al reported the sensitivity of frozen-section analysis at detecting SLN metastases was 55/81 (68%) with conventional methods (node bisection followed by freezing half of the node and examining at least three serial sections) and 52/52 (100%) with "exhaustive intraoperative frozen section" (approximately 60 sections per lymph node in conjunction with a rapid staining method for cytokeratin).[44] The investigators stated that the "exhaustive" procedure took 40–50 minutes, during which surgery on the breast was completed.

Frozen-section analysis of SLNs has three potential disadvantages. First, frozen-section analysis could, in theory, lead to delays in the operating room. These intraoperative delays can be averted by performing the SLN biopsy first; while the SLNs are being analyzed by frozen section, the surgeon can proceed with the definitive breast surgery, as in the study of Veronesi et al.[44] A second theoretical disadvantage of frozen-section analysis is the possibility of a false-positive result; however, none has been reported in the literature (to our knowledge). Turner and Giuliano suggest that false-positives can be minimized if "suspicious" (but not positive) intraoperative frozen sections of SLNs do not lead to immediate ALND, but to deferral of that decision until the final histo-logic analysis is complete.[71] It should be remembered that the consequence of a false-positive SLN would be reversion to conventional ALND, which has until recently been the standard of care for treating women with infiltrating breast cancer. A third potential disadvantage of frozen-section analysis is cost. It must be determined whether the cost of frozen-section analysis of SLNs is outweighed by the cost savings due to intraoperative diagnosis, particularly for women with the smallest tumors, who have the least likelihood of axillary metastases. Further work is also necessary to evaluate the use of other techniques such as touch-prep cytology in the intraoperative evaluation of SLNs.

Immunohistochemical analysis of SLNs

Of women with SLN metastases, 11% to 36% are identified on IHC only.[14,20,25,49] There are three lines of evidence that suggest that IHC-detected metastases are clinically important. The first was presented by Dowlatshahi et al,[75] in a review of long-term follow-up studies of women who had conventional ALND with no axillary metastases at routine H&E analysis (see Table 27.2).[76–101] Serial sections, IHC, or both disclosed occult axillary metastases in an average of 15–20% of these women. Except for the study of Wilkinson et al,[78] all studies with 100 or more patients showed that occult axillary metastases detected by serial sectioning, IHC, or both were associated with a decrement in disease-free and/or overall survival (Table 27.10).[73]

The largest retrospective study supporting the use of IHC methods is the recent analysis of data from the International (Ludwig) Breast Cancer Study.[101] In 736 patients with lymph nodes interpreted as negative at conventional ALND, Cote et al found occult nodal metastases by serial sectioning in 52 (7%) and by IHC in 148 (20%).[101] In postmenopausal women, occult metastases by either method were associated with significantly worse disease-free and overall survival. Immunohistochemically

detected metastases were an independent and highly significant predictor of tumor recurrence independent of tumor grade, size, estrogen-receptor status, and treatment protocol.

A second line of evidence supporting the clinical relevance of IHC-detected metastases is derived from analysis of studies of SLN biopsy with correlative ALND.[10–52] In the study of Weaver et al, use of IHC decreased the false-negative rate of SLN biopsy by 18%.[54] Turner et al found SLN biopsy with IHC analysis had a high negative predictive value: if SLNs were tumor-free by H&E and IHC, tumor was present in non-SLNs in only 1 of 60 (1.7%) women and in only 1 of 1087 (<0.1%) non-SLNs.[58] Other studies that used IHC analysis of the SLNs report significantly higher sensitivity, negative predictive value, and accuracy, and a significantly lower false-negative rate compared with studies that did not: sensitivity, 97% vs 92% ($p < 0.01$); negative predictive value, 98% vs 96% ($p < 0.05$); accuracy, 99% vs 97% ($p < 0.03$); and false-negative rate, 3% vs 8% ($p < 0.01$) (Table 27.11).[73]

The clinical importance of IHC-detected metastases is also supported by the frequency of non-SLN metastases in women with IHC-positive SLNs. Approximately half of all women with SLN metastases have tumor in non-SLNs at subsequent ALND (see Table 27.2). In the study of Weaver et al, ALND revealed additional metastases in 41% of women with SLN metastases detected by conventional pathologic analysis and in 21% of women with IHC-detected SLN metastases.[54] Hill et al reported that ALND revealed additional metastases in 39% of women with SLN metastases and in 16% of women with IHC-detected SLN metastases.[57] Krag et al found that the likelihood of finding tumor in a non-SLN related to tumor size and to the tumor burden in the SLNs.[23]

The existing data suggest that the frequency of non-SLN metastases (and prognosis) in women with IHC-detected SLN metastases may be between that of women with tumor-free SLNs and women with a larger SLN tumor burden. Dowlatshahi et al have suggested that the presence of a large (>10-celled) colony of

Table 27.10 Occult micrometastases in lymph nodes interpreted as negative at conventional ALND: frequency and significance

Investigator/year	No. of patients	No. of patients with occult micrometastases n (%)	Follow-up (yr)	Disease-free survival	Overall survival
Serial sections					
Neville/1991[76]	921	83 (9)	6	$p = 0.0008$	$p = 0.0009$
Ludwig/1990[77]	921	83 (9)	5	$p = 0.003$	$p = 0.002$
Cote/1999[101]	736	52 (7)	12	$p = 0.001$	$p = 0.0005$
Wilkinson/1982[78]	525	89 (17)	15	NS	NS
Fisher/1978[79]	78	19 (24)	5	NS	NS
Pickren/1961[80]	51	11 (22)	5	NS	NS
Sedmak/1989[81]	45	5 (11)	10	Not determined	NS
Saphir/1948[82]	30	10 (33)	3	Not determined	Not determined
Rosen/1982[83]	28	9 (32)	10	NS	NS
Immunohistochemistry					
Cote/1999[101 a]	736	148 (20)	12	$p = 0.09$	NS
Hainsworth/1993[84]	343	41 (12)	6.5	$p < 0.05$	NS
De Mascarel/1992[85 b]	129	13 (10)	10	$p = 0.01$ (recurrences)	$p = 0.07$
Trojani/1987[86 b]	122	13 (11)	10	$p < 0.003$	$p = 0.02$
Trojani/1987[87 c]	91	37 (41)	10	NS	NS
De Mascarel/1992[85 c]	89	37 (42)	10	NS	NS
Chen/1991[88 d]	80	23 (29)	3.2	$p < 0.05$	Not determined
Sedmak/1989[81]	45	9 (20)	10	Not determined	$p < 0.02$
Wells/1984[89 e]	45	7 (16)	0	Not determined	Not determined
Byrne/1987[90]	40	4 (10)	5	NS	NS
Berry/1988[91 f]	31	4 (13)	2	Not determined	Not determined
Sloane/1980[92]	31	0 (0)	0	Not determined	Not determined
Raymond/1989[93]	30	7 (23)	0	Not determined	Not determined
Immunohistochemistry and serial sections					
McGuckin/1996[94]	208	53 (25)	5	$p = .007$	$p = 0.02$
Nasser/1993[95]	159	50 (31)	11	$p = 0.04^g$	$p = 0.07^g$
Galea/1991[96]	98	9 (9)	14	NS	NS
Clare/1997[97]	86	11 (13)	6.7	$p < 0.05$	NS
Bussolati/1986[98]	50	12 (24)	3.5	Not determined	Not determined

Adapted from Dowlatshahi et al[75] and Liberman,[73] with permission.

Numbers in parentheses are percentages. NS, not significant. The p values give the statistical significance of the decrease in disease-free or overall survival among women with micrometastases when compared with women without metastases.

[a]Immunohistochemically detected metastases were associated with a significant decrease in disease-free and overall survival for postmenopausal women but not for premenopausal women. Among 736 women, 45 (6%) had metastases detected by both IHC and serial sections and 581 (79%) were negative by both methods. In the 110 cases for which there was disagreement, metastases were found by IHC in 103 and serial sections in 7; in the latter 7 cases, IHC stains of deeper sections showed tumor. In 64 patients with infiltrating lobular carcinoma, occult metastases were found by IHC in 39% and by H&E in 3%.

[b]Infiltrating ductal carcinomas.

[c]Infiltrating lobular carcinomas.

[d]Occult micrometastases were observed in 21/76 (28%) infiltrating ductal carcinomas and 2/4 (50%) infiltrating lobular carcinomas.

[e]Occult micrometastases were found in 3/33 (9%) infiltrating ductal carcinomas and 4/12 (33%) infiltrating lobular carcinomas.

[f]Immunohistochemistry increased detection of metastases by 17%, including 13% for infiltrating ductal carcinomas and 38% for infiltrating lobular carcinomas.

[g]Data for patients with micrometastases larger than 0.2 mm. No decrement in disease-free or overall survival was observed in patients with micrometastases measuring 0.2 mm or less.

Table 27.11 Validation studies of SLN biopsy: impact of immunohistochemistry

Investigator/year	Technique	Sensitivity	NPV	Accuracy	False-negative rate
Immunohistochemistry					
Borgstein/1998[20]	Radioisotope	44/45 (98)	59/60 (98)	103/104 (99)	1/45 (2)
Offodile/1998[25]	Radioisotope	18/18 (100)	22/22 (100)	40/40 (100)	0/18 (0)
Snider/1998[29] [a]	Radioisotope	13/14 (93)	56/57 (98)	69/70 (99)	1/14 (7)
Veronesi/1999[44] [b]	Radioisotope	52/55 (95)	64/67 (96)	116/119 (97)	3/55 (5)
Giuliano/1997[14]	Blue dye	42/42 (100)	58/58 (100)	100/100 (100)	0/42 (0)
Kapteijn/1998[34]	Blue dye	10/10 (100)	16/16 (100)	26/26 (100)	0/10 (0)
Kern/1999[47]	Blue dye	15/15 (100)	24/24 (100)	39/39 (100)	0/15 (0)
Morgan/1999[48]	Blue dye	10/12 (83)	20/22 (91)	30/32 (94)	2/12 (17)
Czerniecki/1999[45]	Radioisotope + blue dye	15/15 (100)	26/26 (100)	41/41 (100)	0/15 (0)
van der Ent/1999[42]	Radioisotope + blue dye	26/27 (96)	43/44 (98)	69/70 (99)	1/27 (4)
SUBTOTAL		*245/253 (97)*	*388/396 (98)*	*633/641 (99)*	*8/253 (3)*
No immunohistochemistry					
Krag/1993[10]	Radioisotope	7/7 (100)	11/11 (100)	18/18 (100)	0/7 (0)
Pijpers/1997[17]	Radioisotope	11/11 (100)	19/19 (100)	30/30 (100)	0/11 (0)
Roumen/1997[18]	Radioisotope	22/23 (96)	34/35 (97)	56/57 (98)	1/23 (4)
Galimberti/1998[19]	Radioisotope	109/115 (95)	123/129 (95)	232/238 (97)	6/115 (5)
Krag/1998[23]	Radioisotope	39/41 (95)	78/80 (98)	117/119 (98)	2/41 (5)
Miner/1998[24]	Radioisotope	7/8 (88)	33/34 (97)	40/41 (98)	1/8 (12)
Crossin/1998[27]	Radioisotope	7/8 (88)	34/35 (97)	41/42 (98)	1/8 (12)
Krag/1998[28]	Radioisotope	101/114 (89)	291/304 (96)	392/405 (97)	13/114 (11)
Rubio/1998[31]	Radioisotope	15/17 (88)	36/38 (95)	51/53 (96)	2/17 (12)
Gulec/1998[38]	Radioisotope	8/8 (100)	22/22 (100)	30/30 (100)	0/8 (0)
Feldman/1999[43]	Radioisotope	17/21 (81)	49/53 (92)	66/70 (94)	4/21 (19)
Veronesi/1999[44] [b]	Radioisotope	116/125 (93)	127/136 (93)	243/252 (96)	9/125 (7)
Moffat/1999[46]	Radioisotope	18/20 (90)	42/44 (95)	60/62 (97)	2/20 (10)
Giuliano/1994[11]	Blue dye	37/42 (88)	72/77 (94)	109/114 (96)	5/42 (12)
Guenther/1997[16]	Blue dye	28/31 (90)	72/75 (96)	100/103 (97)	3/31 (10)
Flett/1998[26]	Blue dye	15/18 (83)	38/41 (93)	53/56 (95)	3/18 (17)
Koller/1998[30]	Blue dye	48/51 (94)	45/48 (94)	93/96 (97)	3/51 (6)
Ratanawichitrasin/1998[40]	Blue dye	7/9 (78)	26/28 (93)	33/35 (94)	2/9 (22)
Imoto/1999[41]	Blue dye	25/29 (86)	36/40 (90)	61/65 (94)	4/29 (14)
Dale/1998[39]	Blue dye	5/5 (100)	9/9 (100)	14/14 (100)	0/5 (0)
Morrow/1999[49]	Blue dye (+radioisotope in 42)	28/32 (88)	78/82 (95)	106/110 (96)	4/32 (13)
Albertini/1996[12]	Radioisotope + blue dye	18/18 (100)	39/39 (100)	57/57 (100)	0/18 (0)
Borgstein/1997[13]	Radioisotope + blue dye	14/14 (100)	11/11 (100)	25/25 (100) (f)	0/14 (0)
O'Hea/1998[21]	Radioisotope + blue dye	17/20 (85)	35/38 (92)	52/55 (95)	3/20 (15)
Barnwell/1998[22]	Radioisotope + blue dye	15/15 (100)	23/23 (100)	38/38 (100)	0/15 (0)
Nwariaku/1998[36] [c]	Radioisotope + blue dye	26/27 (96)	69/70 (99)	95/96 (99)	1/27 (4)
Schneebaum/1998[35]	Radioisitope + blue dye	11/13 (85)	15/17 (88)	26/28 (93)	2/13 (15)
Canavese/1998[37]	Radioisotope + blue dye	28/33 (85)	63/68 (93)	91/96 (95)	5/33 (15)
Bass/1999[50]	Radioisotope + blue dye	53/54 (98)	119/120 (99)	172/173 (99)	1/54 (2)
Burak/1999[51]	Radioisotope + blue dye	14/14 (100)	31/31 (100)	45/45 (100)	0/14 (0)
Jaderborg/1999[52]	Radioisotope + blue dye	19/20 (95)	44/45 (98)	63/64 (98)	1/20 (5)
SUBTOTAL		*885/963 (92)*	*1724/1802 (96)*	*2609/2687 (97)*	*78/963 (8)*
TOTAL	**ALL**	**1130/1216 (93)**	**2112/2198 (96)**	**3242/3328 (97)**	**86/1216 (7)**

Adapted from Liberman,[73] with permission. Numbers in parentheses are percentages. All studies report 100% specificity and 100% positive predictive value.
NA, not applicable; NPV, negative predictive value.
[a] Immunohistochemistry done in 56 patients; data from those done with and without immunohistochemistry analyzed together.
[b] Study of 371 patients, of whom 119 had immunohistochemistry. Data presented separately in their study and in this table.
[c] Fifteen sections taken per node.

metastatic cells in an SLN may be of prognostic importance, while perhaps a single malignant cell or a small (<10) group of cells may not be;[55] this hypothesis should be tested in future work. The appropriate management of women with SLN metastases detected only by IHC needs further investigation.[55,69,102] Additional study is also needed to determine the relative value of serial sections versus IHC in histologic analysis of SLNs.

OTHER ISSUES IN SLN BIOPSY

Accuracy

Early studies suggested that SLN biopsy is most accurate in women with small infiltrating carcinomas. Veronesi et al reported an accuracy of 100% (45/45) for tumors measuring less than 1.5 cm, versus 97% (111/115) for larger tumors.[15] Galimberti et al reported an accuracy of 100% (38/38) for tumors measuring less than 1.2 cm, versus 97% (194/200) for larger lesions.[19] O'Hea et al reported an accuracy of 100% (19/19) for tumors measuring 1 cm or less, 98% (43/44) for T1 lesions, and 82% (9/11) for T2–3 lesions.[21] More recent work has shown that SLN biopsy can be accurate in larger tumors as well: in a study of SLN biopsy using radioisotope and blue dye, Olson et al reported accuracy of 97% (141/145) and false-negative rate of 8% (4/57) for 145 T1 tumors, versus accuracy of 98% (58/59) and a false-negative rate of 3% (1/35) for 59 T2 tumors.[103]

In analyzing results of SLN biopsy, it is important to evaluate not only the detection accuracy [true positive + true negative]/[true positive + true negative + false positive + false negative]) but also other parameters including sensitivity (true positive/[true positive + false negative]).[104,105] In women with T1 breast carcinoma, approximately 75% of whom are free of axillary metastases, an SLN biopsy procedure that resulted in the interpretation of every SLN as free of tumor would have 0% sensitivity but would be 75% accurate. The "false-negative rate" of SLN biopsy should be reported as the proportion of women with axillary metastases

in whom the SLNs are free of tumor (i.e., false negative/[true positive + false negative], or 1 minus sensitivity); in the published literature, the false-negative rate of SLN biopsy has averaged 6% (range 0–12%) (see Table 27.1).[10-52] During the initial "validation" work with backup ALND upon commencing an SLN biopsy program, it is important to include an adequate number of women with axillary metastases in order to determine the procedure's sensitivity (and false-negative rate) in one's own hands.

SLN biopsy in women with ductal carcinoma in situ

Ductal carcinoma in situ (DCIS) accounts for approximately 10–20% of all breast cancers. Axillary lymph-node dissection has not been part of the standard of care for DCIS owing to the low (<1%) frequency of axillary metastases in these women. Furthermore, controversy exists regarding the need for ALND in women with DCIS with microinvasion, in whom the frequency of axillary metastases is 0–5%. With the introduction of SLN biopsy, however, the issue of the need for surgical assessment of the axilla in these women has been revisited for two reasons. First, the morbidity of SLN biopsy is lower than that of ALND. Second, SLN biopsy allows the pathologist to focus intensive scrutiny on the smaller number of nodes most likely to contain tumor, potentially increasing the yield. For these reasons, the risk–benefit ratio of SLN biopsy may be preferable to that of ALND for women with DCIS.

Klauber-Demore et al evaluated the results of SLN biopsy in a highly selected group of 76 women with DCIS suspected to have a higher likelihood of invasion based on mammographic or histologic criteria, as well as in 31 women who had DCIS with microinvasion.[106] Sentinel lymph node metastases were found in 9 (12%) of the 76 women with DCIS and also in 3 (10%) of the women who had DCIS with microinvasion. Sentinel lymph-node metastases have been reported in 5 (6%) of 87 patients with DCIS in a study by Pendas et al,[107] and in 2

(14%) of 14 patients with DCIS with microinvasion reported by Zavotsky et al.[108] Further work is necessary to determine which patients with DCIS or DCIS with microinvasion are most likely to benefit from SLN biopsy, and to determine the clinical significance of SLN metastases in these women.

Radiation safety

The dose of radioactivity injected in studies that used radioisotope methods for identifying SLNs has ranged from 0.1 mCi to 1.6 mCi (5–60 MBq), which is substantially less than the 25 mCi (925 MBq) dose routinely given for a bone scan. No special radiation precautions are necessary for patients, operating-room staff, or pathologists handling the SLN biopsy specimens.

In a series of 100 consecutive SLN biopsy procedures after intraparenchymal injection of 5–10 MBq (0.1–0.3 mCi) of Tc-99m-colloidal albumin the day before surgery, Veronesi et al reported that the mean residual activity was 9×10^{-3} (range 0.7×10^{-3} to 15×10^{-3}) MBq in excised SLNs and 0.9 (range 0.4–1.1) MBq in removed breast tissue.[44] The doses absorbed by staff in 100 operations were substantially lower than the recommended annual dose limits for the general population according to the International Commission on Radiological Protection (ICRP) recommendations. The highest total absorbed dose, to the surgeon's hands, was 450 ± 20 microsieverts in 100 operations, less than 1% of the 50 000 μSv annual limit for the general population recommended as safe by the IRCP.[44] Considering that each surgical team performs an average of 50 operations involving SLN biopsy per year, these personnel can be classified as nonexposed workers as defined by the IRCP.[44]

Follow-up

Sentinel lymph-node biopsy is a relatively recent procedure, and therefore postsurgical follow-up data are limited. The hypothesis that the morbidity of SLN biopsy is less than that of ALND must be validated in clinical studies. Schrenk et al compared outcome in 70 patients, half of whom had SLN biopsy (follow-up 15.4 months) while the remainder had ALND (follow-up 17.0 months).[109] They reported a significantly lower upper and forearm circumference of the operated arm and significantly lower subjective rates of lymphedema, pain, numbness, and motion restriction in the SLN group. No difference was observed in arm stiffness or strength or in daily living. Further work is needed to assess long-term outcome, including rates of axillary recurrence after SLN biopsy, an event which has not (to our knowledge) been reported.

Future directions: percutaneous evaluation of the SLN?

Parker et al described 20 women who had injection of 0.5–1.0 mCi (18.5–37 MBq) Tc-99m-SC adjacent to their primary breast cancer, followed 1 hour later by LSG.[110] The skin overlying the area of increased activity in the axilla was marked, and the area was then examined using a hand-held gamma detector and real-time sonography. A localizing wire was placed in the SLN and the area was surgically excised along with other areas of increased activity in the axilla. In 19 (95%) of 20 women, at least one SLN was correctly identified and localized; in the one woman in whom the SLN was not found preoperatively, none was found at surgery either. This study suggests that percutaneous histologic assessment of the SLN may be possible in the future.

CONCLUSION

The American Cancer Society estimates that over half of the 182 800 American women diagnosed with infiltrating breast cancer in 2000 will be free of axillary metastases.[111] Sentinel lymph-node biopsy may spare many women with small infiltrating breast carcinomas the need to undergo ALND. Currently, clinical use of SLN biopsy in lieu of ALND may be best reserved for the following:

(a) high-volume health centers with close coordination of surgery, nuclear medicine, and pathology
(b) smaller tumors
(c) implementation after a preliminary trial with correlative ALND to document the performance of SLN biopsy in one's own institution
(d) use in the context of a carefully designed protocol, with informed consent, careful recording of technical factors, and follow-up.[112–114]

With such an approach, SLN biopsy technique may be refined and standardized, allowing more women to benefit from this minimally invasive approach to the treatment of breast carcinoma.

REFERENCES

1. Harris JR, Morrow M, Local management of invasive breast cancer. In: Harris JR, Lippman ME, Morrow M, Hellman S, eds, *Diseases of the Breast*, 487–547. Lippincott-Raven: Philadelphia, 1996.
2. Liberman L, Cody HS III, Hill ADK et al, Sentinel lymph node biopsy after percutaneous diagnosis of nonpalpable breast cancer. *Radiology* 1999; **211**:835–44.
3. Kopans DB, Screening for breast cancer. In: Kopans DB, ed, *Breast Imaging*, 2nd edn, 55–106. Lippincott-Raven: Philadelphia, 1998.
4. Fleming ID, Cooper JS, Henson DE et al, eds, *AJCC Cancer Staging Manual*, 5th edn, 171–80. Lippincott-Raven: Philadelphia, 1997.
5. Carter CL, Allen C, Henson DE, Relation of tumor size, lymph node status, and survival in 24 740 breast cancer cases. *Cancer* 1989; **63**:181–7.
6. Cody HS III, Laughlin EH, Trillo C, Urban JA, Have changing treatment patterns affected outcome for operable breast cancer? Ten year follow-up in 1288 patients, 1965 to 1978. *Ann Surg* 1991; **213**:297–307.
7. Silverstein MJ, Gierson ED, Waisman JR et al, Axillary lymph node dissection for T1a breast carcinoma: is it indicated? *Cancer* 1994;

73: 664–7.
8. Mustafa IA, Cole B, Wanebo HJ et al, The impact of histopathology on nodal metastases in minimal breast cancer. *Arch Surg* 1997; **132**:384–91.
9. Port ER, Tan LK, Borgen PI, Van Zee KJ, Incidence of axillary lymph node metastases in T1a and T1b breast carcinoma. *Ann Surg Oncol* 1998; **5**:23–7.
10. Krag DN, Weaver DL, Alex JC, Fairbank JT, Surgical resection and radiolocalization of the sentinel lymph node in breast cancer using a gamma probe. *Surg Oncol* 1993; **2**:335–40.
11. Giuliano AE, Kirgan DM, Guenther JM, Morton DL, Lymphatic mapping and sentinel lymphadenectomy for breast cancer. *Ann Surg* 1994; **220**:391–401.
12. Albertini JJ, Lyman GH, Cox C et al, Lymphatic mapping and sentinel node biopsy in the patient with breast cancer. *JAMA* 1996; **276**:1818–22.
13. Borgstein PJ, Meijer S, Pijpers R, Intradermal blue dye to identify sentinel lymph node in breast cancer. *Lancet* 1997; **349**:1668–9.
14. Giuliano AE, Jones RC, Brennan M, Statman R, Sentinel lymphadenectomy in breast cancer. *J Clin Oncol* 1997; **15**:2345–50.
15. Veronesi U, Paganelli G, Galimberti V et al, Sentinel-node biopsy to avoid axillary dissection in breast cancer with clinically negative lymph-nodes. *Lancet* 1997; **349**:1864–7.
16. Guenther JM, Krishnamoorthy M, Tan LR, Sentinel lymphadenectomy for breast cancer in a community managed care setting. *Cancer J Sci Am* 1997; **3**:336–40.
17. Pijpers R, Hoekstra OS, Collet GJ et al, Impact of lymphoscintigraphy on sentinel node identification with technetium-99m-colloidal albumin in breast cancer. *J Nucl Med* 1997; **38**:366–8.
18. Roumen RMH, Valkenburg JGM, Geuskens LM, Lymphoscintigraphy and feasibility of sentinel node biopsy in 83 patients with primary breast cancer. *Eur J Surg Oncol* 1997; **23**:495–502.
19. Galimberti V, Zurrida S, Zucali P, Luini A, Can sentinel node biopsy avoid axillary dissection in clinically node-negative breast cancer patients? *Breast* 1998; **7**:8–10.
20. Borgstein PJ, Pijpers R, Comans EF et al, Sentinel lymph node biopsy in breast cancer: guidelines and pitfalls of lymphoscintigraphy and gamma probe detection. *J Am Coll Surg* 1998; **186**:275–83.

21. O'Hea BJ, Hill ADK, El-Shirbiny AM et al, Sentinel lymph node biopsy in breast cancer: initial experience at Memorial Sloan-Kettering Cancer Center. *J Am Coll Surg* 1998; **186**:423–7.

22. Barnwell JM, Arredondo MA, Kollmorgen D et al, Sentinel node biopsy in breast cancer. *Ann Surg Oncol* 1998; **5**:126–30.

23. Krag DN, Ashikaga T, Harlow SP, Weaver DL, Development of sentinel node targeting technique in breast cancer patients. *Breast J* 1998; **4**:67–74.

24. Miner TJ, Shriver CD, Jaques DP et al, Ultrasonographically guided injection improves localization of the radiolabeled sentinel lymph node in breast cancer. *Ann Surg Oncol* 1998; **5**:315–21.

25. Offodile R, Hoh C, Barsky SH et al, Minimally invasive breast carcinoma staging using lymphatic mapping with radiolabeled Dextran. *Cancer* 1998; **82**:1704–8.

26. Flett MM, Going JJ, Stanton PD, Cooke TG, Sentinel node localization in patients with breast cancer. *Br J Surg* 1998; **85**:991–3.

27. Crossin JA, Johnson AC, Stewart PB, Turner WW, Gamma-probe-guided resection of the sentinel lymph node in breast cancer. *Am Surg* 1998; **64**:666–9.

28. Krag D, Weaver D, Ashikaga T et al, The sentinel node in breast cancer: a multicenter validation study. *N Engl J Med* 1998; **339**:941–6.

29. Snider H, Dowlatshahi K, Fan M, Bridger WM, Sentinel node biopsy in the staging of breast cancer. *Am J Surg* 1998; **176**:305–10.

30. Koller M, Barsuk D, Zippel D et al, Sentinel lymph node involvement—a predictor for axillary node status with breast cancer—has the time come? *Eur J Surg Oncol* 1998; **24**:166–8.

31. Rubio IT, Korourian S, Cowan C, Krag DN et al, Sentinel lymph node biopsy for staging breast cancer. *Am J Surg* 1998; **176**:532–7.

32. De Cicco C, Cremonesi M, Luini A et al, Lymphoscintigraphy and radioguided biopsy of the sentinel axillary node in breast cancer. *J Nucl Med* 1998; **39**:2080–4.

33. De Cicco C, Chinol M, Paganelli G, Intraoperative localization of the sentinel node in breast cancer: technical aspects of lymphoscintigraphic methods. *Semin Surg Oncol* 1998; **15**:268–71.

34. Kapteijn BAE, Nieweg OE, Petersen JL et al, Identification and biopsy of the sentinel lymph node in breast cancer. *Eur J Surg Oncol* 1998; **24**:427–30.

35. Schneebaum S, Stadler J, Cohen M et al, Gamma probe-guided sentinel node biopsy— optimal timing for injection. *Eur J Surg Oncol* 1998; **24**:515–19.

36. Nwariaku FE, Euhus DM, Beitsch PD et al, Sentinel lymph node biopsy, an alternative to elective axillary dissection for breast cancer. *Am J Surg* 1998; **176**:529–31.

37. Canavese G, Gipponi M, Catturich A et al, Sentinel lymph node mapping opens a new perspective in the surgical management of early-stage breast cancer: a combined approach with vital blue dye lymphatic mapping and radioguided surgery. *Semin Surg Oncol* 1998; **15**:272–7.

38. Gulec SA, Moffat FL, Carroll RG et al, Sentinel lymph node localization in early breast cancer. *J Nucl Med* 1998; **39**:1388–93.

39. Dale PS, Williams JT IV, Axillary staging utilizing selective sentinel lymphadenectomy for patients with invasive breast carcinoma. *Am Surg* 1998; **64**:28–31.

40. Ratanawichitrasin A, Levy L, Myles J, Crowe JP, Experience with lymphatic mapping in breast cancer using isosulfan blue dye. *J Womens Health* 1998; **7**:873–7.

41. Imoto S, Hasebe T, Initial experience with sentinel node biopsy in breast cancer at the National Cancer Center Hospital East. *Jpn J Clin Oncol* 1999; **29**:11–15.

42. Van der Ent FWC, Kengen RAM, van der Pol HAG, Hoofwijk AGM, Sentinel node biopsy in 70 unselected patients with breast cancer: increased feasibility by using 10 mCi radiocolloid in combination with a blue dye tracer. *Eur J Surg Oncol* 1999; **25**:24–9.

43. Feldman S, Krag DN, McNally RK et al, Limitation in gamma probe localization of the sentinel node in breast cancer patients with large excisional biopsy. *J Am Coll Surg* 1999; **188**:248–54.

44. Veronesi U, Paganelli G, Viale G et al, Sentinel lymph node biopsy and axillary dissection in breast cancer: results in a large series. *J Natl Cancer Inst* 1999; **91**:368–73.

45. Czerniecki BJ, Scheff AM, Callans LS et al, Immunohistochemistry with pancytokeratins improves the sensitivity of sentinel lymph node biopsy in patients with breast carcinoma. *Cancer* 1999; **85**:1098–103.

46. Moffat FL, Gulec SA, Sittler SY et al, Unfiltered sulfur colloid and sentinel node biopsy for breast cancer: technical and kinetic considerations. *Ann Surg Oncol* 1999; **6**:746–55.

47. Kern KA, Sentinel lymph node mapping in breast cancer using subareolar injection of blue dye. *J Am Coll Surg* 1999; **189:**539–45.

48. Morgan A, Howisey RL, Aldape HC et al, Initial experience in a community hospital with sentinel lymph node mapping and biopsy for evaluation of axillary lymph node status in palpable invasive breast cancer. *J Surg Oncol* 1999; **72:**24–31.

49. Morrow M, Rademaker AW, Bethke KP et al, Leaning sentinel node biopsy: results of a prospective randomized trial of two techniques. *Surgery* 1999; **126:**714–22.

50. Bass SS, Cox CE, Berman C, Reintgen DS, The role of sentinel lymph node biopsy in breast cancer. *J Am Coll Surg* 1999; **189:**183–94.

51. Burak WE, Walker MJ, Yee LD et al, Routine preoperative lymphoscintigraphy is not necessary prior to sentinel node biopsy for breast cancer. *Am J Surg* 1999; **177:**445–9.

52. Jaderborg JM, Harrison PB, Kiser JL, Maynard SL, The feasibility and accuracy of the sentinel lymph node biopsy for breast carcinoma. *Am Surg* 1999; **65:**699–705.

53. Winchester DJ, Sener SF, Winchester DP et al, Sentinel lymphadenectomy for breast cancer: experience with 180 consecutive patients: efficacy of filtered technetium 99m sulphur colloid with overnight migration time. *J Am Coll Surg* 1999; **188:**597–603.

54. Weaver DL, Kag DN, Ashikaga T et al, Pathologic analysis of sentinel and nonsentinel lymph nodes in breast carcinoma: a multicenter study. *Cancer* 2000; **88:**1099–107.

55. Dowlatshahi K, Fan M, Bloom KJ et al, Occult metastases in the sentinel lymph nodes of patients with early stage breast carcinoma: a preliminary study. *Cancer* 1999; **86:**990–6.

56. Cox CE, Pendas S, Cox JM et al, Guidelines for sentinel node biopsy and lymphatic mapping of patients with breast cancer. *Ann Surg* 1998; **227:**645–51.

57. Hill ADK, Tran KN, Akhurst T et al, Lessons learned from 500 cases of lymphatic mapping for breast cancer. *Ann Surg* 1999; **229:**528–35.

58. Turner RR, Ollila DW, Krasne DL, Giuliano AE, Histopathologic validation of the sentinel lymph node hypothesis for breast carcinoma. *Ann Surg* 1997; **226:**271–8.

59. Schreiber RH, Pendas S, Ku NN et al, Microstaging of breast cancer patients using cytokeratin staining of the sentinel lymph node. *Ann Surg Oncol* 1999; **6:**95–101.

60. Cody HS III, Fey J, Akhurst T et al, Complementarity of blue dye and isotope in sentinel node localization for breast cancer: univariate and multivariate analysis of 966 procedures. *Ann Surg Oncol* 2001; **8:**13–19.

61. Shen P, Glass EC, DiFronzo LA et al, Dermal vs intra-parenchymal lymphoscintigraphy of the breast. In: *Society of Surgical Oncology 53rd Annual Cancer Symposium Abstract Book,* 13. Society of Surgical Oncology: Arlington Heights, 2000 (Abstract).

62. Linehan DC, Hill ADK, Tran KN et al, Sentinel lymph node localization in breast cancer: unfiltered radioisotope is superior to filtered. *J Am Coll Surg* 1999; **188:**377–81.

63. Linehan DC, Akhurst T, Yeung H, Yeh SDJ, Intradermal radiocolloid and intraparenchymal blue dye injection optimizes sentinel node identification in breast cancer patients. *Ann Surg Oncol* 1999; **6:**450–4.

64. Boolbol SK, Fey J, Borgen PI et al, Intradermal isotope injection: a highly accurate method of lymphatic mapping in breast carcinoma. *Ann Surg Oncol* 2001; **8:**20–4.

65. Cody HS III, Hill ADK, Tran KN et al, Credentialing for breast lymphatic mapping: how many cases are enough? *Ann Surg* 1999; **229:**723–8.

66. Cox C, Bass S, McCann C et al, Learning curves for sentinel lymph node mapping in breast cancer based on surgical volume analysis. In: *Society of Surgical Oncology 53rd Annual Breast Cancer Symposium Abstract Book,* 27. Society of Surgical Oncology: Arlington Heights, 2000 (Abstract).

67. Cox CE, Bass SS, Boulware D et al, Implementation of new surgical technology: outcome measures for lymphatic mapping of breast carcinoma. *Ann Surg Oncol* 1999; **6:**553–61.

68. Cody HS III, Urban JA, Internal mammary node status: a major prognosticator in axillary node-negative breast cancer. *Ann Surg Oncol* 1995; **2:**32–7.

69. Weiser MR, Montgomery LL, Tan LK et al, Lymphovascular invasion enhances the prediction of non-sentinel node metastases in breast cancer patients with positive sentinel nodes. In: *Ann Surg Oncol* 2001; **8:**145–9.

70. Giuliano AE, Dale PWS, Turner RR et al, Improved axillary staging of breast cancer with sentinel lymphadenectomy. *Ann Surg* 1995; **222:**394–9.

71. Turner RR, Giuliano AE, Intraoperative pathologic examination of the sentinel lymph node. *Ann Surg Oncol* 1998; **5**:670–2.

72. Turner RR, Ollila DA, Stern S, Giuliano AE, Optimal histopathologic examination of the sentinel lymph node for breast carcinoma staging. *Am J Surg Pathol* 1999; **23**:263–7.

73. Liberman L, Pathologic analysis of sentinel lymph nodes in breast cancer (editorial). *Cancer* 2000; **88**:971–7.

74. Weiser MR, Montgomery LL, Susnik B et al, Is routine intraoperative frozen-section examination of sentinel lymph nodes in breast cancer worthwhile? *Ann Surg Oncol* 2000; **7**:651–5.

75. Dowlatshahi K, Fan M, Snider HC, Habib FA, Lymph node micrometastases from breast carcinoma: reviewing the dilemma. *Cancer* 1997; **80**:1188–97.

76. Neville AM, Price KN, Gelber RD, Goldhirsch A, Axillary node micrometastasis and breast cancer (letter). *Lancet* 1991; **337**:1110.

77. International (Ludwig) Breast Cancer Study Group, Prognostic importance of occult axillary lymph node micrometastases from breast cancer. *Lancet* 1990; **335**:1565–8.

78. Wilkinson EJ, Hause L, Hoffman RG et al, Occult axillary lymph node metastases in invasive breast carcinoma: characteristics of the primary tumor and significance of the metastases. *Pathol Ann* 1982; **17**:67–91.

79. Fisher ER, Swamidoss S, Lee CH et al, Detection and significance of occult axillary node metastases in patients with invasive breast cancer. *Cancer* 1978; **42**:2025–31.

80. Pickren JW, Significance of occult metastases: a study of breast cancer. *Cancer* 1961; **14**:1266–71.

81. Sedmak D, Meinecke TA, Knechtges DS, Anderson J, Prognostic significance of cytokeratin-positive breast cancer metastases. *Mod Pathol* 1989; **2**:516–20.

82. Saphir O, Amromin GD, Obscure axillary lymph-node metastasis in carcinoma of the breast. *Cancer* 1948; **1**:238–41.

83. Rosen PP, Saigo PE, Braun DW et al, Occult axillary lymph node metastases from breast cancers with intramammary lymphatic tumor emboli. *Am J Surg Pathol* 1982; **6**:639–41.

84. Hainsworth PJ, Tjandra JJ, Stillwell RG et al, Detection and significance of occult metastases in node-negative breast cancer. *Br J Surg* 1993; **80**:459–63.

85. De Mascarel I, Bonichon F, Coindre JM, Trojani M, Prognostic significance of breast cancer axillary lymph node micrometastases assessed by two special techniques: reevaluation with longer follow-up. *Br J Cancer* 1992; **66**:523–7.

86. Trojani M, de Mascarel I, Bonichon F et al, Micrometastases to axillary lymph nodes from carcinoma of the breast: detection by immunohistochemistry and prognostic significance. *Br J Cancer* 1987; **55**:303–6.

87. Trojani M, de Mascarel I, Coindre JM et al, Micrometastases to axillary lymph nodes from invasive lobular carcinoma of the breast: detection by immunohistochemistry and prognostic significance. *Br J Cancer* 1987; **56**:838–9.

88. Chen ZL, Wen DR, Coulson WF et al, Occult metastases in the axillary lymph nodes of patients with breast cancer node-negative by clinical and histologic examination and conventional histology. *Dis Markers* 1991; **9**:239–48.

89. Wells CA, Heryet A, Brochier J et al, The immunocytochemical detection of axillary micrometastases in breast cancer. *Br J Cancer* 1984; **50**:193–7.

90. Byrne J, Waldron R, McAvinchey D, Dervan P, The use of monoclonal antibodies for the histopathologic detection of mammary axillary micrometastases. *Eur J Surg Oncol* 1987; **13**:409–11.

91. Berry N, Jones DB, Marshall R et al, Comparison of the detection of breast carcinoma metastases by routine histological diagnosis and by immunohistochemical staining. *Eur Surg Res* 1988; **20**:225–32.

92. Sloane JP, Ormerod MG, Imrie SF, Coombes RC, The use of antisera to epithelial membrane antigen in detecting micrometastases in histological sections. *Br J Cancer* 1980; **42**:392–8.

93. Raymond WA, Leong ASY, Immunoperoxidase staining in the detection of lymph node metastases in stage I breast cancer. *Pathology* 1989; **21**:11–15.

94. McGuckin MA, Cummings MC, Walsh MD et al, Occult axillary node metastases in breast cancer: their detection and prognostic significance. *Br J Cancer* 1996; **73**:88–95.

95. Nasser IA, Lee AKC, Bosari S et al, Occult axillary lymph node metastases in "node-negative" breast carcinoma. *Hum Pathol* 1993; **24**:950–7.

96. Galea MH, Athanassiou E, Bell et al, Occult regional lymph node metastases from breast carcinoma: immunohistochemical detection with antibodies CAM 5.2 and NCRC-11. *J Pathol* 1991; **165**:221–7.

97. Clare SE, Sener SF, Wilkens W et al, Prognostic

significance of occult lymph node metastases in node-negative breast cancer. *Ann Surg Oncol* 1997; **4**:447–51.

98. Bussolati G, Gugliotta P, Morra I et al, The immunohistochemical detection of lymph node metastases from infiltrating lobular carcinoma of the breast. *Br J Cancer* 1986; **54**:631–6.

99. Chu KU, Turner RR, Hansen NM et al, Do all patients with sentinel node metastasis from breast carcinoma need complete axillary node dissection? *Ann Surg* 1999; **229**:536–41.

100. Jannink I, Fan M, Nagy S et al, Serial sectioning of sentinel nodes in patients with breast cancer: a pilot study. *Ann Surg Oncol* 1998; **5**:310–14.

101. Cote RJ, Peterson HF, Chaiwun B et al, for the International Breast Cancer Study Group. Role of immunohistochemical detection of lymph-node metastases in management of breast cancer. *Lancet* 1999; **354**:869–900.

102. Chu KU, Turner RR, Hansen NM et al, Do all patients with sentinel node metastasis from breast carcinoma need complete axillary node dissection? *Ann Surg* 1999; **229**:536–41.

103. Olson J, Fey J, Winawer J et al, Sentinel lymphadenectomy accurately predicts nodal status in T2 breast cancer. *J Am Coll Surg* 2000; **191**:593–9.

104. Lopchinsky RA, Tartter PL, Sentinel lymph node biopsy (letter). *J Am Coll Surg* 1998; **187**:337.

105. Hill ADK, Borgen PI, Cody HS, Sentinel lymph node biopsy: reply (letter). *J Am Coll Surg* 1998; **187**:337–8.

106. Klauber-Demore N, Tan LK, Liberman L et al, Sentinel lymph node biopsy: is it indicated in patients with high-risk ductal carcinoma-in-situ and ductal carcinoma-in-situ with microinvasion? *Ann Surg Oncol* 2000; **7**:636–42.

107. Pendas S, Dauway E, Giuliano R et al, Sentinel node biopsy in ductal carcinoma in situ patients. *Ann Surg Oncol* 2000; **7**:15–20.

108. Zavotsky J, Hansen N, Brennan MB et al, Lymph node metastasis from ductal carcinoma in situ with microinvasion. *Cancer* 1999; **85**: 2439–43.

109. Schrenk P, Rieger R, Shamiyeh A, Wayand W, Morbidity following sentinel lymph node biopsy versus axillary lymph node dissection for patients with breast carcinoma. *Cancer* 2000; **88**:608–14.

110. Parker SH, Klaus AJ, Dennis MA, Ultrasound identification of the sentinel node in breast cancer. *Radiology* 1997; **205**(P):490 (Abstract).

111. Greenlee RT, Murray T, Bolden S, Wingo PA, Cancer statistics, 2000. *CA Cancer J Clin* 2000; **50**:7–33.

112. Morton DL, Intraoperative lymphatic mapping and sentinel lymphadenectomy: community standard care or clinical investigation? *Cancer J Sci Am* 1997; **3**:328–30 (commentary).

113. McMasters KM, Giuliano AE, Ross MI et al, Sentinel-lymph-node biopsy for breast cancer—not yet the standard of care (Sounding Board). *N Engl J Med* 1998; **339**:990–5.

114. Veronesi U, Zurrida S, Galimberti V, Consequences of sentinel node in clinical decision making in breast cancer and prospects for future studies. *Eur J Surg Oncol* 1998; **24**:93–5.

28

The significance of micrometastases

Kambiz Dowlatshahi

CONTENTS Definition of micrometastases • Detection of micrometastases in lymph nodes •
Immunohistochemical staining of lymph nodes • Micrometastases in SLNs • Serial sectioning of lymph
nodes • Micrometastases in bone marrow • Micrometastases in peripheral blood • Discussion

Malignant cells from breast cancer disseminate to regional nodes through lymphatic channels, and to distant sites through blood vessels. Most information about the significance of these metastases has been derived from evaluation of the lymph nodes. With the introduction of more sophisticated technology and the application of immunocytochemical techniques, however, investigators are now reporting on detection of malignant cells in the bone marrow and the peripheral blood. This information will assist the practitioner in formulating a better strategy for treatment of a subset of patients at greater risk for disease recurrence.

DEFINITION OF MICROMETASTASES

A review of the literature indicated that tumor deposits detected in the lymph nodes draining breast cancer were arbitrarily categorized as either micrometastasis or macrometastasis, with the cutoff point ranging from 0.2 mm to 2.0 mm.[1] The American Joint Committee on Cancer staging manual defines micrometastases of any clinical significance to be ≤2 mm.[2] This is based upon the histological examination of a single section of a lymph node stained with hematoxylin and eosin (H&E).

DETECTION OF MICROMETASTASES IN LYMPH NODES

Traditionally, the pathologist reports on the presence of malignant cells in 15 to 20 lymph nodes surgically removed from the axilla in conjunction with lumpectomy or mastectomy. Each node is bivalved, and a single 5-μm section is stained with H&E. This technique has two disadvantages. First, the examined section represents less than 0.1% of a lymph node. Second, small clusters of malignant cells may be overlooked because of close staining resemblance between malignant cells and normal cellular components of the lymph node. This is especially true in the case of lobular carcinoma cells that measure slightly larger than the lymphocytes. The combination of these two factors appears to account for underestimation of nodal metastases in 9–33% of "node-negative" breast-cancer patients who subsequently experience disease recurrence within 10 years.

In order to overcome these two problems,

researchers began to examine multiple sections of the lymph nodes and to use special stains. In 1948, Saphir and Amromin detected additional metastatic disease in 10 of 30 patients (33%) with primary invasive breast carcinoma when the "negative nodes" were serially sectioned and stained with H&E.[3] In 1961, Pickren noted metastatic disease in 21 of 97 (22%) node-negative patients when the lymph nodes were sectioned at 12-μm intervals.[4] In 1971, Huvos et al introduced an arbitrary distinction between axillary lymph-node micrometastases (<2 mm) and macrometastases (>2 mm).[5] In 1978, Fisher et al sectioned the "negative nodes" at 5-μm intervals, staining every fourth section with H&E.[6] The rationale for choosing these intervals was that the average size of tumor cells is greater than 20 μm. Fisher and colleagues noted that 19 of 78 node-negative patients (24%) converted to a positive nodal status upon H&E staining.[6] These investigators reported that in 10 of 19 patients (53%), tumor emboli were seen in subcapsular lymphatic spaces and in 9 of 19 (47%), in the lymph-node parenchyma. The size of the metastases ranged from 0.2 mm to 1.3 mm.[6] Using 2-mm serial sections and H&E staining, Friedman et al found occult tumor emboli in the sinus margins of lymph nodes in 43 of 456 cases (9.4%).[7] In 1990, the International (Ludwig) Breast Cancer Study Group examined the axillary lymph nodes of 921 patients with node-negative breast cancer.[8] Sections were taken from six levels, and 30-μm intervals of paraffin blocks were stained with H&E. Micrometastases were found in 83 of 921 (9%). These patients had a poor disease-free ($p = 0.003$) and overall ($p = 0.002$) survival at the 5-year median follow-up.

From this brief review of the literature, it appears that micrometastases may be detected in those lymph nodes initially reported negative in patients with invasive breast cancer if additional sections are examined. It should also be noted that in all of these reports, only a *small portion* of the lymph nodes was examined.

IMMUNOHISTOCHEMICAL STAINING OF LYMPH NODES

In the early 1990s, investigators began to report a higher detection rate of occult metastases in lymph nodes stained with immunohistochemical (IHC) methods. A variety of cytokeratin-specific monoclonal antibodies were used. Hainsworth et al evaluated 343 cases with IHC (BC2-BC3 and 3E 1.2), finding occult metastases in 41 cases (12%), 10 of which also were noted when H&E-stained sections were reviewed.[9] Thirty-one of these micrometastases were smaller than 2 mm. At a median follow-up of 6.5 years, patients with micrometastases had a higher disease-recurrence rate (32% versus 17%; $p = 0.05$). Elson et al re-cut the "negative nodes" of 97 patients and stained them with AE1:AE3 and DF3.[10] Twenty per cent of negative cases were converted into positive cases as a result. Nasser et al took five sections from negative lymph nodes at 150-μm intervals and evaluated them with H&E and IHC.[11] Fifty of 159 patients (31%) had metastases, 28 of which were detected by H&E staining and an additional 22 by IHC alone. In 19 patients metastases were greater than 0.2 mm in size, and in 31 patients they were 0.2 mm or smaller. Patients with metastases greater than 0.2 mm had a higher recurrence rate and shorter disease-free and overall survival. More recently, McGuckin et al, in a retrospective series of 208 axillary node-negative patients, used a combination of step-sectioning from four levels, 100 μm apart, and staining with IHC. They detected occult metastases in 53 patients (25%).[12] The presence and greater size of occult metastases were significantly associated with poorer disease-free survival. In 1999, Cote et al reported on 736 of 921 patients previously studied by the Ludwig Group in 1990.[13] Sections were taken from six levels, comparing the effect of H&E with IHC. Occult metastases were detected in 52 of 736 patients (7%) when the sections were stained by H&E, versus 148 (20%) when the sections were stained by IHC. Furthermore, only 2 of 64 (3%) invasive lobular or mixed invasive lobular and ductal cancers had their micrometastases detected by H&E,

versus 25 (39%) by IHC. Occult metastases were associated with significantly poorer disease-free and overall survival rates in postmenopausal women. These investigators concluded that the current method of lymph-node examination of patients with breast cancer is no longer clinically tenable.

MICROMETASTASES IN SLNs

With the emergence of sentinel lymph-node biopsy as an alternative to axillary lymph-node dissection (ALND) for staging of breast cancer, a more detailed pathological evaluation of an average of two sentinel lymph nodes (SLNs) instead of 15–20 ALND-derived nodes has become practical. Review of many reports correlating the results of SLN biopsy with those of ALND reveals an average sensitivity of 94%, specificity of 100%, positive predictive value of 100%, negative predictive value of 96%, and accuracy of 98%.[14–18] The pathologist has time to expeditiously and efficiently survey cytokeratin-stained slides under low power to exclude metastases. A small group of cells that would require scrutiny under high power for detection with H&E staining is immediately obvious under low power with cytokeratin stains (Figure 28.1).

Schreiber et al reported on 210 patients with invasive breast cancer staged with SLN biopsy.[19] Forty-seven patients were found to have metastases. In 17 cases, the metastases were detected with unspecified serial sections and IHC only. This finding upstaged 9.4% of their patients from Stage I to Stage II. Weaver et al examined the SLNs as well as non-SLNs of 214 node-negative participants in a multicenter trial.[20] Additional sections taken at 100 μm and 200 μm deeper levels from the paraffin blocks of node-negative cases revealed occult metastases in 10%, all of which were smaller than 1 mm. The authors concluded that the significance of these occult metastases and their impact on patient survival should be evaluated further, and this is now the subject of an ongoing clinical trial by the National Surgical Adjuvant Breast and Bowel Project (NSABP).

SERIAL SECTIONING OF LYMPH NODES

Review of the literature reveals that investigators who attempted to detect occult or micrometastases in the lymph nodes of patients with breast cancer took *additional and not serial sections* at arbitrary intervals from archival tissues. The intervals between sections varied from 5 μm to 2 mm, and the number of

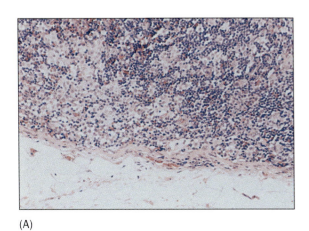

(A)

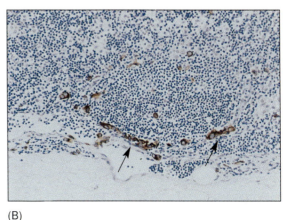

(B)

Figure 28.1 Section of an SLN stained with H&E (A) and cytokeratin (B). Micrometastases are readily visible (arrows) in B. Magnification ×100.

Table 28.1 Review of literature reporting on occult metastases in the lymph nodes of patients with breast cancer

Year	Author	Serial-sectioning intervals	Staining Technique used	Incidence of occult metastases (%)
1948	Saphir[3]	Alternate sections	H&E	33
1961	Pickren[4]	12-μm intervals	H&E	22
1978	Fisher[6]	5-μm intervals	H&E	24
1988	Friedman[7]	2-mm intervals	H&E	9.4
1990	Ludwig Group[8]	Six levels at 30-μm intervals	H&E	9
1993	Nasser[11]	Five levels at 150-μm intervals	IHC	31
1996	McGuckin[12]	Four levels at 100-μm intervals	IHC	28
1999	Cote[13]	Six levels at 30-μm intervals	H&E	7
			IHC	20
1998	Jannink[21]	500-μm intervals (entire SLN)	IHC	23
1999	Dowlatshahi[22]	250-μm intervals (entire SLN)	IHC	46
2000	Dowlatshahi[23]	250-μm intervals (entire SLN)	IHC	26.5

H&E, Hematoxylin-and-eosin; IHC, immunohistochemistry.

recorded sections taken varied from four to six (Table 28.1). Routine practice was to retain only half of each bivalved lymph node in paraffin blocks for future studies; the other half was discarded. Therefore, the serial section reports in the literature refer in each case to examination of a small portion of one-half of a lymph node.

Jannink et al, reporting on 13 patients with invasive breast cancer, examined entire SLNs sectioned at 0.5-mm intervals and stained with IHC (CAM 5.2).[21] They detected three additional occult metastases in the same SLNs that had been initially sectioned at 2.0-mm intervals and stained with H&E. The largest micrometastasis measured 1.0 mm in diameter. Dowlatshahi et al reported 46% additional occult micrometastases when the entire SLNs of 52 patients with invasive breast cancer were sectioned at 0.25-mm intervals and stained with IHC (CAM 5.2).[22] The same investigators, reporting on an extended experience, noted 41 of 155 patients (26.5%) with occult metastases either as single cells or

colonies of several thousand cells detected in subcapsular lymphatic channels or in the lymph-node follicles (Table 28.2).[23] Although some of the isolated tumor cells may not survive and become clinically significant, a colony of several hundred or thousand cells exhibiting growth and multiplication in the immunologically hostile environment of the lymph node suggests a good chance of similar growth in other organs such as the liver and bone marrow, leading to disease recurrence in that patient. The larger metastases were revisualized when the adjacent sections were restained with H&E (Figure 28.2), strongly suggesting that they had been missed by the pathologist's knife, which did not cut that part of the node. In one patient with a 1.5-cm invasive lobular carcinoma who had been initially reported tumor-free on 2-mm sections stained with H&E, numerous single cells were found by cytokeratin stains, underscoring the need for IHC in all cases of lobular carcinoma (Figure 28.3).

Table 28.2 Distribution of tumors by stage and SLN metastases in 155 patients with invasive breast cancer

Tumor		SLN metastases			
Stage	No. (%)	2 mm/H&E	0.25-mm colonies	IHC cells	Negative
T1a	18 (11.6)	0	2	6	10
T1b	46 (29.7)	5	4	7	30
T1c	62 (40)	11	7	7	37
T2	29 (18.7)	12	7	1	9
Total	155 (100)	28 (18%)	20 (13%)	21 (13.5%)	86 (55.5%)

Sentinel lymph nodes were sectioned at 2-mm intervals stained with H&E and at 0.25-mm intervals stained with IHC.

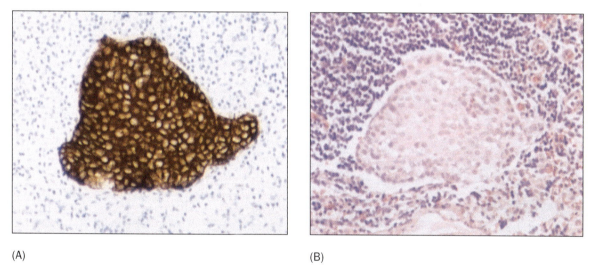

(A) (B)

Figure 28.2 A colony of malignant cells detected on 0.25-mm sectioning and cytokeratin staining (A) of the entire SLN. The metastases were also seen by H&E staining of the adjacent section (B).

MICROMETASTASES IN BONE MARROW

Cytokeratin-positive micrometastases, either as single cells or small cluster of cells, have been observed in the bone-marrow aspirates of patients with breast cancer. In a prospective study of 552 patients with Stages I, II, and III breast cancer, Braun et al reported 199 patients (36%) to have occult metastases, with means of 5, 9, and 86 tumor cells respectively per 2 million examined bone-marrow cells.[24] Samples were taken from the iliac crest of patients while under general anesthesia prior to surgical treatment of the breast cancer. Specimens were processed and stained with cytokeratin-specific antibody A45-B/B3. After 4 years of follow-up, 49 of 199 patients with bone-marrow metastases died of cancer, in contrast to 22 of 353 patients

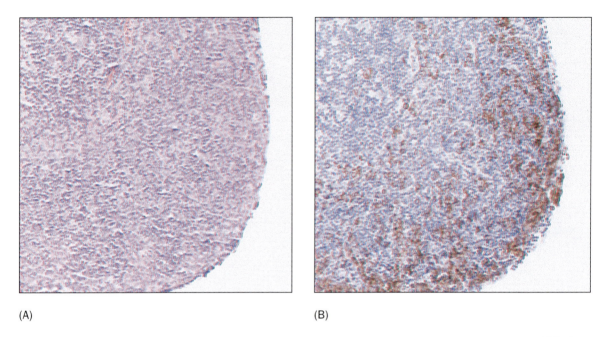

(A)   (B)

Figure 28.3 Adjacent sections of an SLN from a patient with invasive lobular carcinoma, stained with H&E (A) and cytokeratin (B) and revealing innumerable malignant cells. The patient was upstaged on the basis of the cytokeratin stain.

without such cells ($p < 0.001$). The investigators warn that not all detected micrometastases are clinically significant. For example, patients with T1a and T1b tumors had 23% and 35% occult metastases. Since the long-term survival of patients with primary tumors smaller than 1 cm is 90–95%, it appears that only a fraction of these micrometastases are clinically significant; an observation analogous to that of cytokeratin-positive cells found on ultrathin sections of SLNs. Analysis of the results also showed that if both regional lymph nodes and bone marrow were negative for metastases, the disease-free survival and overall survival of patients at 4 years was 99%.[25]

MICROMETASTASES IN PERIPHERAL BLOOD

An intriguing and important new technique has been described that detects malignant cells in the peripheral blood.[26,27] Antibodies to surface antigens of cancer cells are attached to colloidal iron compounds and mixed with the patient's blood. The mixture is exposed to a magnetic field that separates cancer cells attached to iron particles. A second set of antibodies specific for cytokeratin are used to further separate the malignant cells from mononuclear cells in the blood. The isolated cells are then stained with IHC. In a pilot study, 18 of 19 patients with breast carcinoma had cancer cells detected in their peripheral-blood samples before surgery, but the incidence rapidly declined during the 2 postoperative days; however, 30% of patients still exhibited malignant cells in the peripheral blood 2 weeks later.[28] Successful application of this technique may be helpful in early detection and monitoring of patients with systemic micrometastases.

DISCUSSION

The search for micrometastases or occult metastases stems largely from the observation that up to 25% of patients with node-negative invasive breast cancer experience disease recurrence after definitive therapy. Initially, this search led to the detection of malignant cells in the regional lymph nodes and, more recently, in the bone marrow and the peripheral blood. With the advent of annual mammography as a means of mass screening for early detection of breast cancer, more tumors smaller than 1 cm are being detected. This development has led to yet another observation and related question, namely, the paucity of metastases in T1a tumors and whether ALND is justified in such cases.[29] With the introduction of SLN biopsy in lieu of ALND, the dilemma was temporarily resolved. The central question of the significance of micrometastases remained, however, and indeed was magnified, because it was now possible to evaluate in detail an average of two SLNs with multiple sections and IHC. Several investigators began to report the presence of micrometastases in SLNs and suggested that a subset of such micrometastases would adversely affect the patient's survival. They suggested that these occult metastases are clinically significant and that such patients should be upstaged.[19,22,30] Others cautioned that the prognostic implications of these findings are unknown, and that the evaluation of SLNs in this manner should be avoided in routine clinical practice.[31,32] Carter et al attributed the presence of malignant as well as benign cells in the subcapsular sinus of lymph nodes draining the breast cancer to benign transport without clinical significance.[33]

It seems unlikely, however, that a group of several hundred or several thousand cells can be passively pushed through the small endothelial spaces of terminal lymphatic channels onto the lymph nodes. If tumor-cell dissemination through handling of the tumor at the time of needle biopsy or surgical excision does occur, one would expect passive transport of the malignant cells in all cases. The data from Table 28.2, however, show that 55% of patients were free of micrometastases when the entire SLN was sectioned at 0.25-mm intervals and stained with IHC. There was no demographic, operative or histologic difference between

positive and negative groups. Therefore, one has to consider the active migration of malignant cells into the lymphatic channels and blood vessels as the starting point for dissemination of malignant cells. An equally important observation is that of the total absence of micrometastases in the SLNs subjected to meticulous histologic examination in patients with breast tumors greater than 1 cm. For example, in the series shown in Table 28.2, 46 (37, T1c; 9, T2) patients (29.7%) had no malignant cells in their SLNs, which were examined at 0.25-mm intervals and stained with CAM 5.2. But these patients are recommended to receive chemotherapy based on the size of their tumor alone. If such a subset of patients also had negative bone marrow, as discussed earlier, they might be considered for observation alone.

Hermanek et al recognized the controversy and confusion related to the detection and significance of micrometastases in the lymph nodes, bone marrow, and blood.[34] They suggested that at present all investigators carefully record their methods of data collection, and they proposed a coding schema tabulating the detected isolated tumor cells. Page and colleagues, in a related editorial, emphasized the need for the creation of a specific guideline classifying nodal metastases less than 2 mm (PN1a) as having the same prognostic implication as node-negative tumors.[32] Currently, the guidelines are set by the American Joint Committee on Cancer. These authors agreed with the College of American Pathologists statement that immunohistochemistry or molecular methods to detect metastases are considered investigational.

It is evident that currently there is much controversy over the significance of micrometastases in breast cancer. Rapid technological advances in detection of early-stage breast cancer, as well as the application of newer methodologies, have outstripped the capabilities of the established pathologic classification of tumors. If we accept the dictum "small tumors, small metastases," serial sectioning and application of IHC for the detection of these small metastases would appear logical. The reported detection rate in the regional lymph nodes, bone marrow, and the peripheral blood is 20–30%, which is similar to that of disease recurrence in "node-negative" patients.

In summary, earlier detection of breast cancer has resulted in smaller metastases that escape detection by single-section examination and H&E staining of the lymph node. Step-sectioning of the entire SLN and staining with IHC appears to be a more accurate method of detection and staging of these breast cancers. The significance of either isolated cells or colonies of tumor cells found in SLNs and bone marrow will be determined in clinical trials now being conducted by the American College of Surgeons and the NSABP.

REFERENCES

1. Dowlatshahi K, Fan M, Snider HC et al, Lymph node micrometastases from breast carcinoma: reviewing the dilemma. *Cancer* 1997; **80**:1188–97.
2. Fleming ID, Cooper JS, Henson DE et al, *AJCC Cancer Staging Manual.* Lippincott-Raven: Philadelphia, 1997.
3. Saphir O, Amromin GD, Obscure axillary lymph node metastases in carcinoma of the breast. *Cancer* 1948; **1**:238–41.
4. Pickren JW, Significance of occult metastases. A study of breast cancer. *Cancer* 1961; **14**:1266–71.
5. Huvos AG, Hutter R, Berg JW, Significance of axillary macrometastases and micrometastases in mammary cancer. *Ann Surg* 1971; **173**:44–6.
6. Fisher ER, Swamidoss S, Lee CH et al, Detection and significance of occult axillary node metastases in patients with invasive breast cancer. *Cancer* 1978; **42**:2025–31.
7. Friedman S, Bertin F, Mouriesse H et al, Importance of tumor cells in axillary node sinus margins (clandestine metastases) discovered by serial sectioning in operable breast cancer. *Acta Oncol* 1988; **27**:483–7.
8. International (Ludwig) Breast Cancer Study Group, Prognostic importance of occult axillary lymph node micrometastases from breast cancer. *Lancet* 1990; **335**:1565–8.
9. Hainsworth PJ, Tjandra JJ, Stillwell RG et al, Detection and significance of occult metastases in node-negative breast cancer. *Br J Surg* 1993; **80**:459–63.
10. Elson CE, Kufe D, Johnston WW, Immuno- histochemical detection and significance of axillary lymph node micrometastases in breast carcinoma. A study of 97 cases. *Anal Quant Cytol Histol* 1993; **15**:171–8.
11. Nasser IA, Lee A, Bosari et al, Occult axillary lymph node metastases in "node-negative" breast carcinoma. *Hum Pathol* 1993; **24**:950–7.
12. McGuckin MA, Cummings MC, Walsh MD et al, Occult axillary node metastases in breast cancer: their detection and prognostic significance. *Br J Cancer* 1996; **73**:88–95.
13. Cote RJ, Peterson HF, Chaiwun B et al, Role of immunohistochemical detection of lymph-node metastases in management of breast cancer. *Lancet* 1999; **354**:896–900.
14. Albertini JJ, Lyman GH, Cox C et al, Lymphatic mapping and sentinel node biopsy in the patient with breast cancer. *JAMA* 1996; **276**:1818–22.
15. Giuliano AE, Jones RC, Brennan M et al, Sentinel lymphadenectomy in breast cancer. *J Clin Oncol* 1997; **15**:2345–50.
16. Krag D, Weaver D, Ashikaga T et al, The sentinel node in breast cancer: a multicenter validation study. *N Engl J Med* 1998; **339**:941–6.
17. Snider H, Dowlatshahi K, Fan M et al, Sentinel node biopsy in the staging of breast cancer. *Am J Surg* 1998; **176**:305–10.
18. Veronesi U, Paganelli G, Viale G et al, Sentinel lymph node biopsy and axillary dissection in breast cancer: results in a large series. *J Natl Cancer Inst* 1999; **91**:368–73.
19. Schreiber RH, Pendas S, Ku NN et al, Microstaging of breast cancer patients using cytokeratin staining of the sentinel lymph node. *Ann Surg Oncol* 1999; **6**:95–101.
20. Weaver DL, Krag DN, Ashikaga T et al, Pathologic analysis of sentinel and nonsentinel lymph nodes in breast carcinoma: a multicenter study. *Cancer* 2000; **88**:1099–107.
21. Jannink I, Fan M, Nagy S et al, Serial sectioning of sentinel nodes in patients with breast cancer: a pilot study. *Ann Surg Oncol* 1998; **5**:310–15.
22. Dowlatshahi K, Fan M, Bloom KJ et al, Occult metastases in the sentinel lymph nodes of patients with early stage breast carcinoma: a preliminary study. *Cancer* 1999; **86**:990–6.
23. Dowlatshahi K, Witt TR, Bloom KJ et al, Detection of occult micrometastases by 0.25 mm sectioning and cytokeratin staining of sentinel nodes in early breast cancer. *Proceedings of the American Society of Clinical Oncology*, 36th Annual Meeting, New Orleans 2000 (Abstract 305, vol. 19).

24. Braun S, Pantel K, Müller P et al, Cytokeratin-positive cells in the bone marrow and survival of patients with stage I, II, or III breast cancer. *N Engl J Med* 2000; **342**:525–33.

25. Smith BL, Approaches to breast cancer staging (editorial). *N Engl J Med* 2000; **342**:580–1.

26. Naume B, Borgen E, Beiske K et al, Immunomagnetic techniques for the environment and detection of isolated breast carcinoma cells in bone marrow and peripheral blood. *J Hematother* 1997; **6**:103–14.

27. Racila E, Euhus D, Weiss AJ et al, Detection and characterization of carcinoma cells in the blood. *Proc Natl Acad Sci* USA 1998; **95**:4589–94.

28. Krag DN, Ashikaga T, Moss TJ et al, Breast cancer cells in the blood: a pilot study. *Breast J* 1999; **5**:354–8.

29. Cady B, Stone MD, Schuler JG et al, The new era in breast cancer: invasion, size and nodal involvement dramatically decreasing as a result of mammographic screening. *Arch Surg* 1996; **131**:301–8.

30. Bland Kl, Microstaging of sentinel lymph nodes (editorial). *Ann Surg Oncol* 1999; **6**:15–16.

31. Allred DC, Elledge RM, Caution concerning micrometastatic breast carcinoma in sentinel lymph nodes (editorial). *Cancer* 1999; **86**:905–7.

32. Page DL, Anderson TJ, Carter BA, Minimal solid tumor involvement of regional and distant sites. When is a metastasis not a metastasis? (editorial) *Cancer* 1999; **86**:2589–92.

33. Carter BA, Jensen RA, Simpson JF et al, Benign transport of breast epithelium into axillary lymph nodes post biopsy. *Am J Clin Pathol* 2000; **113**:259–65.

34. Hermanek P, Hutter RVP, Sobin LH et al, Classification of isolated tumor cells and micrometastasis. *Cancer* 1999; **86**:2668–73.

Part IV
Other Applications of Sentinel Lymph-Node Biopsy

29

Head and neck cancers

Snehal Patel and Dennis Kraus

CONTENTS **Anatomical perspectives** • **Technique** • **Results**

The Memorial Sloan-Kettering Cancer Center technique for SLN biopsy for head and neck cancers

Technique	Combination	**Isotope**	*Type*: Tc-99m-SC
Dye	*Type*: Isosulfan blue dye (1%)		*Filtered*: Yes
	Volume: 0.5 ml (cc)		*Dose*: 0.2 mCi (4 injections of 0.05 mCi each)
Injection site	*Isotope*: Intradermal		*Volume*: 0.5 ml (cc)
	Dye: Intradermal		

Unlike squamous-cell carcinoma of the upper aerodigestive tract, which generally spreads to the cervical lymph nodes in an orderly pattern, malignant melanoma of the skin of the head and neck region metastasizes in an unpredictable fashion.[1] Clinical evaluation and prediction of the need for parotidectomy is perhaps equally difficult,[2] and routine subtotal parotidectomy carries higher morbidity and risk compared with elective neck dissection alone. The incidence of nodal metastasis in thin melanomas (generally those less than 1 mm in thickness) of the skin of the head and neck is sufficiently low that elective lymph-node dissection is not recommended. In lesions more than 4 mm thick, dissection of the clinically negative neck may not have an impact on outcome because of the high incidence of distant metastases in this patient population. It is in the intermediate group of lesions, between 1.0 mm and 3.9 mm thick, that elective lymph-node dissection has generally been advocated. However, the yield of metastatic nodes in this

population is approximately 15%, and the remaining 85% are subjected to an unnecessary procedure that carries a small but significant morbidity even in the most experienced hands. A retrospective analysis by Maddox et al combining the experience of the Sydney Melanoma Unit and the University of Alabama, Birmingham, of 534 patients with localized melanoma has demonstrated a survival benefit for elective neck dissection on univariate but not on multivariate analysis for patients with intermediate-thickness melanoma.[3]

Lymphatic mapping and sentinel lymph-node (SLN) biopsy is a relatively simple, effective, and minimally invasive technique that can provide the same staging information as an elective lymph-node dissection without subjecting the patient to the risks and morbidity associated with the more extensive procedure. Apart from the reduced morbidity for the patient, SLN biopsy allows the pathologist to focus attention on a few nodes that are the most likely to harbor metastatic disease, instead of screening the entire nodal basin at risk. Since the pathologic material being examined is limited, step-section examination using routine hematoxylin-and-eosin (H&E) methods and sophisticated techniques such as immunohistochemistry (IHC) and reverse transcriptase–polymerase chain reaction (RT-PCR) become practical and cost-effective. However, the technique entails a learning curve, and the implications of detection of submicroscopic disease in the SLN will need further evaluation and a longer follow-up.

ANATOMICAL PERSPECTIVES

The SLN is defined as the primary node within the regional nodal basin of a primary lesion that is at risk of lymphatic metastasis; it is the SLN that ultimately defines the risk of additional metastatic disease within that basin. The technique of SLN biopsy is based on two principles: (i) lymphatic drainage of a primary melanoma can be accurately followed to an SLN in its regional nodal basin; and (ii) the presence or absence of metastatic disease in the SLN is an accurate and reliable predictor of the status of the entire nodal basin.

An anatomic perspective can be obtained from the prior era in which patients underwent elective lymph-node dissection for high-risk cutaneous melanoma of the head and neck.[1] In 28 patients with positive subclinical nodal disease on final pathology who underwent an elective parotidectomy for high-risk lesions of the ear, face, and anterior scalp, 16 (57%) had metastatic disease in parotid nodes. The remaining 12 (43%) had metastatic disease involving the cervical nodes without parotid involvement.

This same study also attempted to characterize the site of nodal disease by the location of the primary lesion. Involvement of Levels II, III, and IV was common regardless of the primary site. Level I involvement was similar for anterior primary sites (anterior face, scalp, neck, and ear) versus posterior primary sites (posterior scalp and neck): 17% and 14% respectively. In contrast, for posterior primary sites, metasta-

tic disease to Level V occurred in 29%, compared with only 4% for anterior primary sites. The difficulty in predicting nodal involvement based on the site of the primary lesion emphasizes the need for a directed approach to clinically negative regional nodes.

TECHNIQUE

Patients scheduled for SLN biopsy undergo preoperative lymphoscintigraphy (LSG) to facilitate identification of all nodal basins at risk and also to identify in-transit SLNs. At the Memorial Sloan-Kettering Cancer Center (MSKCC), we inject 0.05 mCi of radioactive technetium-99m-sulfur colloid (Tc-99m-SC) in a volume of 0.5 ml (cc) into four quadrants of the lesion or around the biopsy scar, for a total dose of 0.2 mCi. A lead marker is placed in the external auditory canal to provide orientation in interpretation of the images (see Figure 29.2B). The injection is carried out in the nuclear medicine suite on the morning of the planned surgical procedure, and dynamic scans of all nodal basins at risk are obtained beginning 5–10 minutes after injection using a large field-of-view gamma camera set at a 20% window and fitted with a low-energy, high-resolution parallel-hole collimator. Anterior and lateral static images are obtained at 5-minute intervals over a period of 20 minutes to 2 hours. Particular care with this imaging must be taken when the primary site is close to the nodal basin, for example, in an anterior cheek lesion with the parotid bed at risk for metastatic nodal disease.

After LSG, the patient is taken to the operating room for SLN biopsy. This surgical procedure is carried out between 2–4 hours after injection of the radiocolloid, and the images obtained in nuclear medicine are used to guide the procedure in the operating room. The operating-room setup for SLN biopsy includes equipment for injection of 1% isosulfan blue dye and localization of the radioactive colloid. A tuberculin syringe is used to inject the blue dye in an intradermal plane into the four quadrants of the lesion. A volume of 0.5 ml is recommended, as larger volumes tend to dissipate into the subcutaneous tissue and cause artifacts, complicating the interpretation. Do not inject more dye than will be removed with the wide excision, as residual dye may be retained for months or years. Also, injection into deeper subcutaneous tissue not only results in technical failure due to inadequate migration of the dye or radiocolloid, but also in staining of adjacent tissue, which may obscure identification of the SLN.

The operating-room equipment includes a hand-held gamma probe, which is used to localize the SLN guided by the preoperative LSG films. The radioactivity counts over the SLNs and the background levels are noted. When scanning for activity, it is important to avoid pointing the probe in the direction of the injection site, particularly in situations where the SLN is in close proximity to the primary lesion, because the "shine-through" may result in falsely elevated counts, which interfere with or prevent identification of the SLN. This is especially crucial in some locations, such as the cheek, where the nodal basin (e.g., the intraparotid lymph nodes) may be in close proximity to the primary lesion. In such instances, it may become necessary to excise the primary lesion and then proceed with SLN biopsy.

A "hot" node, one containing radioactive colloid, should have an in vivo 10-second count at least 3 times that of the background and should correlate with the preoperative LSG films. After identification of the hot spot, the skin over the node is incised and limited flaps are elevated, first in the direction of the primary lesion, to identify the blue-stained lymphatic channel. It is important in approaching the SLN to use incisions that may be incorporated into the formal incisions for nodal dissection in the case of a positive SLN (Figures 29.1 and 29.2). For example, in patients with a parotid or periparotid SLN, a modified Blair incision should be used in part or in its entirety to access the SLN. In those instances in which a parotidectomy and neck dissection are used for a positive SLN, the entire dissection can be completed through this incision. Similarly, SLN biopsy procedures in the neck should be planned in such a fashion as to incorporate the larger inci-

sions needed for a complete neck dissection, most commonly a trifurcation or "hockey-stick" design. Appropriate incision design will reduce the risk of injury to vital structures, such as the marginal mandibular branch of the facial nerve and spinal accessory nerve, and optimize cosmetic outcome. In elevating the skin flaps, care must be exercised to keep the flaps thin enough to avoid injury to the lymphatic channels, and meticulous hemostasis is crucial. Both the blue-stained channel and radioactivity counts are used to guide dissection and identification of the SLN. Visual dissection of the blue channel can be complemented by the intensity of the audio signal of the gamma probe. After identification of the SLN, the afferent and efferent lymphatics are divided and ligated or clipped, and the node is excised.

The gamma probe is used to measure ex vivo radioactivity of the SLN, and this count should be at least 10 times that of a neighboring non-SLN. A background count is obtained by measuring activity in four quadrants of the nodal basin, and a count is also obtained from the bed of the SLN. A residual radioactive count greater than 10% of that of the hottest node in the basin indicates the presence of additional SLN(s) that should be removed. Once all SLNs are harvested, the activity of the basin should be less than 10% of the hottest SLN.

If dissection and identification of the SLN takes longer than 45 minutes, a repeat injection of the blue dye may become necessary. The half-life of the radioactive sulfur colloid is 6 hours, and although absolute counts drop after that time, the ratios of activity in the SLN versus non-SLN remain similar. It is because of these differences in their dynamics that the isosulfan blue dye and radiocolloid are not administered in a single injection.

The technique of SLN biopsy when used for cervical nodes is similar to that used in the axilla and groin. Considerable controversy exists, however, when the SLN is in the substance of the parotid gland. Options consist of formal parotidectomy with facial-nerve dissection and inspection of the parotid specimen on the back table for the SLN, versus intraparotid gland dissection in vivo with identification and

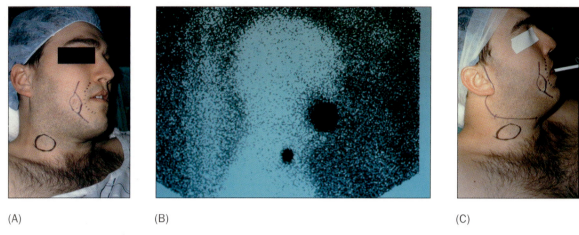

(A) (B) (C)

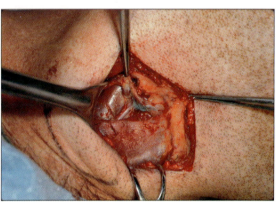

(D)

Figure 29.1 *Case 1*: This patient has a malignant melanoma 2.2 mm thick, involving the right perioral skin (A). The excision of the primary site is marked out, as is the location of the "hot spot" corresponding to the site of the SLN seen on LSG (B). A modified Blair incision allows for a complete parotidectomy and neck dissection in the case of a positive SLN (C). The blue, hot SLN is identified through a smaller incision (D) and proves to be benign on frozen-section analysis. After excision of the primary site, no further surgery is done.

excision of the SLN with preservation of the parotid gland. The latter is associated with the risk of inadvertent facial-nerve injury. The authors' technique has evolved over time from the former to the latter (Figure 29.2). In instances where the lymphoscintigram and gamma probe isolate the parotid gland as the site of the SLN, a formal modified Blair incision is used to obtain broad visual access to the nodal bed. In elevating a thin flap in the parotidomasseteric fascia or superficial musculoaponeurotic system, particular attention must be directed toward identification of SLNs that may be in the periparotid lymph nodes, including those that are situated on the capsule of the gland. In cases where a blue channel is identified, it can be readily followed through the parotid capsule to the SLN with confirmation by the gamma probe both in vivo and ex vivo. In situations where no blue channel is evident, small incisions are made in the parotid fascia to facilitate identification of the intraparotid blue lymphatic channel. The authors feel strongly that the latter technique should be used only by the experienced parotid surgeon who has a sense of the depth and the course of the main trunk of the facial nerve and its subsequent branching. When using this technique, the authors do not use paralytic anesthesia, so that motion in the distribution of the facial nerve can be identified and modifications in dissection directed accordingly. Particular care must be taken when anterior periparotid nodes are being dissected, because damage to both the

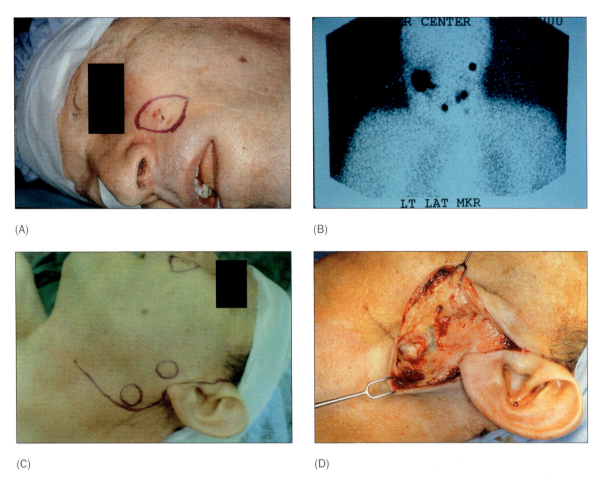

Figure 29.2 *Case 2*: This patient has a malignant melanoma 4 mm thick, involving the left cheek (A). Lymphoscintigraphy shows the primary site with two intraparotid SLNs (B). The most superolateral signal is a lead marker placed in the external auditory canal as an orientation device. A modified Blair incision allows access to both of the intraparotid SLNs, and a parotidectomy if needed (C). Elevation of the anterior skin flap in the parotidomasseteric fascia identifies two blue lymphatic channels leading to two intraparotid SLNs (D). The SLNs are each carefully excised without a facial-nerve dissection or a formal parotidectomy, and both are benign on frozen-section analysis. After excision of the primary site and a local flap closure, no further surgery is done.

distal, terminal facial-nerve branches and the parotid duct can occur. Furthermore, in instances of deep dissection in the stylomastoid foramen region, formal identification of the facial nerve allows the safe and effective delivery of the SLN. The authors are not aware of any instances of deep lobe parotid or parapharyngeal node involvement with an SLN in cases of cutaneous melanoma.

After excision, the SLN is submitted for frozen-section analysis. Alternatively, touch preparation cytology has been shown to be effective for achieving diagnosis while conserving tissue.[4] While acknowledging that frozen-section analysis may detect only 50% of nodes ultimately found to be positive by serial sectioning and IHC, it is felt that if a positive SLN can be identified by frozen-section analysis, immediate completion lymph-node dissection is often safer than delayed completion dissection.

The patients are counselled preoperatively of the potential for a false-negative SLN by frozen-section analysis, which can occur in about 7–9% of cases and will necessitate a secondary nodal dissection. The rationale for obtaining the frozen section is the reduction in morbidity, primarily consisting of facial-nerve and spinal accessory-nerve injury in the primary setting versus the secondary setting. For patients with a positive intraparotid SLN, accurate intraoperative frozen-section analysis is especially important to avoid the need for a secondary procedure through a previously elevated cheek flap. A seasoned pathologist is the surgeon's best ally in this setting. If metastatic disease is identified intraoperatively, a comprehensive nodal dissection consisting of subtotal parotidectomy and/or neck dissection is completed depending upon the site of the primary lesion.

Considerable nuances exist in terms of the extent of comprehensive dissection in the setting of a positive SLN. In cases of positive parotid SLN, a subtotal parotidectomy incorporating all of the periparotid lymph nodes including those over the masseter muscle is performed, leaving only a small tuft of gland deep to the facial nerve. In cases of positive parotid nodes, neck dissection is also indicated, as additional nodal basins are at risk. The authors typically perform a Level I–IV nodal dissection for anterior primaries arising in the face, ear, and anterior scalp. When a parotidectomy is indicated for patients with relatively posterior scalp primaries, which rarely metastasize to the parotid gland, the dissection is extended to Levels II–V, including the postauricular nodes. Finally, for patients with a positive cervical SLN, parotidectomy is only performed in instances where the primary would drain to the parotid gland, such as the anterior scalp, face, or ear. This issue is extremely controversial. The presence of a lymphatic channel on the preoperative lymphoscintigram coursing through the parotid gland adds credence to the decision to incorporate the parotidectomy in the dissection. The authors maintain an aggressive posture toward the issue of parotidectomy in these difficult

situations, given the ability to perform the procedure with limited morbidity. A Level I–V modified neck dissection is routinely performed, with preservation of the internal jugular vein, sternocleidomastoid muscle, and spinal accessory nerve for patients with both anterior and posterior neck cutaneous primaries with a positive SLN identified at any of the cervical levels.

Intraoperatively, isosulfan blue dye injection may rarely result in transient hypotension, which usually responds to a fluid bolus. The dye may also cause falsely depressed oxygen saturation levels intraoperatively. Patients should be warned that they may have blue-green discoloration of the urine for 24–48 hours postoperatively. Other complications attendant with wide excision and lymph-node biopsy or dissection, such as cranial neuropathy, cellulitis, wound infection, and seroma, are rare.

RESULTS

Wells et al reviewed their experience with LSG for melanomas in the head and neck region.[4] These authors used a combination of vital blue-dye and technetium-99m injection, identifying an SLN in 55 of 58 consecutive patients (95%). In the 49 patients with negative SLNs, there was no evidence of metastatic disease in the SLN basin or in other nodal basins with a median follow-up of approximately 1 year. Positive SLNs were detected in 6 patients (11%). Upon completion lymph-nodal dissection, there was no instance of additional metastatic lymph nodes within the lymph-node dissection specimens. The authors did not specifically address the pattern of metastasis and the site of nodal dissection regarding the parotid bed versus the cervical nodes. Likewise, they do not discuss the issue of the primary subsite in the head and neck.

Bostick et al reviewed their experience with 117 patients with primary cutaneous melanoma of the upper chest and head and neck undergoing LSG with SLN biopsy.[5] A total of 82 patients had head and neck primaries and 35 had upper-torso primaries; however, it is not feasible to segregate the patients with head and neck primaries. It should be noted that two different techniques were used; that of blue dye alone and that of blue dye with the use of the gamma probe. For the two groups, the number of SLNs per basin was identical, with a mean of 1.4. Basin identification rate was 92% for the blue dye and 96% for the blue dye plus the probe. The metastasis rate was identical at 11% for each group. The authors conclude that the combination of both blue dye and injection with Tc-99m and the use of the gamma probe may be a more sensitive method to detect SLNs.

O'Brien et al reported a group of 97 patients who underwent LSG for cutaneous melanoma of the head and neck.[6] The primary purpose of the study was to analyze the pattern of SLNs based on the primary subsite in the head and neck region. At least one SLN was identified by preoperative LSG in 95 of 97 patients. There was a mean number of 2.7 SLNs. Fully 21 of 97 patients (22%) demonstrated SLNs in sites other than the parotid gland and the five standard cervical levels. Only a small minority of patients (20) underwent true SLN biopsy procedures. The involved SLNs included a postauricular lymph node in 13 patients, an occipital lymph node in 5 patients, axillary nodes in 2, and 1 patient with an "interval" node from a scalp melanoma. Using a schema of anterior versus posterior primary sites, draining to corresponding anterior posterior nodal basins, a total of 33 of 97 (34%) demonstrated drainage to a site outside the clinically predicted sites of involvement. This confirms the unpredictable drainage pattern of cutaneous primaries. Only 20 of these patients had both a wide excision of the primary and an SLN biopsy procedure. Four patients (20%) had histologically positive SLNs and underwent subsequent completion lymph-node dissection. In 4 of the remaining 16 patients, nodal recurrence developed in the neck, suggesting that the technique of lymph-node mapping with SLN biopsy may have missed half of the patients with positive nodes.

Ollila et al reviewed the experience with parotid regional lymphatic mapping and SLN biopsy for cutaneous melanoma in 39 patients.[7] The authors used the technique of intraparotid

gland dissection without formally identifying the facial nerve. The SLN was identified in 37 of 39 patients (95%). The 2 patients in whom the SLN could not be identified underwent superficial parotidectomy (5%). The mean number of SLNs was 2.3 per patient. A positive lymph node was identified in 4 of 39 patients (10%). The tumor-positive SLN was anterior to the parotid gland in 2 patients, in an intraparotid gland in 1 patient, and at the inferior edge of the gland in 1 patient. Upon completion parotidectomy and modified neck dissection, there was no residual metastatic melanoma of the parotid gland, although 2 of the 4 patients exhibited metastatic melanoma in the modified-neck-dissection specimen. In addition, 6 patients had a second SLN identified in the cervical region. One of these was found to contain metastatic melanoma in the setting of a negative parotid SLN. With a median follow-up of 33 months, in the 33 patients whose parotid SLN was tumor-negative, there has only been 1 recurrence (3%). It should be noted that procedure-related morbidity was minimal, consisting of 1 patient (3%) experiencing temporary facial paresis that resolved completely. There were no cases of permanent facial paralysis, Frey's syndrome, or injury to Stensen's duct. The authors conclude that intra- and peri-parotid lymph-node dissection without formal parotidectomy is a safe and effective SLN procedure.

Kelemen et al have investigated their experience performing lymphatic mapping in SLN biopsy in patients who had undergone previous wide-local excision of the primary melanoma.[8] They performed this mostly in patients who had extremity lesions and in patients who had undergone excision with 2-cm margins. In the 47 patients who underwent the procedure, 11 had positive SLNs, of which 8 were solitary nodal metastases. There was a median follow-up of 36 months, and 3 SLN-negative patients developed nodal recurrence. Two of these patients had positive SLNs on pathology re-review and were felt to be pathologic misses, not failures of the lymphatic mapping technique. The third patient developed in-transit metastasis and delayed nodal recurrence. A fourth patient developed nodal recurrence in the basin opposite that identified by LSG. The overall error rate was 26%, since 4 of 15 patients with positive nodes were missed by the SLN biopsy procedure. The authors have cautioned against the use of this technique in patients who have undergone wide excision, especially with split-thickness skin grafts or closure with flap rotations, and in cases where the melanoma occurs in the head and neck or trunk region.

Between February 1996 and February 2000 at MSKCC, 56 patients underwent lymphatic mapping for a cutaneous malignant melanoma of the head and neck. There were 15 females (27%) and 41 males (73%) among them, and patients ranged in age from 12 years to 86 years, with a median of 62 years. Most patients had had previous surgical manipulation of the primary lesion elsewhere (biopsy in 45% and excision in 52%), while only 3 patients (5%) had unviolated tumors. The site of the primary lesion was the scalp in 19 patients (34%), cheek in 15 patients (27%), ear in 11 patients (20%), neck in 8 (14%) patients, and the face in 3 patients (5%).

Lymphoscintigraphy using Tc-99m-SC was performed in all 56 patients and at least one SLN was identified in 53 of 56 patients (95%). Sentinel lymph nodes were found in the neck in 37 patients (66%), in the parotid gland in 9 (16%), in the neck and parotid in 6 (11%), and in the axilla and neck in 1 patient. No SLN could be identified in 3 (5%) patients. Intraoperative injection of isosulfan blue dye was used in 49 patients; dye failed to migrate to a blue SLN in 14 of these patients (29%), but its combination with LSG improved overall accuracy. One intraparotid node that was not identified on LSG was identified by blue-dye injection. The overall success rate for identifying an SLN using a combination of the two techniques was therefore 93%, with a failure rate of 7%.

Sentinel lymph nodes were identified at and sampled from Level I in 10 patients (18%), Level II in 7 patients (12%), Levels III and IV in 3 patients (5%) each, Level V in 4 patients (7%), the parotid in 15 patients (27%), and occipital in 11 patients (20%). Frozen-section analysis of the SLNs was obtained in 51 patients, while in the remaining 5, it was either not done or not applicable. Sentinel lymph nodes were positive on frozen-section analysis in 4 patients (7%), and these patients were subjected to immediate neck dissection. A total of 134 SLNs were harvested, ranging from 1 to 11 per patient, with a median of 2. Six of the 134 SLNs (4.5%), in 4 patients, were reported to contain metastatic malignant melanoma. All 4 patients with positive SLNs underwent neck dissection, in addition to 3 patients who had negative SLNs. A total of 289 non-SLNs were harvested of which only 2 (0.7%) were positive for melanoma, both of which were in specimens from patients whose necks were dissected for a positive SLN. No positive non-SLNs were detected in patients with negative SLNs. All SLNs were subjected to serial sectioning and IHC for S-100 and HMB-45 in 32 patients; these investigations did not identify any nodal metastases not seen on frozen-section analysis or routine H&E.

With a median follow-up of 13 months (range 1–39 months), 6 of the 56 patients (10.7%) have had a recurrence: two at distant sites, one locally, two locally as well as at distant sites, and one in the neck. One patient with a local recurrence was salvaged surgically, and therefore 51 of the 56 patients (91%) are alive and free of disease at the time of this analysis. All 4 patients who failed SLN mapping are alive and free of disease. One patient had a neck recurrence after SLN mapping that identified an SLN in each of the parotid glands and at Level II. At the index surgery, this patient had been treated with wide-local excision of a previously biopsied left parietal scalp lesion and complex local flap repair with SLN biopsy and superficial parotidectomy. The primary lesion was reported to be Clark's Level 5 and 6.5 mm thick, with no other adverse histological features and negative surgical margins. Frozen-section analysis, permanent analysis, serial step-sectioning, and IHC of the two SLNs showed no evidence of metastatic malignant melanoma, and the patient was kept under observation. One year after index surgery, he developed nodal metastases in the ipsilateral side of the neck at Level II. He underwent a modified radical neck dissection type I, and pathology showed a 2-cm metastatic-node mass at Level II with extracapsular spread; however, all of the remaining 48 nodes were negative. He was not given postoperative radiation therapy. A year later, he developed a soft-tissue recurrence 4.5 cm in diameter spanning Levels II and III, for which he underwent surgical excision and has been recommended postoperative radiation therapy.

As detection techniques become more sophisticated, the relevance of submicroscopic metastasis detected using assays such as RT-PCR for tyrosinase, or one of the other markers such as GP-100, MAGE-3, and MART-1 will need to be determined.[9] The multi-institutional Sunbelt Melanoma Trial is examining this question on a prospective basis, and preliminary results suggest a linear relationship between the Breslow thickness and the rate of positive SLNs by RT-PCR. The clinical significance of node positivity by RT-PCR remains to be clearly defined.[10]

There are some initial reports evaluating the technique of SLN mapping in patients with squamous-cell carcinoma of the head and neck.[11–14] As with cutaneous melanoma, the initial questions to be answered are whether the technique could reliably identify an SLN, and whether the status of this node would accurately reflect that of the remainder of the nodal basin. The largest experience to date comes out of Glasgow in the UK,[13] where a total of 26 patients with a single focus of squamous-cell carcinoma of the head and neck were evaluated using either blue-dye injection alone (13 patients) or a combination of Tc-99m-labeled albumin with blue-dye injection (13 patients). Among the 13 patients who had blue-dye injection alone, an SLN was identified in 5 patients. None of the nodes was found to contain tumor, but 3 of the 5 patients had pathologically positive nodes elsewhere in the neck. During the latter part of that study, blue-dye injection was combined with LSG in evaluating 16 neck sites in 13 patients. Six of the 16 neck sides were clinically positive, but 7 of the remaining 10 were found to be pathologically node-positive. At least one SLN in each of these patients was found to contain tumor. This limited experience suggests the feasibility of the technique in evaluation of head and neck tumors and highlights the importance of combining blue-dye injection with LSG.

In summary, patients with cutaneous melanoma of the head and neck provide a unique anatomic consideration, because they often have multiple SLNs and an unpredictable pattern of involvement. Particular concern exists in terms of intraparotid lymph-node biopsy and ultimate facial-nerve function. Given the incidence of false-negative lymph nodes reported in this and other series, these patients require long-term follow-up, and ultimately, the efficacy of this procedure needs to be better established for head and neck cutaneous sites. Results can be optimized with meticulous attention to detail in the application of the nuclear medicine scan, surgical technique, and pathologic evaluation. It may be concluded that the head and neck region is less "forgiving" than trunk and extremity sites.

REFERENCES

1. Shah JP, Kraus DH, Dubner S, Sarkar S, Patterns of regional lymph node metastases from cutaneous melanomas of the head and neck. *Am J Surg* 1991; **162**:320–3.
2. Caldwell CB, Spiro RH, The role of parotidectomy in the treatment of cutaneous head and neck melanoma. *Am J Surg* 1988; **156**:318–22.
3. Urist MM, Balch CM, Soong SJ et al, Head and neck melanoma in 534 clinical Stage I patients. A prognostic factors analysis and results of surgical treatment. *Ann Surg* 1984; **200**:769–75.
4. Wells KE, Rapaport DP, Cruse CW et al, Sentinel lymph node biopsy in melanoma of the head and neck. *Plast Reconstr Surg* 1997; **100**:591–4.
5. Bostick P, Essner R, Sarantou T et al, Intraoperative lymphatic mapping for early-stage melanoma of the head and neck. *Am J Surg* 1997; **174**:536–9.
6. O'Brien CJ, Uren RF, Thompson JF et al, Prediction of potential metastatic sites in cutaneous head and neck melanoma using lymphoscintigraphy. *Am J Surg* 1995; **170**:461–6.
7. Ollila DW, Foshag LJ, Essner R et al, Parotid region lymphatic mapping and sentinel lym-

phadenectomy for cutaneous melanoma. *Ann Surg Oncol* 1999; **6:**150–4.

8. Kelemen PR, Essner R, Foshag LJ, Morton DL, Lymphatic mapping and sentinel lymphadenectomy after wide local excision of primary melanoma. *J Am Coll Surg* 1999; **189:**247–52.

9. Goscin C, Glass LF, Messina JL, Pathologic examination of the sentinel lymph node in melanoma. *Surg Oncol Clin N Am* 1999; **8:**427–34.

10. Li W, Stall A, Shivers SC et al, Clinical relevance of molecular staging for melanoma: comparison of RT-PCR and immunohistochemistry staining in sentinel lymph nodes of patients with melanoma. *Ann Surg* 2000; **231:**795–803.

11. Pitman KT, Johnson JT, Edington H et al, Lymphatic mapping with isosulfan blue dye in squamous cell carcinoma of the head and neck. *Arch Otolaryngol Head Neck Surg* 1998; **124:**790–3.

12. Koch WM, Choti MA, Civelek AC et al, Gamma probe-directed biopsy of the sentinel node in oral squamous cell carcinoma. *Arch Otolaryngol Head Neck Surg* 1998; **124:**455–9.

13. Shoaib T, Soutar DS, Prosser JE et al, A suggested method for sentinel node biopsy in squamous cell carcinoma of the head and neck. *Head Neck* 1999; **21:**728–33.

14. Alex JC, Sasaki CT, Krag DN et al, Sentinel lymph node radiolocalization in head and neck squamous cell carcinoma. *Laryngoscope* 2000; **110:**198–203.

Urologic cancers

Ramon M Cabanas

SLN Biopsy technique for urologic cancers

Technique	Combination	Isotope	*Type*: Tc-99m-SC
Dye	*Type*: Isosulfan blue dye		*Filtered*: No
	Volume: 0.5–1 ml (cc)		*Dose*: 0.3 mCi (11 MBq)
			Volume: 1–1.5 ml (cc)
Injection site	*Isotope*: Intradermal		
	Dye: Close to tumor		

Today, preoperative and intraoperative lymphatic mapping and sentinel lymph node (SLN) biopsy are important diagnostic and therapeutic tools in urologic surgical oncology, with potential applications in penile, scrotal, prostate, and testicular carcinomas.[1,2] Indeed, despite increasingly wide use in other malignancies, most notably melanoma and breast cancer, the concept of the sentinel lymph node has its origins in the study of penile cancer. The concept was introduced by this author in 1976, and represented the culmination of an 8-year investigation in 100 patients, 80 with penile cancer, 10 with inflammatory conditions, and 10 normal volunteers. Based on the results of lymphangiograms, anatomic dissections, and pathologic findings, the author postulated that the lymphatic system of the penis drains initially to one or a few lymph nodes, the "sentinel lymph nodes," and that these nodes were the primary site of metastases in penile carcinoma. A pathologically negative SLN might predict a negative node basin in general, and might allow the avoidance of an inguinal node dissection.

The importance of lymph-node status as a predictor of survival in patients with early-stage urologic cancers is well documented.[3,4] With clinically localized prostate carcinoma, for example, pelvic lymph-node metastasis is a sign of systematic disease and accurate staging in this setting is crucial.[3-5] Many authors between 1953 and 1983 described the use of radiocolloid injections to image the lymphatic drainage of the prostate gland,[6-11] and all described the potential applications of iliopelvic lymphoscintigraphy (LSG) in urologic malignancies. Horenblas,[12] in 1992, reported the results of pelvic LSG performed by perianal injection of the ischiorectal fossa in 11 patients with locally confined prostatic carcinoma, and concluded that iliopelvic LSG by this technique has low specificity. Significantly, none of the above studies applied the SLN concept.

The SLN concept is a simple one, the mapping agents (blue dye and radioisotopes) are widely available, and the surgical technique is generally straightforward.[1–3,12–19] Horenblas et al have recently validated SLN biopsy for carcinoma of the penis, concluding that "the dynamic sentinel node procedure is a promising staging technique to detect early metastatic dissemination of penile cancer," and that it "enables identification of patients with clinically node negative disease requiring regional lymph node dissection."[17] Other clinical studies of pelvic SLN mapping with LSG, a hand-held intraoperative gamma probe, and blue-dye injection are under way, and the results of these studies are eagerly awaited.[2]

For penile carcinoma, the author recommends bilateral SLN biopsy, and if the SLN proves negative, that no further lymph-node surgery be performed. If the SLN is positive, an inguinofemoroiliac node dissection is done. We recommend a similar approach in patients with squamous-cell carcinomas of the scrotum, performing an ilioinguinal node dissection only if the SLN proves positive.

We presume that the same benefits might apply in prostate cancer, where mapping agents might be injected either intra- or periprostatically, and SLN biopsy be done laparoscopically. Such studies have not yet been done.

THE TECHNIQUE OF SLN BIOPSY

For SLN biopsy in penile and in scrotal cancers, this author recommends a technique that combines preoperative LSG and intraoperative SLN mapping using both blue dye and radioisotope. Both cancers require a wide-local excision of the primary lesion, with preoperative injection of tracer (blue dye and/or isotope) around the primary site. Although the basic treatment of squamous-cell carcinoma of the scrotum is wide-local excision, SLN biopsy allows the surgeon to rule out nodal micrometastasis and therefore the need for a formal ilioinguinal lymphadenectomy.[5] The male genital organ has the advantage of being a midline structure in which both anatomical parameters and lymphatic

mapping (by isotope and blue dye) can be used to identify the SLN.

SLN biopsy using anatomic landmarks

Initial work, based on the injection of contrast agents into the dorsal lymphatics of the penis, demonstrates that these lymphatics drain to the superficial inguinal nodes medially, and to the superomedial inguinal nodes in particular (Figure 30.1). Because this particular technique of lymphangiography proved cumbersome, an alternative method is to identify the SLN by using anatomic parameters alone. Here, a 5-cm incision is made parallel to the inguinal ligament, two fingers'-breadth lateral and two fingers'-breadth distal to the pubic tubercle, overlying the saphenofemoral junction. The SLN is located by inserting the finger under the upper flap toward the pubic tubercle.[1–3,16] The SLN lies among the lymph nodes associated with the superficial epigastric vein (Figure 30.2). The position of the SLN in relation to this vein may vary, but never by more than 1 cm. The superficial epigastric vein is absent in 1.4% of cases, and occasionally there is more than one lymph node in the superficial epigastric group. In this setting, all lymph nodes in this area (generally two or three) should be removed. The true SLN is always the larger and more medially situated.[1–3,15,16]

SLN biopsy using tracers

Modern techniques map the SLN by the preoperative injection of unfiltered technetium-99m-sulfur colloid (Tc-99m-SC). We recommend a dose of 0.3 mCi (11 MBq), injected intradermally either in the foreskin of the penis or proximal to the cancer. The SLN is usually imaged within 30 minutes, using both the conventional gamma camera and a hand-held gamma probe to identify the SLN by its intense isotope uptake.[2] European investigators have used 1.6 mCi (60 MBq) of Tc-99m-colloidal albumin (nanocolloid) to map the SLN. Horenblas et al

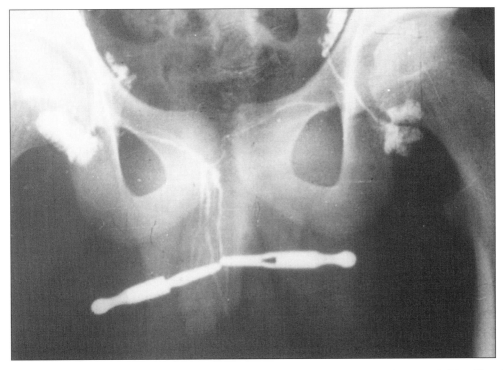

Figure 30.1 Lymphangiogram: direct injection via dorsal lymphatic ducts of the penis identifies the SLN.

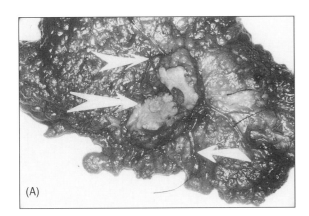

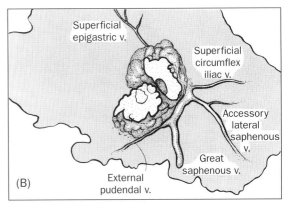

(A)

(B)

Superficial
epigastric v.

Superficial
circumflex
iliac v.

Accessory
lateral
saphenous
v.

Great
saphenous v.

External
pudendal v.

Figure 30.2 Anatomical parameters, indicated by arrows (A) and shown in the accompanying diagram (B), can be used to identify the SLN.

report performing LSG the day before surgery.[17] A focal area of radionuclide accumulation, marking the location of the SLN, is easily discerned, and we recommend leaving a skin marker on this spot (Figure 30.3). Using the same technique, we search the opposite groin for SLNs as well. At the conclusion of the LSG procedure, anterior and lateral images are obtained (Figure 30.4).

We have found that the time between the injection of the Tc-99m-SC and surgery must be at least 2 hours. At surgery, we first inject blue

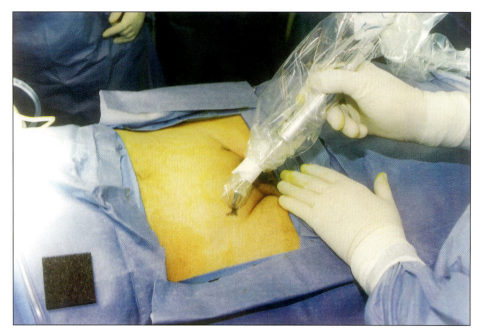

Figure 30.3 The point of maximal emission identifies the SLN, which is then marked.

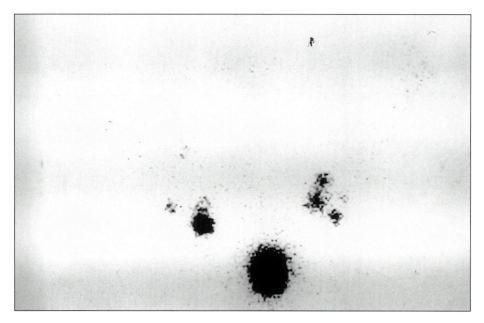

Figure 30.4 Static view of the SLN identified by unfiltered Tc-99m-SC.

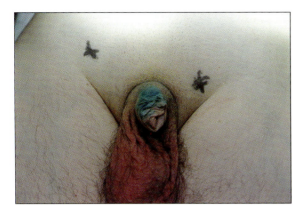

Figure 30.5 Blue dye is injected close to the lesion.

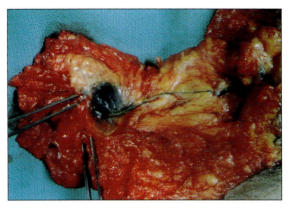

Figure 30.6 Dissecting the lymphatic ducts, which have been dyed blue. The SLN is highlighted.

dye. While we have used Patent Blue-V, Evans blue, and methylene blue in the past, we now use isosulfan blue dye. We inject 5 ml (cc) close to the tumor and gently massage the injection site in order to feel the lymphatic ducts after the blue dye has been injected (Figure 30.5). We then follow the standard steps of the SLN biopsy technique as for other anatomic sites. A skin incision is made at the point correlating with the "hot spot" identified on LSG and/or by the gamma probe.[1,3] Dissection to the level of the radiolabeled SLN(s) is carried out, guided by the gamma probe and by blue staining of the lymphatics as they drain to the SLN (Figure 30.6). Once excised, the SLN can be confirmed by its high ex vivo counts, and by a low level of counts in the surgical bed.

REFERENCES

1. Cabanas RM, The concept of the sentinel lymph node. *Rec Res Cancer Res* 2000; **157**:109–20.
2. Cabanas RM, Application of the sentinel node concept in urogenital cancer. *Rec Res Cancer Res* 2000; **157**:141–9.
3. Cabanas RM, An approach for the treatment of penile carcinoma. *Cancer* 1977; **39**:456–66.
4. Gervasi LA, Mata J, Easley JD et al, Prognostic significance of lymph nodal metastases in prostate cancer. *J Urol* 1989; **142**:332–6.
5. Lowe FC, Squamous-cell carcinoma of the scrotum. *Urol Clin N Am* 1992; **19**:397–405.
6. Gardiner RA, Fitzpatrick JM, Constable AR et al, Human prostatic lymphoscintigraphy. A preliminary report. *Br J Urol* 1979; **51**:300–3.
7. Kaplan WD, Whitmore WF, Gittes RF, Visualization of canine and human prostatic lymph nodes following intraprostatic injection of technetium-99m-antimony sulfide colloid. *Invest Radiol* 1980; **15**:34–8.
8. Kaplan WD, Iliopelvic lymphoscintigraphy. *Semin Nucl Med* 1983; **13**:42–53.
9. Stone AR, Merrick MV, Chisholm GD, Prostatic lymphoscintigraphy. *Br J Urol* 1979; **51**:556–60.
10. Sherman AI, Ter-Pogosian M, Tocus EC, Lymph-node concentration of radioactive colloidal gold following interstitial injection. *Cancer* 1953; **6**:1238–40.
11. Whitmore WF, Blute RD, Kaplan WD, Gittes RF, Radiocolloid scintigraphic mapping of the lymphatic drainage of the prostate. *J Urol* 1980; **124**:62–7.
12. Horenblas S, Nuyten MJ, Hoefnagel CA et al, Detection of lymph node invasion in prostatic carcinoma with iliopelvic lymphoscintigraphy. *Br J Urol* 1992; **69**:180–2.
13. Alex JC, Krag DN, Gamma-probe guided localization of lymph nodes. *Surg Oncol* 1993; **2**:137–43.
14. Boak JL, Agwunobi TC, A study of technetium-labelled sulphide colloid uptake by regional

lymph nodes draining a tumour-bearing area. *Br J Surg* 1978; **65**:374–8.

15. Cabanas RM, *Valoracion quirurgica de la lin-foadenografia facultad de ciencias medicas*. Thesis, University of Asuncion, Paraguay, 1969.

16. Cabanas RM, Anatomy and biopsy of sentinel lymph nodes. *Urol Clin N Am* 1992; **19**:267–76.

17. Horenblas S, Jansen L, Meinhardt W et al, Detection of occult metastasis in squamous cell carcinoma of the penis using a dynamic sentinel node procedure. *J Urol* 2000; **163**:100–4.

18. Morton DL, Wen DR, Wong JH et al, Technical details of intraoperative lymphatic mapping for early stage melanoma. *Arch Surg* 1992; **127**:394–9.

19. Steinbecker KM, Muruve NA, Lympho-scintigraphy for penile cancer. *J Urol* 2000; **163**:1251–2.

31

Gynecologic cancers

Charles Levenback

The MD Anderson Cancer Center technique for SLN biopsy for gynecologic cancers

Technique	*Vulvar*: Dye *Cervical*: Combination	**Isotope**	*Type*: Tc-99m-sulfur colloid *Filtered*: Yes *Dose*: 0.5–1.0 mCi *Volume*: 1.0 ml (cc)
Dye	*Type*: Isosulfan blue dye *Volume*: 1.0 ml (cc)		
Injection site	*Isotope*: Tc-99m-sulfur colloid *Dye*: *Vulvar*: Peritumoral *Cervical*: Peritumoral or 4 quadrants		

Gynecologic surgeons have been using in vivo mapping techniques to study the lymphatic system of the female genital tract for years. Eduard Eichner[1-3] was the first gynecologist to systematically use lymphatic mapping to study both the external and internal female genitalia. He described the complex drainage of the midline structures of the cervix and uterine fundus using the dye Sky Blue. Unfortunately, he used subcutaneous injections of the dye to study the vulva, drawing the incorrect conclusion that vulvar lymphatics drain directly to the pelvis.

More recently, investigators have been adapting sentinel lymph node (SLN) identification methods pioneered in patients with cutaneous melanoma or breast cancer for patients who have gynecologic cancers. Vulvar and cervical cancers are especially attractive targets for lymphatic mapping strategies, because the rate of nodal spread in patients with Stage I tumors is low and the morbidity of regional lym-

phadenectomy is high. In addition, most vulvar and cervical cancer patients with nodal disease do not have systemic disease; therefore, their disease is still curable using radiation or chemoradiation. Accurate identification of patients with micrometastases that were missed using other methods could improve the overall outcome of patients who have these diseases.

This chapter reviews the rationale for lymphatic mapping in patients who have vulvar or cervical cancers and current techniques of SLN identification at each disease site.

VULVAR CANCER

Background

Vulvar cancers account for only 1–2% of all female cancers (Table 31.1). In addition, many studies have confirmed the presence of two

Table 31.1 Estimated number of new cancer cases in the USA in 2000, according to Greenlee et al

Site	Total	Female
Breast	184 200	182 800
Colon	93 800	50 400
Melanoma	47 700	20 400
Uterine corpus	36 100	36 100
Ovary	23 100	23 100
Uterine cervix	12 800	12 800
Vulva	3400	3400

Adapted from Greenlee RT, Murray T, Bolden S, Wingo PA, Cancer Statistics, 2000. *CA Cancer J Clin* 2000; **50**:7–33.

different etiologic categories of vulvar cancer.[4] In the first category, the patients are younger, and invasive disease is found with immediately adjacent intraepithelial neoplasia. Human papillomavirus (HPV) DNA is found in a majority of cases. In the second category, the patients are older and there is no association with intraepithelial neoplasia or HPV. The clinical management in both groups is the same.

In the first half of the twentieth century, radical vulvectomy and bilateral inguinal femoral lymphadenectomy were the first successful treatments for vulvar cancer.[5,6] In previous years, vulvar cancer was considered a particularly gruesome and cruel disease because death occurred slowly and painfully due to local extension to the bladder and anus. Therefore, radical vulvectomy and bilateral inguinal femoral lymphadenectomy were embraced by the surgical community despite their high complication rates. Wound infection and lymphedema, however, occurred almost universally after these procedures; therefore, many investigators sought ways to reduce the radical nature of these operations without compromising outcome.

In 1963, Parry-Jones used intradermal injections of Patent Blue-V dye to study the in vivo anatomy of the vulva.[7] He was able to show that the vulvar lymphatics did not cross the buttocks or labial crural fold *en route* to the inguinal nodes. This was an important observation because radical vulvectomy, as it was practiced at this time, was performed based on the classical description of the vulva in cadaver studies, which stated that the lymphatics of the vulva traversed the buttocks and inner thigh. Parry-Jones had a second goal: to demonstrate direct lymphatic drainage from the vulva to the pelvis. He observed that the blue dye injected into the dermis of the vulva always arrested in the groin and could not be seen in the pelvis. Instead of rejecting his hypothesis, he concluded there was an error in his technique.

Building on the work by Parry-Jones, Morris described the use of hemivulvectomy in patients having lateral vulvar carcinomas.[8] Additionally, DiSaia et al were the first to emphasize the devastating impact of vulvectomy on body image and sexual function.[9] They emphasized the use of partial vulvectomy, regardless of the location of the primary tumor, for selected patients.

DiSaia et al were also the first gynecologists to attempt to incorporate the SLN concept into the management of gynecologic cancers.[9] They noted that they never observed a patient having positive femoral nodes who had negative superficial inguinal nodes. At the same time, Riveros et al and Cabanas described lymphatic mapping of penile cancers using a lymphography technique.[10,11] They observed that the SLN in penile cancer patients was invariably in the superficial inguinal nodes. Also, DiSaia et al described the eight to ten superficial inguinal nodes as the SLNs of the vulva.[9] Unlike the method of the Cabanas study, these SLNs were identified by their anatomic location instead of through the use of a mapping technique.

Since the original description of radical partial vulvectomy and superficial inguinal lymphadenectomy, there have been several series reporting relapse rates ranging from 0% to 7.3% following a negative superficial inguinal lymphadenectomy.[12–14] The most interesting comparison has been between Gynecologic Oncology Group (GOG) protocols 37 and 74.[15,16]

In the GOG study, 385 patients underwent a full radical vulvectomy and inguinal femoral lymphadenectomy, and were found to have histologically negative nodes. Only one of these patients had a recurrence in the groin. In the GOG 75 group, 121 patients with negative nodes underwent radical partial vulvectomy and superficial inguinal lymphadenectomy. Nine patients had a relapse in the groin in this study. Short-term surgical morbidity was acceptable in both studies. Long-term lymphedema was not described, although its incidence was probably much higher in the earlier study.

The inguinal femoral lymph-node dissection technique has continued to evolve, reducing the morbidity of the procedure. In the 1970s, it included complete removal of all of the fat and fascia of the groin, exposing the femoral artery and vein. A sartorius muscle transposition was necessary to cover the vessels and prevent hemorrhage in the event of a wound breakdown. Gynecologic oncologists have gradually reduced the extent of this dissection by eliminating removal of the fascial covering of the muscular boundaries of the femoral triangle. In addition, in cadaver studies, Borgno et al determined that the femoral lymph nodes are almost exclusively medial to the femoral vein.[17] Superficial inguinal and medial femoral lymphadenectomy accomplishes the goal of removing the eight to ten superficial inguinal nodes and two to three femoral nodes without requiring sartorius transposition.[18]

The current standard surgical treatment of a labial early vulvar carcinoma is a partial radical vulvectomy along with ipsilateral superficial inguinal and medial femoral lymphadenectomy and bilateral groin dissections for patients who have midline tumors. The rate of lymph-node metastasis is less than 1% in patients with an invasion depth of less than 1 mm, and in the 20–30% range in patients with an invasion of 3–5 mm (Table 31.2). Also, patients who have more advanced disease are considered good candidates for chemoradiation.[19,20] This is especially true when surgical margins of 1–2 cm around the tumor would compromise anal or bladder function. Preoperative chemoradiation

Table 31.2 Depth of invasion and risk of nodal metastases in patients with squamous-cell cancer of the vulva

Depth (mm)	%
<1	0
1.1–2	7.6
2.1–3	8.4
3.1–5	26.7
>5	34.2

Adapted from Berek JS, Hacker NF, eds, *Practical Gynecologic Oncology*, 3rd edn. Lippincott Williams & Wilkins: Philadelphia, 2000.

Table 31.3 Five-year survival rate versus stage for patients treated with curative intent

Clinical stage	5-year survival rate (%)
I	90.4
II	77.1
III	51.3
IV	18
Total	**69.7**

Adapted from Berek JS, Hacker NF, eds, *Practical Gynecologic Oncology*, 3rd edn. Lippincott Williams & Wilkins: Philadelphia, 2000.

allows a reduction in the extent of surgery, sparing desired organ function without sacrificing long-term survival.

Finally, the overall survival rate in patients with negative nodes is around 90%, whereas the rate in patients with positive nodes is around 50% (Table 31.3).

Lymphatic mapping using blue dye alone

Intraoperative lymphatic mapping has been described in published reports in patients having vulvar cancer. Owing to the infrequency of this disease (3500 new cases in the United States per year), however, experience with this procedure has grown slowly. At the University of Texas MD Anderson Cancer Center, our initial efforts at mapping included peritumoral injections of isosulfan blue 35 minutes prior to the inguinal incision. This incision is made parallel to and just below the inguinal ligament. In patients with labial lesions, the afferent lymphatic channel is usually found first, traversing the inguinal fat pad to the SLN. A hemostat or similar instrument is used to separate the fat lobules in order to identify the afferent channel and then the SLN. In patients with clitoral or perineal tumors, it is not uncommon to find the SLN first, with the afferent lymphatic channel entering the SLN from below. In addition, in patients with midline tumors, the SLN may be found at the extreme medial border of the femoral triangle, just lateral to the adductus longus and just above the pectineus muscle. We think this is important, because nodes in that extreme location can be missed when performing a groin dissection without the aid of lymphatic mapping.

In our series, we have identified the SLN in 88% of the patients and 76% of the lymphatic basins without any false-negative results.[21–23] We found that a prior wide-local excision, midline location, and procedure performed in the first 2 years of the series were associated with failure to identify the SLN. Following an initial 2-year learning period, and studying well-selected patients (those having squamous-cell carcinoma, a tumor limited to the vulva, no gross infection, and normal nodes according to palpation), we have identified the SLNs in 95% of the patients using blue dye alone.

The results obtained by Ansink et al from the Netherlands using blue dye alone are not as encouraging, however.[24] In this series, the SLN was identified in only 56% of the 93 groins dissected, and 2 patients had false-negative results. Additionally, although this was a multi-institu-tional study, 80% of the cases originated from one center; three other centers participated in the study, each with 6 or fewer cases. The proportion of cases performed by physicians early on in the learning curve is not clear. Despite these findings, the use of blue dye alone is an attractive option for patients who have vulvar cancer: because the SLN is found exclusively in the groin, the technique is simple and easy to perform, and the cost is minimal.

Preoperative lymphoscintigraphy and intraoperative radiolocalization

Preoperative lymphoscintigraphy (LSG) has proven to be highly valuable in disease sites that have ambiguous drainage patterns. For example, Krag et al found that 6% of breast-cancer patients undergoing surgical management had nonaxillary SLNs identified using LSG.[25] Using blue dye alone with an axillary incision would have missed the SLN in all of these patients. Similarly, patients with truncal or head and neck melanomas can have SLNs in one or more of a number of lymphatic basins; preoperative knowledge of this information is crucial to surgical planning.

There have been several series of patients with vulvar cancer who have undergone preoperative LSG.[26–28] The LSG techniques used in these patients are very similar to those used in patients with cutaneous melanoma. In addition, the application of the eutectic mixture of local anesthetic cream 1 hour prior to the injection of radiocolloid appears to be important to reduce the pain associated with the injection.

De Cicco et al used a preoperative perilesional injection of technetium-99m-labeled human albumin colloid to identify SLNs in all 37 patients studied.[28] The following day, an intraoperative hand-held gamma probe was used successfully to identify the SLNs in all of the patients. Interestingly, in just 5 of the 18 patients believed to have midline lesions on clinical grounds, only unilateral SLNs were identified. None of these patients had metastatic disease in the groin. The authors suggested using preoperative LSG to select patients for unilateral or bilateral groin dissection procedures. Another series of 59 patients from The Netherlands resulted in a similar finding.[29,30] Twelve patients had tumors primarily involving the labium; however, these tumors were defined as midline because of their encroachment to within 1 cm of the midline. Preoperative LSG showed ipsilateral SLNs only in all 12 cases. All 12 patients underwent bilateral groin dissections, and none of them had contralateral metastases. Eleven patients had clearly unilateral lesions, and none had SLNs identified in the contralateral groin using preoperative LSG.

In the operating room, the hand-held gamma probe is used to scan through the skin and locate the SLN. Following the skin incision, the probe is inserted into the wound, and the SLNs are localized and removed. The radioactivity measured in the node ex vivo should be at least 10 times greater than background counts for it to be considered an SLN. The SLN can be close to the primary tumor, especially in patients having a clitoral primary tumor, and the "shine-through" from the primary injection can interfere with SLN identification.[27,31] Using maximal collimation with the gamma probe and directing it away from the vulva helps to prevent this difficulty. Another alternative is to perform the vulvectomy portion of the procedure first. Although this conflicts with the traditional approach of proceeding from the cleaner wound (groin) to the less clean wound (vulva), it is not a serious problem in the era of modern antibiotic therapy and wound-care.

Combined SLN identification using blue dye and radiolocalization

Combining the blue dye and radiolocalization techniques appears to bring together the advantages of both. In other disease sites, it appears that in the vast majority of cases, the blue and "hot" SLNs are in fact the same nodes. In the series of 59 patients referred to above, 107 groins were dissected; the SLN was identified using at least one technique in 95 groins (89%).[29] The authors stated that the SLN was stained with blue dye in only 60% of the cases. Also, none of the patients had a false-negative SLN. Of additional interest, they found positive nodes in 20 patients using standard hematoxylin-and-eosin (H&E) staining, while an additional 102 SLNs were found to be negative for metastatic disease using H&E staining. Upon further step-sectioning of these nodes, the authors found four nodes (4%) that had micrometastases: three nodes came from one patient, while the fourth came from a patient who had another SLN that was positive according to H&E staining. The combined approach is demonstrated in Figures 31.1 through 31.4.

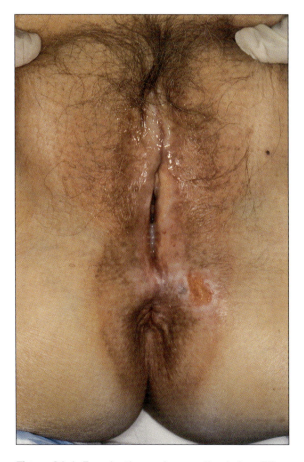

Figure 31.1 Examination under anesthesia in a 75-year-old with a slowly progressive ulcerative lesion. A punch biopsy revealed squamous-cell carcinoma. The medial border of the tumor is within 2 cm of the midline.

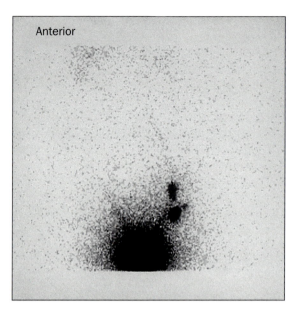

Figure 31.4 Intraoperative localization of the SLN
with blue dye and gamma probe. Note afferent
channel entering at the medial border of the field.

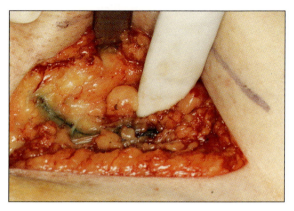

Figure 31.2 Preoperative lymphoscintigram showing
left SLNs. No significant tracer uptake on the right.

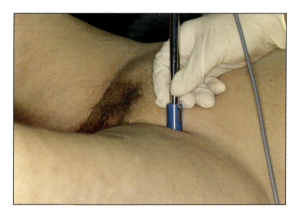

Figure 31.3 Transcutaneous localization of the SLN
using the gamma probe.

Vulvar cancer: summary

In summary, vulvar cancer is an excellent target
for SLN identification. Single-institution studies
conducted by surgeons familiar with the techniques and using well-selected patients have
indicated that using blue dye alone is adequate
to identify the SLN in almost all patients. Multi-

institution series, however, have found that
using blue-dye techniques alone is not as reliable.

Although the data are preliminary, it does
appear that preoperative LSG can determine
the need for unilateral versus bilateral groin
dissections in cases where the laterality of lymphatic drainage is ambiguous based on tumor
location alone. When preoperative LSG is performed, the hand-held gamma probe should be
used in the operating room to help localize the
SLN.

One word of caution to gynecologic oncologists: although SLN identification is clearly feasible in patients with vulvar cancer, the full
mapping concept has not yet been validated for
this disease site. It should be remembered that
knowledge of the SLN status of patients with
melanoma or breast cancer is frequently used to
select an adjuvant therapy, not to determine the
need for adjuvant therapy. Additionally,
because all patients will go on to receive further
treatment, clinicians are willing to accept a
higher false-negative rate. In patients having
vulvar cancer, a very low false-negative rate is
desirable because those having a false-negative
SLN may miss an opportunity for curative therapy. Gynecologic Oncology Group protocol 173
is in progress to determine the validity of the
SLN concept in vulvar cancer patients;

however, results of this study are still some years off. In the meantime, gynecologic oncologists should gain experience in using lymphatic mapping in patients who have vulvar cancer while continuing to perform inguinal femoral lymph-node dissection unless surgical contraindications exist.

CERVICAL CANCER

Rationale for lymphatic mapping

There are approximately 12 800 new cases of cervical cancer a year in the United States, making it the third most common gynecologic cancer after endometrial cancer and ovarian cancer. Cervical cancer is the most common female cancer in many parts of the world where screening by Papanicolaou (Pap) smear is not widely available. In well-screened populations, the incidence of cervical cancer has dropped since the introduction of the Pap smear in the 1940s. The disease has not been eliminated, however. In the United States, 50% of the women with invasive cervical cancer have not had a Pap smear within 5 years of diagnosis.

Cervical cancer was the first type of cancer to be cured using radiation therapy. After loading, tandem and cylinders placed in the uterus and vagina can be used to situate radioactive sources very close to the tumor. The cervix, bladder, and rectum are all relatively radioresistant, allowing the delivery of a high dose of radiation to the cervix without damaging the other organs. Radiation remains the mainstay for patients who have tumors too large to be removed using radical hysterectomy with maintenance of adequate margins.

Radiation therapy has been the standard treatment in patients with large tumors or regional metastases since the 1940s. In 1999, however, several published Phase III studies[32–34] demonstrated a 50% improvement in survival with the addition of cisplatin-based chemotherapy concurrent with radiation therapy. Postoperative chemoradiation also improves survival in patients with positive nodes found at the time of radical hysterectomy.

The currently preferred treatment in patients with small tumors (less than 4 cm in diameter) who are good surgical candidates is radical hysterectomy and bilateral pelvic lymph-node dissection. Radical hysterectomy provides a cure rate equal to that provided by radiation therapy alone (about 90%),[35] with fewer long-term complications in this group of patients. Radical hysterectomy is especially favorable in young patients. Ovarian metastases from cervical cancer are extremely rare, and so the ovaries can be preserved. In addition, radiation therapy can result in reduction of the length and caliber of the vagina to a much greater degree than radical hysterectomy.

A recent treatment innovation is radical trachelectomy for patients with very small lesions (usually less than 2 cm in diameter) who wish to preserve their fertility. For this procedure, the patient undergoes a laparoscopic pelvic lymphadenectomy. If the nodes are negative, a radical trachelectomy with preservation of the uterine fundus and approximately 0.5 cm of the cervix, just enough to seat a cerclage suture, is performed. Several successful pregnancies have been reported following this technique.[36–38]

The triage of patients to the most appropriate therapy is a major clinical challenge for gynecologic oncologists. The majority clinical opinion is that the combination of radical hysterectomy and radiation therapy should be avoided because cost and morbidity are increased.[39,40] Also, as is the case with other solid tumors, noninvasive imaging fails to identify small-volume or microscopic metastases. Most gynecologic oncologists perform frozen-section analysis of clinically suspicious lymph nodes intraoperatively and abort a radical hysterectomy if metastases are found. Accurate SLN identification in patients with cervical cancer could facilitate triage of patients to the most appropriate treatment and reduce the morbidity from that associated with radical surgery combined with radiation therapy.

There are several potential routes of lymphatic drainage of the cervix. The major routes are along the uterine vessels toward the pelvic side-wall; however, the obturator, common iliac, and presacral nodes all may be sites of

Site	Right	Left	Total	Per cent		
Table 31.4 Incidence of lymph-node group involvement and location in carcinoma of the uterine cervix						
Paracervical	3	3	3	2		
Obturator	34	31	65	20		
External iliac						76
medial	50	53	103	31	74	
anterior	15	17	32	10		
lateral	10	9	19	6		
Hypogastric	15	9	24	7		
Common iliac	28	18	46	14		
Periaortic	14	17	31	10		
Total number of involved node groups	169	157	323	—		
Total number of cases	91	—	—	—		
Average number of node groups per case	—	—	3.5	—		

From Graham JB, Sotto LSJ, Paoloucek FP, *Carcinoma of the Cervix*. Lippincott Williams & Wilkins: Philadelphia, 2000.

metastases in patients with cervical cancer. Para-aortic metastases are considered very rare in the absence of pelvic node metastases (Table 31.4).

Lymphatic mapping using blue dye alone

O'Boyle et al have reported a series of 20 patients who underwent mapping using blue dye alone.[41] They identified the SLN in 60% of the patients and in 43% of the lymphatic basins. Sentinel lymph-node identification was more successful in patients with Stage IB1 disease (<4 cm in diameter) than in those with Stage IB2 disease (>4 cm in diameter). Patients with larger tumors are more likely to have nodes and lymphatic channels congested with tumor or inflammatory debris, altering lymphatic flow. Of the four patients with nodal metastases in the study by O'Boyle et al, three had a positive SLN and one had an inadequate study.[41]

Experience at the MD Anderson Cancer Center has confirmed these previous observations. We have found that the dye is not visible for very long in the pelvis (only about 30 minutes). Presumably, this is due to the high volume of lymph flowing through the pelvis. The short duration of dye visibility is confounded by the time it takes to reach the nodal basin and the requirement of bilateral dissection.

In contrast, Dargent et al, working in France, have found SLN identification using blue dye alone to be highly successful.[42] Dargent is a well-known champion in gynecologic oncology of minimally invasive surgery and has extensive experience with laparoscopically assisted radical vaginal hysterectomy and pelvic lymph-node dissection. The reason for their greater success at SLN identification using laparoscopy versus laparotomy is unknown. One possible explanation is that the increased intra-abdominal pressure slows the diffusion of dye, causing it to remain in the SLN longer. Another possible explanation is that Dargent's radical vaginal surgery is tailored to patients with small tumors. In any event, blue dye is injected into the stroma of the cervix in four quadrants. The vast majority of cervical cancers are midline; therefore, this is a peritumoral injection. The efferent lymphatic channel is found in the retroperitoneum exiting the cervix and then passing adjacent to the uterine artery and vein and over the ureter. Blue nodes are most commonly found in the parametrium, external iliac vessels, and occasionally, in the common iliac vessels.

Preoperative lymphoscintigraphy

Verheijen et al are the first to report using preoperative LSG in patients with cervical cancer who were scheduled to undergo radical hysterectomy.[43] Preoperative lymphoscintigrams identified the SLN in 6 of 10 patients undergoing a four-quadrant injection of radioactive Tc-99m-colloidal albumin in the cervix. In two additional patients, SLNs were identified using an intraoperative hand-held gamma probe.

At the MD Anderson Cancer Center, along with the University of Texas Southwestern Medical Center, preoperative LSG has been performed as part of a clinical trial prior to radical hysterectomy. Typically, an SLN is found on each side of the basin, and a parametrial SLN is found very close to the primary tumor. Lateral and oblique views can help distinguish the SLN from the primary injection site.

Combined intraoperative mapping

Verheijen et al demonstrated the feasibility of the combined-technique intraoperative mapping in the 10 patients described above.[43] In their study, the SLN was identified using blue dye in 4 patients. In each of these cases, the node was also identified by the hand-held gamma probe.

Additionally, a feasibility trial of combined intraoperative lymphatic mapping has been initiated in patients undergoing radical hysterectomy at MD Anderson and the University of Texas Southwestern Medical Center. In this trial, radionuclide is injected into four quadrants of the cervix, and the patient is then scanned (Figure 31.5). If the preoperative lymphoscintigram is obtained more than 18 hours

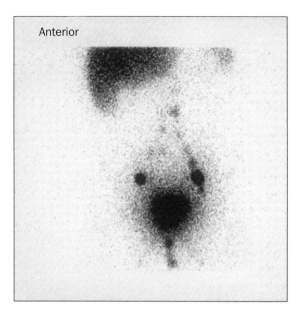

Figure 31.5 Preoperative lymphoscintigram in a patient with cervical cancer demonstrating bilateral SLNs.

prior to surgery, we reinject radionuclide into the cervix the morning of the procedure. In the operating room, the patient is placed in Allen stirrups to allow access to the perineum. After the abdomen is open and explored, a retractor is placed, and the bowel is packed out of the pelvis. At this point, 1 ml (cc) of isosulfan blue dye is injected into each quadrant of the cervix using a spinal needle or needle extender. The cervix is then massaged, and the pelvis is observed for about 5 minutes. Frequently, the blue dye can be seen through the peritoneum (Figures 31.6 and 31.7). The retroperitoneum is then opened, and the SLN is identified using staining with blue dye or with the gamma probe (Figure 31.8). A preoperative lymphoscintigram is also obtained in certain cases. In more than 20 patients, we have found the SLN using either blue dye or the gamma probe. So far, all the patients with positive nodes have had a positive SLN. Finally, whereas with well-selected vulvar cancer patients we are confident in our ability to find the SLN using blue dye

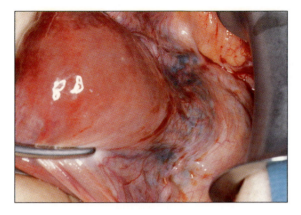

Figure 31.6 Blue dye can be seen taken up into paracervical lymphatics following intraoperative injection into the cervix.

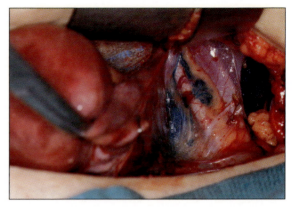

Figure 31.8 The left external iliac SLN is easily seen with blue dye alone in this patient. Additionally, lymphatic channels are going to second-echelon common iliac nodes.

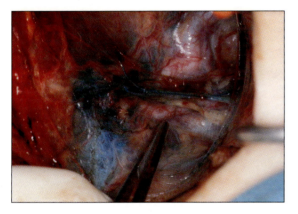

Figure 31.7 The pick-ups are pointing at the uterine artery. The afferent lymphatic channel is seen exiting the cervix on the left and traveling towards the iliac nodes on the right. The ureter is seen passing under the afferent channel and uterine artery.

only, we have found the hand-held gamma probe to be invaluable in finding the SLN in patients with cervical cancer.

Cervical cancer: summary

The data regarding SLN identification are very premature; however, there is great promise for the technique. Lymphatic drainage of the cervix is complex, and the morbidity of radical surgery is high. Nonsurgical alternatives such

as chemoradiation are preferable for patients who have lymph-node metastases. On the other hand, surgery is preferable for patients without lymph-node metastases to avoid the late complications of radiation therapy. If the negative predictive value of SLNs proves to be acceptable, lymphatic mapping will become an integral part of the management of cervical cancer.

REFERENCES

1. Eichner E, Bove ER, In vivo studies on the lymphatic drainage of the human ovary. *Obstet Gynecol* 1954; **3**:287–97.
2. Eichner E, Goldberg I, Bove ER, In vivo studies with direct sky blue of the lymphatic drainage of the internal genitals of women. *Am J Obstet Gynecol* 1954; **67**:1277–86.
3. Eichner E, Mallin LP, Angell ML, Further experience with direct sky blue in the in vivo studies of gynecic lymphatics. *Am J Obstet Gynecol* 1955; **69**:1019–26.
4. Trimble CL, Hildesheim A, Brinton LA et al, Heterogeneous etiology of squamous carcinoma of the vulva. *Obstet Gynecol* 1996; **87**:59–64.
5. Way S, Carcinoma of the vulva. *Am J Obstet Gynecol* 1960; **79**:692.
6. Taussig FJ, Cancer of the vulva: an analysis of 155 cases. *Am J Obstet Gynecol* 1940; **40**:764.

7. Parry-Jones E, Lymphatics of the vulva. *J Obstet Gynaecol Br Commonw* 1963; **70**:751–65.

8. Morris JM, A formula for selective lymphadenectomy: its application to cancer of the vulva. *Obstet Gynecol* 1977; **50**:152–8.

9. DiSaia PJ, Creasman WT, Rich WM, An alternate approach to early cancer of the vulva. *Am J Obstet Gynecol* 1979; **133**:825–32.

10. Riveros M, Garcia R, Cabanas R, Lymphadenectomy of the dorsal lymphatics of the penis. *Cancer* 1967; **20**:2026–31.

11. Cabanas RM, An approach for the treatment of penile carcinoma. *Cancer* 1977; **39**:456–66.

12. Burke TW, Levenback C, Coleman RL et al, Surgical therapy of T1 and T2 vulvar carcinoma: further experience with radical wide excision and selective inguinal lymphadenectomy. *Gynecol Oncol* 1995; **57**:215–20.

13. Berman ML, Soper JT, Creasman WT et al, Conservative surgical management of superficially invasive stage I vulvar carcinoma. *Gynecol Oncol* 1989; **35**:352–7.

14. Stehman FB, Bundy BN, Dvoretsky PM, Creasman WT, Early stage I carcinoma of the vulva treated with ipsilateral superficial inguinal lymphadenectomy and modified radical hemivulvectomy: a prospective study of the Gynecologic Oncology Group. *Obstet Gynecol* 1992; **79**:490–7.

15. Homesley HD, Bundy BN, Sedlis A, Adcock L, Radiation therapy versus pelvic node resection for carcinoma of the vulva with positive groin nodes. *Obstet Gynecol* 1986; **68**:733–40.

16. Homesley HD, Bundy BN, Sedlis A et al, Assessment of current International Federation of Gynecology and Obstetrics staging of vulvar carcinoma relative to prognostic factors for survival (a Gynecologic Oncology Group study). *Am J Obstet Gynecol* 1991; **164**:997–1004.

17. Borgno G, Micheletti L, Barbero M et al, Topographic distribution of groin lymph nodes. *J Reprod Med* 1990; **35**:1127–9.

18. Micheletti L, Borgno G, Maggiorino B et al, Deep femoral lymphadenectomy with preservation of the fascia lata. *J Reprod Med* 1990; **35**:1130–3.

19. Russell AH, Mesic JB, Scudder SA et al, Synchronous radiation and cytotoxic chemotherapy for locally advanced or recurrent squamous cancer of the vulva. *Gynecol Oncol* 1992; **47**:14–20.

20. Eifel PJ, Morris M, Burke TW et al, Preoperative continuous infusion cisplatinum and 5-fluorouracil with radiation for locally advanced or recurrent carcinoma of the vulva. *Gynecol Oncol* 1995; **59**:51–6.

21. Levenback C, Burke TW, Morris M et al, Potential applications of intraoperative lymphatic mapping in vulvar cancer. *Gynecol Oncol* 1995; **59**:216–20.

22. Levenback C, Intraoperative lymphatic mapping of the vulva with blue dye. *Proceedings of the Society of Gynecologic Oncologists*, 31st Annual Meeting, San Diego, 2000 (Abstract 17).

23. Burke T, Munkarah A, Kavanagh J et al, Treatment of advanced or recurrent endometrial carcinoma with single-agent carboplatin. *Gynecol Oncol* 1993; **51**:397–400.

24. Ansink AC, Sie-Go DM, van der Velden J et al, Identification of sentinel lymph nodes in vulvar carcinoma patients with the aid of a patent blue V injection: a multicenter study. *Cancer* 1999; **86**:652–6.

25. Krag D, Weaver D, Ashikaga T et al, The sentinel node in breast cancer. *N Engl J Med* 1998; **339**:941–6.

26. Iversen T, Aas M, Lymph drainage from the vulva. *Gynecol Oncol* 1983; **16**:179–89.

27. DeCesare SL, Fiorica JV, Roberts WS et al, A pilot study utilizing intraoperative LSG for identification of the sentinel lymph nodes in vulvar cancer. *Gynecol Oncol* 1997; **66**:425–8.

28. De Cicco C, Sideri M, Bartolomei M et al, Sentinel node biopsy in early vulvar cancer. *Br J Cancer* 2000; **82**:295–9.

29. De Hullu JA, Hollema H, Piers DA et al, Sentinel lymph node procedure is highly accurate in squamous cell carcinoma of the vulva. *J Clin Oncol* 2000; **18**:2811–16.

30. De Hullu JA, Doting E, Piers DA et al, Sentinel lymph node identification with technetium-99m-labeled nanocolloid in squamous cell cancer of the vulva. *J Nucl Med* 1998; **39**:1381–5.

31. Grendys ECJ, Salud C, Durfee JK, Fiorica JV, Lymphatic mapping in gynecologic malignancies. *Surg Oncol Clin N Am* 1999; **8**:541–53.

32. Morris M, Eifel PJ, Lu J et al, Pelvic radiation with concurrent chemotherapy compared with pelvic and paraaortic radiation for high-risk cervical cancer. *N Engl J Med* 1999; **340**:1137–43.

33. Rose PG, Bundy BN, Watkins J et al, Concurrent cisplatin-based chemotherapy and radiotherapy for locally advanced cervical cancer. *N Engl J Med* 1999; **340**:1144–53.

34. Keys HM, Bundy BN, Stehman FB et al, Cisplatin, radiation, and adjuvant hysterectomy for bulky stage IB cervical carcinoma. *N Engl J Med* 1999; **340**:1154–61.

35. Eifel PJ, Radiotherapy versus radical surgery for gynecologic neoplasms: carcinomas of the cervix and vulva. *Front Radiat Ther Oncol* 1993; **27**:130–42.

36. Dargent D, Brun JL, Roy M et al, Pregnancies following radical trachelectomy for invasive cervical cancer. *Gynecol Oncol* 1994; **52**:105.

37. Roy M, Plante M, Renaud MC et al, Vaginal radical hysterectomy versus abdominal radical hysterectomy in the treatment of early-stage cervical cancer. *Gynecol Oncol* 1996; **62**:336–9.

38. Renaud M, Plante P, Roy M, Combined laparoscopic and vaginal radical surgery in cervical cancer. *Gynecol Oncol* 2000; **79**:59–63.

39. Eifel P, Morris M, Irradiation alone or combined with surgery in carcinoma of the cervix: when will we know the answer? (editorial) *Int J Radiat Oncol Biol Phys* 1995; **31**:1007–8.

40. Russell A, Truth and consequences. *Gynecol Oncol* 1999; **73**:175–6.

41. O'Boyle JD, Coleman RL, Flowers LC et al, Intraoperative lymphatic mapping with isosulfan blue in patients undergoing radical hysterectomy: a pilot study. *Gynecol Oncol* 1999; **74**:322.

42. Dargent D, Martin X, Roy M, Mathevet P, Identification of a sentinel node with laparoscopy in cervical cancer. *Proceedings of the Society of Gynecologic Oncologists*, 31st Annual Meeting, San Diego, 2000, p. 128.

43. Verheijen R, Pijpers R, van Diest P et al, Sentinel node detection in cervical cancer. *Obstet Gynecol* 2000; **96**:135–8.

32

Colorectal cancer*

Sukamal Saha, Anton Bilchik and David Wiese

CONTENTS **Personal series** • **Patients and methods** • **Pathologic evaluation** • **Results** • **Role of laparoscopy in SLN mapping for colorectal cancer** • **Ultrastaging by immunohistochemistry and RT-PCR** • **Conclusion**

Colorectal cancer remains the fourth leading cause of cancer-related death worldwide, with the most recent published account of 783 000 new cases in 1990 causing about 437 000 deaths globally.[1] In the USA, it is the third most common cause of cancer-related mortality, with an estimated 129 400 new cases diagnosed in 1999 and 56 600 deaths.[2]

Lymph-node metastasis remains one of the most powerful and predictive prognostic factors for survival in most solid tumors, including colorectal cancer. Success of treatment is greatly influenced by appropriate staging of the disease. The basis of colorectal cancer staging depends upon evaluation of the primary tumor in the bowel as well as assessment of the regional lymph nodes in the adjacent mesentery for the presence of metastasis. Although the extent of resection for a particular tumor in the large bowel is fairly standardized, nodal staging is highly dependent on harvesting the lymph nodes from the adjacent mesentery and their pathologic assessment for metastatic disease. This undoubtedly varies greatly between pathologists and laboratories. Small (<5 mm) lymph nodes often may be missed, and lymph nodes draining directly from the primary tumor may not be harvested at all.[3] Although a technician can take over 1000 6 μm-thick sections from a 10 mm lymph node, usually only one or two such sections per lymph node are examined by the pathologist – and this is often considered the standard of care. Thus, there is a great probability that small metastatic lymph nodes, as well as those containing micrometastases, are being missed by routine pathologic examination.

About 55% of patients with colorectal cancers initially present with disease confined to the bowel wall (American Joint Committee on Cancer (AJCC) Stage I or II disease). These patients are usually not treated with adjuvant chemotherapy outside a protocol, because of the paucity of data showing a survival advantage.[4] Nonetheless, about 20–30% of patients with so-called localized disease (AJCC Stage I or II) develop systemic metastases within 5 years of diagnosis.[4] It is possible that failure to

* Reprinted from Saha S et al, Sentinel lymph-node mapping in colorectal cancer. In Colorectal Cancer: A Clinical Guide to Therapy (eds H Bleiberg, N Kemeny, Ph Rougier, H-J Wilke). London: Martin Dunitz, 2002.

identify micrometastatic disease by routine pathologic examination of the lymph nodes may play a role in understaging the disease. Thus, patients with missed nodal disease may not receive chemotherapy, and this may have a negative impact on their survival. Various methods have been described in order to increase the yield of occult micrometastases in the lymph nodes (i.e. serial sectioning,[5] the fat clearing technique,[6] the pinning and stretching method,[7] immunohistochemistry,[8] etc). Although such techniques are useful, they remain extremely labor-intensive and costly, and thus have not been adapted as standard pathologic practice.

The "sentinel lymph node" (SLN) concept was originally proposed by Cabanas in 1977 for patients with carcinoma of the penis,[9] and was popularized by Morton and his colleagues for patients with melanoma.[10] The SLN is the first node on the direct lymphatic pathway from the primary tumor. Thus, the SLN is the first one (or few) lymph nodes most likely to harbor metastatic cells when a regional nodal metastasis takes place. Numerous publications in the last seven or eight years have described the usefulness of the SLN mapping technique for the diagnosis of nodal micrometastases in melanoma and breast cancers.[11-13] Morton and colleagues have shown that in patients with malignant melanoma, the status of SLNs reflects the histologic features of the remainder of the lymphatic basin with more than 98% accuracy.[10] Many authors have confirmed since then the validity of accurate staging by the SLN mapping technique in melanoma and breast cancer.[11-13] The identification of one to four such SLNs in the direct lymphatic pathway from the primary tumor allows the pathologist to perform meticulous histologic and immunohistochemical studies by multilevel microsections. Such a detailed analysis of all the lymph nodes resected would be extremely cost-prohibitive. Yet analysis of these few "high-risk" SLNs would greatly enhance the diagnosis of nodal micrometastases that could have been missed by routine pathologic examinations. Patients who are upstaged by the diagnosis of occult micrometastases in the SLNs may then receive adjuvant chemotherapy, and this may lead to an increase in survival.

PERSONAL SERIES

For the first time in the world, our group has performed a prospective study for SLN mapping in patients with colorectal cancer.[14] The purpose of the study was fourfold: (1) to determine the feasibility of SLN mapping using isosulfan blue dye (Lymphazurin 1%; United States Medical Corp., Norwalk, CT); (2) to assess the accuracy of the SLNs in determining the status of regional nodes; (3) to identify any aberrant mesenteric lymphatic drainage patterns; (4) to assess the limitations of the technique in patients with colorectal cancer.

PATIENTS AND METHODS

From October 1996 to March 1999, 101 consecutive patients with the diagnosis of colorectal cancer were prospectively entered into the study. There were 48 males and 53 females, with ages ranging from 36 to 97 years (mean 71 years). Preoperative evaluation included a complete history and physical examination, complete blood counts, liver function study, carcinoembryonic antigen (CEA), colonoscopy, and computed tomography of the abdomen and pelvis. At operation, the abdomen was explored to confirm the site of the primary tumor and any distant metastases. Some mobilization of the bowel away from the tumor was needed to deliver the bowel adjoining the tumor near the surface. Mesenteric dissection was kept at a minimum to prevent disruption of the lymphatic pathway. With a tuberculin syringe, 1–2 ml (cc) of isosulfan blue dye was injected subserosally around the tumor in a circumferential manner without injecting into the lumen (Figure 32.1). For low- and mid-rectal lesions, the tumor was visualized through a proctoscope, and approximately 2 ml of the dye was injected transanally in the submucous layer using a spinal needle. Within 5–10 minutes of injection, the dye then travels via the lymphat-

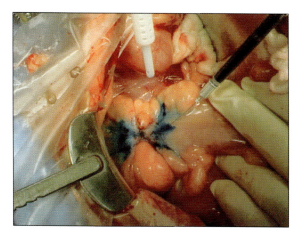

Figure 32.1 Isosulfan blue dye being injected in the subserosal layer of a sigmoid colon cancer.

ics to the nearby lymph nodes and turns them pale to dark blue. The first one to four such blue nodes near the tumor with the most direct drainage from the primary tumor are considered as SLN(s). The SLNs, as they turn blue, can be better visualized on the posterior or retroperitoneal surface of the mesentery (Figure 32.2), usually lying along the main feeding vessels. They are marked with sutures as 1st, 2nd, 3rd, or 4th SLN(s), and are not removed imme-

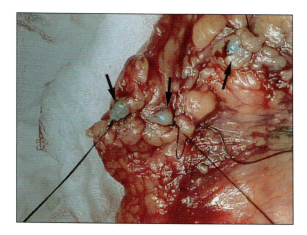

Figure 32.2 Three blue SLNs seen on the retroperitoneal surface of the sigmoid colon.

diately. Once these nodes have been marked with suture, a standard oncologic resection with segmental colectomy and regional lymphadenectomy is performed. The identification of the SLNs may be difficult in patients with thick mesentery, where some cautery dissection may be needed to expose the SLNs. For mid- to low-rectal lesions, immediate bedside dissection of the specimen to identify the most directly draining blue lymph node(s) adjacent to the tumor is done to mark the SLN(s).

PATHOLOGIC EVALUATION

Pathologic examination of the SLNs is critical for accurate staging of the disease. Once the SLNs have been tagged with suture in the operative suite, the entire specimen is sent to the pathology laboratory. The SLNs are dissected free from the specimen. These lymph nodes are sectioned grossly at about 2–3 mm intervals, and are blocked separately in individual cassettes. The remainder of the specimen is dissected and sampled for routine evaluation by standard pathologic methods. It is recommended that pericolic mesenteric tissue be postfixed in Carnoy's fluid for 2–14 hours to assist in the identification of additional non-SLNs. On average, a total of 15–20 lymph nodes should be recovered from a standard colorectal resection specimen.

For each SLN, usually a total of 10 sections are cut through the blocks, at a thickness of 4 μm each about 20–40 μm apart. One of the sections, usually at the 5th level, is immunostained for the demonstration of low-molecular-weight cytokeratin (AE-1; Ventana, Tucson, AZ). The other sections are stained routinely with hematoxylin and eosin (H&E).

RESULTS

Of the 101 consecutive patients in this study, 90 had colon and 11 had rectal cancer. The numbers and actual locations of the primary tumors were as follows: cecum 17; right colon 28; transverse colon 11; splenic flexure 2; left colon 2;

Table 32.1 Distribution of numbers and incidence of metastases in the SLNs

Total number of patients with SLN(s)	100/101 (99%)
Total number of lymph nodes	1642 (16.4 per patient)
Total number of SLNs	165 (1.6 per patient)
One SLN	46%
Two SLNs	44%
Three SLNs	9%
Four SLNs	1%
Patients with negative SLN	61%
Patients with positive SLN	39%
Patients with negative SLN and positive non-SLNs	3% (skip metastases)
Patients with solitary metastasis in SLN	19%
Patients with isolated micrometastases in SLN	10%
Patients with positive immunohistochemistry and negative H&E	4%

sigmoid colon 20; rectosigmoid colon 10; rectum 11. The SLN mapping technique successfully identified one to four SLN(s) in 100 (99%) of the 101 patients. One patient with a low rectal cancer was treated with preoperative chemo-radiotherapy. No SLN was identified in this patient, although 1 of 43 lymph nodes was positive for metastasis. The analysis that follows is based on results for the remaining 100 consecutive patients, in all of whom at least one SLN was identified. A total of 1642 lymph nodes (mean 16.4 per patient) were examined, of which 165 (mean 1.6 per patient) lymph nodes were identified as SLN(s). The distribution and pattern of nodal metastases are shown in Table 32.1. As in melanoma and breast cancer, more than one SLN was found in 54% of patients. In 58 (95%) of the 61 patients, the SLNs, as well as all non-SLNs, were without any metastasis. In the other three patients, the SLNs were negative, but five non-SLNs were positive for metastases (skip metastases). In 39 patients, the SLNs had metastases; of these, in 19 patients, the SLNs were the only site of

metastasis, with all other non-SLNs being negative. In 10 of these 39 patients, micrometastases were found only in one or two microsections of a single SLN (four were confirmed only by immunohistochemistry). These 10% of patients therefore had occult micrometastases.

In two patients, the SLN mapping technique detected an aberrant lymphatic pathway, thus altering the extent of surgery. Overall, the specificity of SLN mapping for colorectal cancer in our series of 100 patients was 100%, with a sensitivity of 93% and a negative predictive value of 95%. Solitary metastasis in one SLN, as was found in 19% of patients, may have upstaged these patients from AJCC Stage I/II to Stage III, and they may then benefit from adjuvant chemotherapy.

To evaluate whether the higher incidence of micrometastases in the SLNs, as opposed to the non-SLNs, might be due to an increased number of microsectionings of the SLNs, all non-SLNs, as well as SLNs from the first 25 consecutive patients, were sectioned at 10 levels. Of the 390 lymph nodes examined (average 15.6 per patient), 13 (36%) of the 36 SLNs were positive for metastases, while only 24 (7%) of the 354 non-SLNs had metastases. When all the initially negative non-SLNs were sectioned at 10 levels and reexamined, only 0.6% (2 of 330 lymph nodes) revealed previously undetected micrometastases.[15] These results not only confirm the well-known fact that the distribution of metastases is reflective of the lymphatic drainage, but also confirm that there may be no further benefit in performing multilevel sections of the non-SLNs in standard practice.

ROLE OF LAPAROSCOPY IN SLN MAPPING FOR COLORECTAL CANCER

Laparoscopic colon surgery is increasingly being used for benign conditions. The reported benefits for this technique include reduction in cost and improvement in quality of life. Its role in malignancy is unclear. Inadequate resection, leaving behind metastatic lymph nodes, and port-site recurrences are among the arguments given against laparoscopic colon resection for colorectal cancer. We therefore evaluated the potential role of lymphatic mapping in laparoscopic colon resection for cancer. Seven patients with early colon cancer (malignant polyps, T1–T2 lesions) underwent lymphatic mapping. After the abdomen was insufflated to a pressure of 15 mmHg, a laparoscope was inserted into the abdominal cavity. A colonoscope was then introduced transrectally and the lumen of the colon was transilluminated. An endobabcock was placed around the colon distal to the tip of the colonoscope to facilitate visualization of the tumor or primary site. Isosulfan blue dye 0.5–1 ml was then injected submucosally at the periphery of the tumor or the polypectomy site at four quadrants via the colonoscope. The primary site was then identified and the blue lymphatic channel followed to the SLN(s) by the laparoscope. The SLN(s) were identified and marked with a suture or a clip. Following this, a standard laparoscopic colectomy was performed, including the tagged SLN(s) within the resected specimen.

Colonoscopic injection and the lymphatic mapping added approximately 20 minutes to the operating time. In all seven cases, the primary site and an average of two SLNs per patient were identified. The SLN correctly identified the nodal status of the entire resected specimen in all cases. In one case, the mapping demonstrated aberrant drainage that altered the margins of resection. In another case, the SLN was negative by H&E but positive by cytokeratin, thereby upstaging this patient from AJCC Stage I to Stage III disease. Thus, this laparoscopic technique may be used to identify the primary site, demonstrate aberrant lymphatic pathways, and identify the most important lymph node (SLN) draining the primary site.

ULTRASTAGING BY IMMUNOHISTOCHEMISTRY AND RT-PCR

Although H&E staining is the gold standard for the diagnosis of metastasis in the lymph nodes, 15–20% of the cases of occult micrometastasis may be missed by routine H&E examination.

Multiple studies have been published[7,16–18] regarding the method of immunostaining with cytokeratin for the diagnosis of occult nodal micrometastasis. Immunohistochemical studies can be performed on paraffin-imbedded tissue samples. The interpretation of a positive reaction requires that the positive staining be present in cells that exhibit a malignant cytologic feature, preferably in cellular clusters in a subcapsular sinus location (Figure 32.3). The possibility of benign epithelial inclusions must be eliminated before accepting a positive staining result.

An even more sensitive molecular technique using the reverse-transcriptase polymerase chain reaction (RT-PCR) has been developed to further upstage node-negative patients.[19] It is extremely important to avoid contamination of the SLNs by tumor cells at the time of pathologic dissection in order to avoid a false-positive result.

Since it is not practical to perform RT-PCR on all resected lymph nodes, we applied this technology to the SLNs. Specific primers targeting mRNA expression of tumor markers expressed in colon cancer were used. The

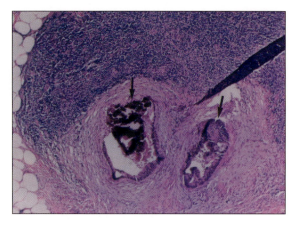

Figure 32.3 Micrometastasis in the subscapular layer of an SLN (arrows) (×200).

advantage of this multiple-marker RT-PCR assay is that even though these tumors can be heterogeneous, the possibility of detection of micrometastases is increased. We have demonstrated concordance between the primary tumor and the SLNs, and 30% of patients were upstaged in this study.[20]

CONCLUSIONS

Multiple studies have confirmed the high accuracy of the SLN mapping technique in correctly predicting the presence of micrometastases in regional lymph nodes of patients with malignant melanoma and breast cancer.[10–13]

The first report of the SLN mapping technique in colorectal cancer was given by our group in 1997 at the annual meeting of the Society of Surgical Oncology.[21] Since then, our studies have further confirmed that, as in melanoma and breast cancer, SLNs can be localized in a high (99%) number of cases with a high degree of accuracy (97%) in colorectal cancer patients. The only failure of identification of an SLN in a patient with low-rectal cancer may be due to submucosal fibrosis of the lymphatics resulting from neoadjuvant radiotherapy. Despite the technical difficulty associated with peritumoral injection of the dye in

rectal tumors, SLN mapping was successful in 10 (91%) of 11 patients with rectal cancer as compared with all patients with colon cancer. Three patients with skip metastases in this series included one patient with two closely situated primary tumors, one patient with perforated carcinoma, and one patient with previous colon surgery. Thus, potential limitations of this technique in colorectal cancer may include previous surgery, radiation therapy, perforation, and possibly multiple primaries.

In both melanoma and breast cancer, a combination of radionuclide dye and isosulfan blue dye is used for optimal SLN mapping in most reported series. Radionuclide dye was unnecessary for SLN mapping in colorectal cancer, which reduces the cost of the procedure ($31 per vial of the dye). Furthermore, the majority of the SLNs were found within 7 cm of the primary tumor site within the mesentery. The proximity to the primary site could lead to a "shine-through" effect, reducing the sensitivity of the radioactivity of the SLNs. Owing to this and other logistic problems involved with the use of radiolabeled material in the operating room, no attempt was made to use this for SLN mapping in colorectal cancer. Unlike melanoma and breast cancer, a much shorter learning curve is anticipated in performing this technique because of the ease in identifying the blue nodes and most general surgeons' relative familiarity with performing routine colorectal surgery.

One of the main advantages of SLN mapping in patients with melanoma and breast cancer is that it allows the surgeon to avoid routine radical lymphadenectomy in patients with negative SLNs. In our study, no attempt was made to perform less than a standard oncologic colon resection. Instead, our focus was to identify the few "high-risk" SLNs that have the highest probability of harboring micrometastases. Pathologists can then perform more meticulous examinations on these few nodes by means of multilevel microsections. Indeed, 19% of patients may have been upstaged to AJCC Stage III disease. In particular, micrometastases seen in one or two microsections of a single SLN, in 10% of patients, most probably would have been missed by conventional pathologic examination. Thus, these patients truly were upstaged from AJCC Stage I/II to Stage III. Patients whose disease is upstaged on discovery of such micrometastases can be offered adjuvant chemotherapy, with the potential for improved survival.

The prognostic significance of occult micrometastases has been confirmed in many studies for breast cancer[22] and melanoma.[11] As this technique identifies a significant number (19%) of cases of colorectal cancer with occult micrometastases, we believe that effective systemic chemotherapy may play an important role in changing the prognosis of these patients. The implication of RT-PCR analysis for micrometastasis in colorectal cancer is evolving. Liefers et al[23] have shown a significant survival advantage for RT-PCR-negative patients with stage II colorectal cancer as opposed to RT-PCR-positive patients (5-year survival rates of 75% versus 36%). Owing to its potential in predicting this survival advantage, an ongoing RT-PCR study is being done for patients undergoing SLN mapping, the results of which will be published soon.

As the application of SLN mapping is being expanded for other solid neoplasms,[24] we hope that its use in colorectal cancer will become part of the standard practice of the general surgeon, given its simplicity, high accuracy, and low cost, and its aid to pathologists in focusing their attention on one to four nodes for detailed analysis, thereby upstaging a significant number of patients. A larger multi-institution study is warranted to evaluate the potential implications of the SLN mapping technique in colorectal cancer patients for appropriate therapeutic planning and to determine its impact on survival.

REFERENCES

1. Parkin DN, Pisani P, Ferlay J, Global cancer statistics. *CA Cancer J Clin* 1999; **49**:33–64.
2. Landis SH, Murray T, Bolden S et al, Cancer statistics 1999. *CA Cancer J Clin* 1999; **49**:8–31.
3. Rodriguez-Bigas MA, Maamoun S, Weber TK et al, Clinical significance of colorectal cancer: metastases in lymph nodes <5 mm in size. *Ann Surg Oncol* 1996; **3**:124–30.
4. Cohen AM, Kelsen D, Saltz L et al, Adjuvant therapy for colorectal cancer. *Curr Prob Cancer* 1998; **22**:5–77.
5. Pickreen JW, Significance of occult metastases, a study of breast cancer. *Cancer* 1961; **14**:1261–71.
6. Cawthorn SJ, Gibbs NM, Marks CG, Clearance technique for the detection of lymph nodes in colorectal cancer. *Br J Surg* 1986; **73**:58–60.
7. Crucitti F, Doglietto GB, Bellantone R et al, Accurate specimen preparation and examination is mandatory to detect lymph nodes and avoid understaging in colorectal cancer. *J Surg Oncol* 1992; **51**:153–8.
8. Greenson JK, Isenhart CE, Rice R et al, Identification of occult micrometastases in pericolic lymph nodes of Dukes' B colorectal cancer patients using monoclonal antibodies against cytokeratin and CC49. *Cancer* 1994; **73**: 563–9.
9. Cabanas RM, An approach for treatment of penile carcinoma. *Cancer* 1977; **39**:456–66.
10. Morton DL, Wen DR, Wong JH et al, Technical details of intraoperative lymphatic mapping for early stage melanoma. *Arch Surg* 1992; **127**: 392–9.
11. Reintgen D, Haddad F, Pendas S et al, Lymphatic mapping and sentinel lymph node biopsy. *Sci Am* 1998; **17**:1–17.
12. Guiliano AE, Kirgan DM, Guenther JM et al, Lymphatic mapping and sentinel lymphadenectomy for breast cancer. *Ann Surg* 1994; **220**: 391–401.
13. Cox CE, Haddad F, Bass S et al, Lymphatic mapping in the treatment of breast cancer. *Oncology* 1998; **12**:1283–98.
14. Saha S, Accurate staging of colorectal cancer by SLN mapping – a prospective study. In: Post Graduate Course 22, *Annual Meeting American College of Surgeons*, 1999: 34–7.
15. Wiese D, Saha S, Badin J, Sentinel lymph node mapping in staging of colorectal cancer. *Am J Clin Pathol* 1999; **112**:542 (abstract).
16. Bertoglio S, Percivale P, Gambini C et al, Cytokeratin immunostaining reveals micrometastasis in negative hematoxylin–eosin lymph nodes of resected stage I–II (PT2–pT3) colorectal cancer. *J Chemother* 1997; **9**:119–20.
17. Oberg A, Stenling R, Tavelin B, Lindmark G, Are lymph node micrometastases of any clinical significance in Dukes' stages A and B colorectal cancer? *Dis Colon Rectum* 1998; **41**:1244–9.
18. Broll R, Schauer V, Schimmelpenning H et al, Prognostic relevance of occult tumor cells in

lymph nodes of colorectal carcinomas. *Dis Colon Rectum* 1997; **40:**1465–71.

19. Mori M, Mimori K, Inoue H et al, Detection of cancer micrometastases in lymph nodes by reverse transcriptase polymerase chain reaction. *Cancer Res* 1995; **55:**3417–20.

20. Bilchik AJ, Saha S, Wiese D et al, Molecular staging of early colon cancer on the basis of sentinel node analysis: a multicenter phase II trial. *J Clin Oncol* 2001; **19:**1128–36.

21. Saha S, Ganatra BK, Gauthier J et al, Localizations of sentinel lymph node (SLN) in colon cancer – a feasibility study. In: *Cancer Symposium (Abstract Book – Society of Surgical Oncology)*, 1997: 54.

22. International Ludwig Breast Cancer Study Group, Prognostic importance of occult axillary lymph node micrometastases from breast cancers. *Lancet* 1990; **335:**1565–8.

23. Liefers G, Cleton-Jansen C, Van de Velde C et al, Micrometastases and survival in stage II colorectal cancer. *N Engl J Med* 1998; **339:**223–8.

24. Bilchik A, Giuliano A, Essner R et al, Universal application of intraoperative lymphatic mapping and sentinel lymphadenectomy in solid neoplasms. *Cancer J Sci Am* 1998; **4:**351–8.

Index